Fundamentals of Toxicology

Fundamentals of Toxicology

Essential Concepts and Applications

P.K. Gupta

Director, Toxicology Consulting Services;
Patron and Founder, Society of Toxicology of India;
President, Academy of Sciences for Animal Welfare,
Bareilly, UP, India

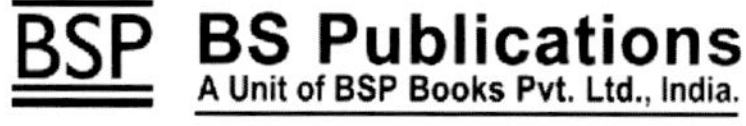

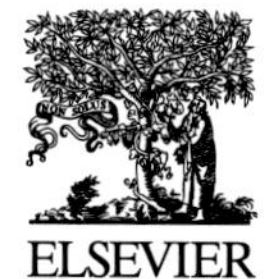

AMSTERDAM • BOSTON • HEIDELBERG • LONDON
NEW YORK • OXFORD • PARIS • SAN DIEGO
SAN FRANCISCO • SINGAPORE • SYDNEY • TOKYO
Academic Press is an imprint of Elsevier

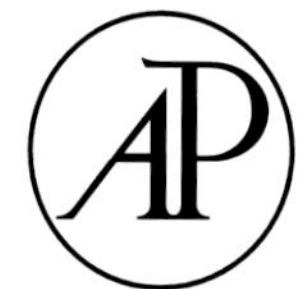

Academic Press is an imprint of Elsevier
125 London Wall, London EC2Y 5AS, United Kingdom
525 B Street, Suite 1800, San Diego, CA 92101-4495, United States
50 Hampshire Street, 5th Floor, Cambridge, MA 02139, United States
The Boulevard, Langford Lane, Kidlington, Oxford OX5 1GB, United Kingdom

Notices

Knowledge and best practice in this field are constantly changing. As new research and experience broaden our understanding, changes in research methods, professional practices, or medical treatment may become necessary.

Practitioners and researchers must always rely on their own experience and knowledge in evaluating and using any information, methods, compounds, or experiments described herein. In using such information or methods they should be mindful of their own safety and the safety of others, including parties for whom they have a professional responsibility.

To the fullest extent of the law, neither the Publisher nor the authors, contributors, or editors, assume any liability for any injury and/or damage to persons or property as a matter of products liability, negligence or otherwise, or from any use or operation of any methods, products, instructions, or ideas contained in the material herein.

British Library Cataloguing-in-Publication Data
A catalogue record for this book is available from the British Library

Library of Congress Cataloging-in-Publication Data
A catalog record for this book is available from the Library of Congress

ISBN: 978-0-12-805426-0

For Information on all Academic Press publications
visit our website at https://www.elsevier.com/

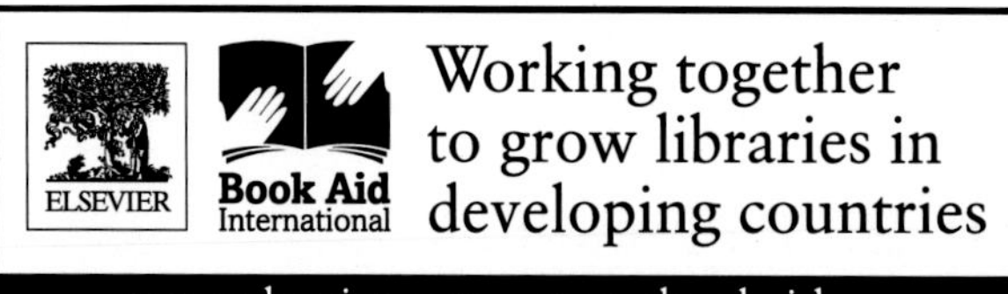

Publisher: Mica Haley
Acquisition Editor: Erin Hill-Parks
Editorial Project Manager: Tracy Tufaga
Production Project Manager: Lucía Pérez
Designer: Mark Rogers

Typeset by MPS Limited, Chennai, India

Contents

About the Author

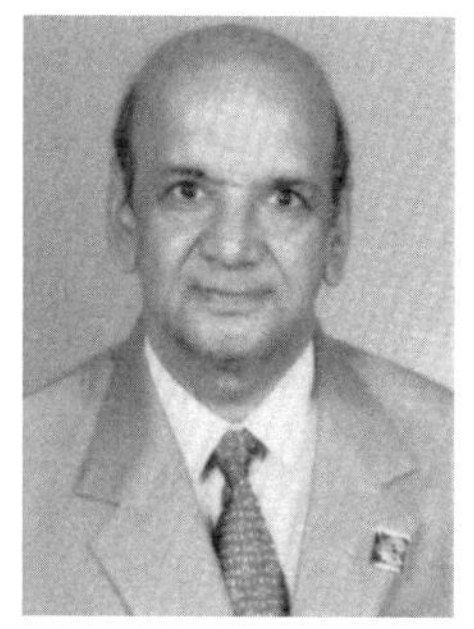

Prof Dr P.K. Gupta
PhD (Toxicology), Postdoctorate in Toxicology (USA), PGDCA, FACVT (USA), FAEB, FST, FASc AW, FNAVS
Director, Toxicology Consulting Services; Patron and Founder, Society of Toxicology of India; President, Academy of Sciences for Animal Welfare, Bareilly, UP, India

Prof Dr Gupta is an internationally known toxicologist with 48 years of experience in the fields of teaching, research, and research management. He has guided many postgraduate students in their thesis work in toxicology and has been honored with several national and international awards, including best teacher, best researcher, Alarsin award, lifetime achievement awards, and IUTOX-Astra Zeneca Award (USA). To his credit, he has written several books, book chapters (Elsevier, Academic Press, John Wiley, Merck Manual, etc.), and scientific research publications (550) that have been published in national and international peer-reviewed journals of repute. His contributions to the publication *Indian Veterinary Pharmacopeia* are highly praiseworthy. He is the Founder Editor-in-Chief of the peer-reviewed scientific journal *Toxicology International*; Book Review Editor for Marcel Dekker, USA; Expert Member Consultant and Advisor to WHO, Geneva; Consultant to the United Nations FAO, Rome, and to IAEA, Vienna; Founder of the Academy of Sciences for Animal Welfare; Founder and Past President of the Society of Toxicology of India; Adjunct Professor at SRMS; Founder Director and member of the nominating committee of the International Union of Toxicology; Founder President of the Society of Toxicology of India; and has held several prominent positions in scientific organizations in India and abroad.

In addition, Dr. Gupta has also been biographer for several WHO's WHO all over the world, including Marquis WHO's WHO (USA), IBC (UK), and other leading publications around the world. At present, Dr. Gupta is the Director of Toxicology at Consultant Group, Patron and Founder President of the Society of Toxicology of India, and President of the Academy of Sciences for Animal Welfare.

Foreword

Toxicology is the study of chemicals in biological systems. This science was born to deal with the safe use of chemicals, which cause more pain and danger than the illnesses being treated. In recent years, toxicology has evolved into a modern science. Further, new governmental legislations designed to safeguard against a variety of chemical substances have brought a large demand for trained toxicologists all over the world. Advances in the field of toxicology during the past several decades are widely scattered because of their multidisciplinary character. Very few of today's toxicologists and environmentalists are primarily trained in toxicology or environmental science. As such, scientists from other closely related disciplines, such as nutrition, biochemistry, pharmacology, chemistry, or bioengineering, are entrusted with the task of tackling toxicology problems. In addition, to meet the demand of safety evaluations of a large variety of compounds, a good number of multinational organizations have established their laboratories worldwide to perform contract research in toxicology. In the past, toxicology has been a branch of the pharmacology discipline. However, keeping in mind the demand for trained toxicologists, many universities have started offering courses or degrees in the field of toxicology.

Toxicology is a wide and vast subject that needs to be explored by overburdened students in the short time available to them. There are a number of reference books available on the market, but many of them provide only archaic information that is of little to no relevance at the present time. The subject matter of toxicology is rapidly changing and new laws and principles are being enforced. The concept of Good Laboratory Practice has been introduced. As such, there is a need to look at toxicology from a current perspective. I have known the author of this eminently readable book, Professor P.K. Gupta, for more than four decades. His three-volume set about modern toxicology is an excellent reference that is very concise and caters to the needs of students in developing countries. His other publications include his book entitled *Essential Concepts in Toxicology* and a peer-reviewed toxicology journal entitled *Toxicology International*, which is under his stewardship. The journal is a PubMed-indexed scientific research publication. From time to time, he also contributes chapters to various international books of repute published in Western countries. His contribution and commitment to science in general and toxicology in particular are praiseworthy.

For a long time, we were all waiting to have a book that examined toxicology from a fresh angle, and I had no doubt that it was Dr. Gupta who could do it. I am happy to know that he has shown his rich experience as a teacher in writing this book, which is primarily important to those who want first-hand knowledge of toxicology. His present book, *Fundamentals of Toxicology: Essential Concepts and Applications*, is very crisp and concise but covers all vital aspects of toxicology, such as nanomaterial toxicology, chemoinformatics including Good Laboratory Practice, and regulatory toxicology. This book contains very useful information and is intended to provide a better understanding of the subject for formal courses in graduate toxicology programs or self-study by those individuals who wish to be accredited by various organizations concerned with toxicology. We hope that this book will facilitate the training of toxicologists who are required to have multidisciplinary knowledge in areas like environmental health and clinical and forensic toxicology (detection of intentional or unintentional toxic substances). This book will be useful in private commercial laboratories, in material science toxicology (biomedical and engineering disciplines), in education (courses in pharmacy, medicine, dentistry, agricultural, and veterinary practice), and, finally, for collecting, storing, and retrieving toxicology information. As such, I feel that this book will be an asset for all pharmacy, pharmacology, and medical students and for other concerned groups of readers with an interest in toxicology.

The formatting and printing of this book are of high order. Photographs, line drawings, flow charts, and tables in the book are relevant and extremely useful. The language of the book is simple and easily understandable. Dr. Gupta deserves our compliments for preparing this very readable text, which I hope will become popular among a wide range of readers with an interest in toxicology. I wish this book all success.

R.C. Gupta
Murray State University, Hopkinsville, KY, United States

Preface

Toxicology is a very complex and fascinating subject that deals with a wide variety of poisons and toxicants from a variety of sources such as chemicals, plants, fungi, and animals. Presently, synthetic compounds constitute the largest class of chemicals that are most frequently encountered in poisoning cases and are responsible for environmental contamination and occupational health hazards. My earlier three-volume set on modern toxicology, published in 1985, was designed with the objective of offering a comprehensive reference source to research toxicologists. The encouraging response given to this publication has led to the reprint of the three-volume set in 2010. In addition, there was great demand for a book that can meet the requirements of students from various universities and research institutions offering courses in toxicology. I am experienced in creating and presenting courses in toxicology at various Universities in India and abroad. My experience as a teacher of toxicology over the past five decades has shown me that there is a dearth of readily accessible text material that can provide basic toxicological information to students who wish to specialize in toxicology. Several requests for a well-illustrated book with precise and specific information with relevance to India that can serve the need of beginners in the area of toxicology were received. This encouraged me to write a book entitled *Essential Concepts in Toxicology*, which was published in 2014. While preparing that book, several universities and institutes offering courses in toxicology were consulted so that it may better serve their requirements.

The present book, *Fundamentals of Toxicology: Essential Concepts and Application*, has been designed to meet the requirements of the international market. Keeping this in mind, a short and lucid text that is easily understandable and supported with simple figures and self-explanatory tables has been prepared.

The book is subdivided into five units consisting of 34 chapters. Unit I includes six chapters that provide extensive coverage of general information, including basic concepts, definitions, historical perspectives, and scope of toxicology. These chapters may be useful for understanding the fundamental principles, including natural laws and approaches to toxicology.

Unit II comprises three chapters (chapters 7–9) dealing with absorption, distribution, excretion, biotransformation, and basic principles of toxicokinetics of xenobiotics.

Unit III is specifically focused on regulatory requirements in the United States and REACH regulation of European countries, the role of animal testing, the use of alternate approaches, Good Laboratory Practices, and current trends in toxicology such as chemoinformatics and nanomaterial toxicology. This unit has seven chapters (chapters 10–16) with many novel sections on recent topics such as toxicology testing, in vivo and in vitro test procedures used during assessment of the toxic potential of chemicals, including developmental and reproduction toxicity, genotoxicity studies, preclinical testing procedures for pharmaceuticals, safety evaluation of biotechnology-derived products, and regulatory toxicology of biomaterials and medical devices used in medical practice.

The main focus of Unit IV (chapters 17–30) is on toxic agents derived from different sources, such as pesticides, drugs, plant and animal toxins, neurotoxins, irritant poisons, cardiotoxicants, asphyxiants, food poisonings, and therapeutic drugs of abuse. The latest information on problems related to adverse effects of radioactive materials on the health is presented.

Unit V is devoted to analytical, forensic, and diagnostic toxicology, which includes basic principles of specific and nonspecific therapeutic measures of common poisonings.

Each chapter is well supported with concise tables, illustrations, diagrams, and important images of plants whenever necessary.

This book is intended to provide a better understanding for those involved in formal courses in graduate programs in toxicology and for those individuals who wish to partake in self-study to be accredited by various toxicology organizations. I hope that this book will facilitate the training of toxicologists who are required to have multidisciplinary knowledge in areas like environmental health and clinical and forensic toxicology (detection of intentional or unintentional toxic substances). In addition, this book will be useful in private commercial laboratories, for material science toxicology (biomedical and engineering disciplines), for educators (courses in pharmacy, medicine, dentistry, agricultural, and veterinary practice), and, finally, for collecting, storing, and retrieving toxicology information.

I hope that this book will find a favorable response from all pharmacy and medical students and other concerned groups of readers, that it will find a suitable place in toxicology literature, and that it will benefit all scientists with an interest in toxicology.

The author welcomes suggestions, constructive criticism, thoughts, and comments from readers for improving this book. Kindly e-mail them to drpkg_brly@yahoo.co.in or to drpkg1943@gmail.com.

P.K. Gupta

UNIT

I

CHAPTER

Introduction and historical background

1

CHAPTER OUTLINE

1.1 INTRODUCTION

The word "toxicology" is derived from the Greek word "toxicon," which means "poison," and logos, which means to study. Thus, toxicology literally means the study of poisons. It can thus be defined as the "study of poisons that include their physical and chemical properties, detection and identification, biological effects, treatment, and prevention of disease conditions produced by them." It also includes the study of special effects of toxicant developmental toxicity, teratogenicity, carcinogenicity, mutagenesis, immunotoxicity, neurotoxicity, and endocrine disruption.

1.2 HISTORICAL BACKGROUND

1.2.1 ANTIQUITY

The knowledge of poisons is as old as human civilization. Early poisons were almost exclusively plant and animal toxins and some minerals. They were used mainly for hunting. Some were used as "ordeal poisons," such as physostigmine from *Physostigma venenosum* (Calabar bean) and amygdalin from peach pits. Arrow and dart poisons were very popular for hunting animals (and sometimes fellow humans!). Common arrow poisons included strophanthin, aconitine, and extracts from hellebores (a cardiotoxic plant) and történelmi venoms. Since ancient times, people have learned how to protect themselves from the harmful

Fundamentals of Toxicology. DOI: http://dx.doi.org/10.1016/B978-0-12-805426-0.00001-9

effects of plants and animals. They also knew how to use poisons to destroy their enemies. The earliest records are available in the form of ancient books on mythology and legendry, archeological literature, and history books. The Ebers Papyrus (1550 BC) is perhaps the earliest medical record that contains a number of disease conditions and prescriptions; it was previously used in Egyptian medicine. Many of these contain recognized poisons such as aconite, an arrow poison of ancient times, and opium (both as a poison and antidote).

Hippocrates (460–375 BC) is regarded as the "Father of Rational Medicine." The Hippocrates School was formed by a group of physicians to provide an ethical basis for the practice of therapeutics by those who have knowledge of lead, mercury, copper, antimony, and others as poisons and who have some knowledge of their properties. They advocated hot oil as an antidote to poisoning and induced vomiting to prevent absorption of the poisons. Hemlock, which contains the alkaloid coniine, was one of the poisons used during that time. Socrates (470–390 BC) was sentenced to death by hemlock. Theophrastus (371–287 BC), the most dedicated pupil of Aristotle, provided an early treatise on plant poisons. Experimental toxicology perhaps began with Nicander (204–135 BC). Homicidal poisoning has also had a hoary past. One of the earliest laws against the murderous use of poisons was the *Lex Cornelia* passed in Rome in 81 BC.

During AD 40–80, Pedanius Dioscorides, a Greek army physician, classified poisons according to their origin (animal, vegetable, or mineral). His classification of natural substances as being toxic or therapeutic is still valid today. Dioscorides is famous for writing a five-volume book, *De Materia Medica*, that is a precursor to all modern pharmacopeias and is one of the most influential herbal books in history.

1.2.2 MIDDLE AGES

After the fall of the Roman empire, there was a lull in the development of toxicology until 1198, when a famous Swiss Philosopher, Maimonides (Moses ben Maimon) (1135–1204), published his classic work *Treatise on Poisons and Their Antidotes* in 1198, which describes the treatment of poisonings from insects, snakes, and dogs. During the early Renaissance, the Italians, with characteristic pragmatism, brought the art of poisoning to its zenith. The poisoner became an integral part of the political scene. The records of the city councils of Florence, particularly those of the infamous Council of Ten of Venice, contain ample testimony about the political use of poisons. Victims were named, prices were set, and contracts were recorded; when the deed was accomplished, payment was made. An infamous figure of the time was a lady named Toffana, who peddled specially prepared arsenic-containing cosmetics (*Agua Toffana*).

Unfortunately, during this period, poisoning as a method of homicide became increasingly popular in several parts of Europe, particularly Italy and France, where schools actually existed for teaching the art of poisoning. Among the notorious poisoners, Madame Guilia Toffana killed more than 600 people with white arsenic solution called aqua Toffana that was freely sold as a cosmetic in Italy. Toward the end of the 16th century, the wave was spread from Italy to France, where poisons were commonly used by all classes of society to get rid of enemies or persons considered undesirable. Criminal poisoning continued in many parts of the world during the 18th and 19th centuries.

1.2.3 AGE OF ENLIGHTENMENT

A significant figure in the history of science and medicine in the late Middle Ages was the renaissance man Philippus Aureolus Theophrastus Bombastus von Hohenheim-Paracelsus (1493–1541), who referred to himself as Paracelsus because of his belief that his work was beyond the work of Celsus, a first-century Roman physician who was perhaps the first to promote a focus on toxicon, a toxic agent, as a chemical entity. He recognized the dose–response concept and, in one of his writings, stated: "All substances are poisons, there is none which is not a poison. The right dose differentiates a poison and a remedy." Paracelsus advanced many views that were revolutionary for his time and that are now accepted as fundamental concepts for the field of toxicology. In contrast to previous emphasis on mixtures, he focused on toxicon as a specific primary chemical entity that was toxic. Paracelsus advanced four fundamental concepts:

1. Experimentation is required for examining responses to chemicals.
2. A distinction should be made between the therapeutic and toxic properties of chemicals.
3. The therapeutic and toxic properties are closely related and distinguished by dose.
4. It is possible to ascertain a degree of specificity for chemicals and their therapeutic or toxic effects.

Modern toxicology is a relatively young science based on scientific work performed by numerous dedicated workers. It is the outcome of rational thinking, experimentation, the relationship between dose and therapeutics (as compared with toxic), and the responses to chemicals. Advances made in all allied disciplines contributed to the better understanding of effects of a number of toxicants in humans and animals. Modern toxicology began with Friedrich Serturner (1783–1841), a German pharmacist who isolated the specific narcotic substance from opium and named it morphine after Morpheus, the Roman God of sleep. Subsequently, Mattie Josesph Benaventura Orfila (MJB; 1787–1853), a Spanish physician who is considered the "Father of Toxicology," established toxicology as a discipline distinct from others and defined toxicology as the study of poisons. He advocated the practice of autopsy followed by chemical analysis of viscera to prove that poisoning had taken place. His treatise *Traite des Poisons* published in 1814 laid the foundation for forensic toxicology. In 1829, one of his students, Robert Christison (1797–1882), published a simplified English version titled *A Treatise on Poisons*. The first published work (published in 1848) on clinical toxicology was *A Practical Treatise on Poisons*, written by O. Costill.

Francois Magendie (1783–1855), a pioneer French physiologist and toxicologist, studied the mechanism of action of emetine, morphine, quinine, strychnine, and other alkaloids, for which he is also called the "Father of Experimental Pharmacology" Magendie passed on his interest to his famous student Claude Bernard (1813–78), who continued to study arrow poisons and used these toxicants to learn more about the mechanism of body functions.

Louis Lewin (1854–1929) was a German scientist who accepted the task of classifying drugs and plants in accordance with their psychological effects. He also published many articles and books dealing with toxicology of methyl alcohol, ethyl alcohol, chloroform, opium, and some other chemicals. His important publications are *Toxicologist's View of World History* and *A Textbook of Toxicology*. Development occurred rapidly in the 20th century with the development of dimercaprol (BAL) as an antidote for arsenic and the discovery of insecticidal properties of DDT by Paul Hermann Muller in 1939. He was awarded a Nobel Prize in 1948 "for his discovery of the high efficiency of DDT as a contact poison against several arthropods."

Gerhard Schrader (1903–90) was a German chemist who accidentally developed the toxic nerve agents serin, tabun, soman, and cyclosarin while attempting to develop new insecticides. Schrader and his team therefore introduced a new class of synthetic insecticides, the organophosphorus insecticides (OP), and defined the structural requirements for insecticidal activity of anticholinesterase (anti-ChE) compounds. He is called the "Father of Nerve Agents."

1.3 MODERN TOXICOLOGY

Toxicology has evolved rapidly during the 1900s. The exponential growth of the discipline can be traced to the World War II era, with its marked increase in the production of drugs, pesticides, synthetic fibers, and industrial chemicals. It also marked the beginning of understanding in-depth the nature and mechanism of the effects of poisons and the invention of their specific antidotes. Along with other sciences, toxicology contributes to the development of safer chemicals to be used as drugs, food additives, pesticides, industrial chemicals, and several other chemicals required for use in everyday life.

Because of the need for an affluent society to protect itself from injurious effects resulting from the introduction of new chemicals, physical agents, and various industrial and consumer products, there has been an expansion of the various facets of toxicology. Therefore, application of the discipline of toxicology to safety evaluation and risk assessment is of utmost importance in today's modern world.

1.3.1 AFTER WORLD WAR II

The mid 1950s witnessed the strengthening of the US Food and Drug Administration's commitment to toxicology under the guidance of Arnold Lehman. Lehman, Fitzhugh, and their co-workers formalized the experimental program for the appraisal of food, drug, and cosmetic safety in 1955, and it was updated by the US FDA in 1982. The Delaney clause (1958) of these amendments stated broadly that any chemical found to be carcinogenic in laboratory animals or humans could not be added to the US food supply. Regardless of one's view of Delaney, it has served as an excellent starting point for understanding the complexity of the biological phenomenon of carcinogenicity and the development of risk assessment models.

The end of the 1960s witnessed the discovery of TCDD as a contaminant in the herbicide Agent Orange (the original discovery of TCDD toxicity, the "Chick Edema Factor," was reported in 1957). The expansion of legislation, journals, and new societies involved with toxicology was exponential during the 1970s and 1980s and shows no signs of slowing down. Currently, in the United States, there are dozens of professional, governmental, and other scientific organizations with thousands of members and more than 120 journals dedicated to toxicology and related disciplines. As an example of this diversification, one now finds toxicology graduate programs in medical schools, schools of public health, and schools of pharmacy, as well as programs in environmental science and engineering and undergraduate programs in toxicology at several institutions. Surprisingly, courses in toxicology are now being offered in several liberal arts undergraduate schools as part of their biology and chemistry curricula. Some important developments in the field of toxicology are summarized in Table 1.1.

Table 1.1 Some Important Developments in the Field of Toxicology

F. Magendie, 1809: study of "arrowpoisons," mechanism of action of emetine and strychnine
Marsh, 1836: development of method for arsenic analysis
Reinsh, 1841: combined method for separation and analysis of As and Hg
Fresenius, 1845 and von Babo, 1847: development of screening method for general poisons
Stas-Otto, 1851: detection and identification of phosphorus
C. Bernard, 1850: carbon monoxide combination with hemoglobin, study of mechanism of action of strychnine, site of action of curare
Friedrich Gaedcke, 1855: first isolated cocaine from leaves of Erthroxylon coca
Oswald Schmiedeberg, 1869: isolated muscarine from Amanita muscaria
R. Bohm, approximately 1890: active anthelmintics from fern, action of croton oil catharsis, poisonous mushrooms
C. Voegtlin, 1923: mechanism of action of As and other metals in the SH groups
K.K. Chen, 1934: demonstrated antagonistic effect of sodium nitrite and sodium thiosulphate in cyanide poisoning
P. Müller, 1944–46: introduction and study of DDT (dichlorodiphenyltrichloroethane) and related insecticide compounds
R.A. Peters, L.A. Stocken, and R.H.S. Thompson, 1945: development of British anti-Lewisite (BAL) as a relatively specific antidote for arsenic
Judah Hirsch Quastel, 1946: developed 2,4-D, the first widely used systemic herbicide
G. Schrader, 1952: introduction and study of organophosphorus compounds
Rachel Carson, 1962: started crusade against the use of DDT and published the great book, *Silent Spring*

CHAPTER

Definitions and scope of toxicology

2

CHAPTER OUTLINE

2.1 DEFINITIONS

Toxicology: To a lay person, toxicology is the study of adverse effects of chemicals on various biological systems, including humans. However, in modern times, toxicology is considered a scientific discipline and, like medicine, an art that is practiced. Thus, it is the study of poisons, including their physical and chemical properties, detection and identification, biological effects, treatment, and prevention of disease conditions produced by them.

Xenobiotic: Xenobiotic (xeno is a Greek word that means strange or alien) are the substances that are foreign to the body and are biologically active. These cannot be broken down to generate energy or assimilated into a biosynthetic pathway. It is a very wide class of structurally adverse agents, including both natural and synthetic chemicals such as drugs, industrial chemicals, pesticides, alkaloids, secondary plant metabolites and toxins of molds, plants, and animals, and environmental pollutants.

Fundamentals of Toxicology. DOI: http://dx.doi.org/10.1016/B978-0-12-805426-0.00002-0

2.2 SUB-DISCIPLINES OF TOXICOLOGY

Forensic Toxicology: Forensic toxicology deals with medical and legal aspects of the harmful effects of the chemicals.

Clinical Toxicology: Clinical toxicology refers to health problems caused by or associated with abnormal exposure to chemical substance. In other words, it deals with the cause, diagnosis, treatment, and clinical management of health problems/diseases that are caused by or are associated with toxic substance(s).

Nutritional Toxicology: The study of toxicological aspects of food/feed stuffs and nutritional products/habits.

Reproductive Toxicology: The study of the occurrence of adverse effects on the male and female reproductive system due to exposure to chemicals or physical agents.

Development Toxicology: The study of harmful effects of chemicals and drugs on the development of an organism; manifestations of development toxicity include structural malformations, growth restriction, functional impairment, and/or death of an organism.

Veterinary Toxicology: This deals with the cause, diagnosis, and management of established poisonings in domestic and wild animals.

Teratology: The study of malformations induced by toxic agents during development between conception and birth.

Environmental Toxicology: This deals with the effects of pollutants on the environment (food, water, air, or soil) and their prevention. Its specialties could include ecotoxicology, aquatic toxicology, and others.

Analytical Toxicology: The application of analytical chemistry tools in the qualitative and quantitative estimation of the agents involved in the process of toxicity.

Aquatic Toxicology: This deals with the study of adverse effects of chemicals discharged into marine and fresh water on aquatic organisms and the aquatic ecosystem. It is largely a study of water pollution and its ecological effects.

Ecotoxicology: A more specialized area of environmental pollution in populations and communities of living organisms. Ecotoxicology, in general, considers effects of pollutants on organisms other than humans.

Food Toxicology: This deals with natural contaminants, food and feed additives, and toxic and chemo-protective effects of compounds in food.

Formal Toxicology: This deals with the formal toxicological studies that are prerequisites for the release of new drugs/chemicals (eg, calculation of LD_{50} and minimum toxic dose).

Genetic Toxicology: This deals with the study of the interaction of toxicants with the process of hereditary.

Industrial Toxicology: This deals with the clinical study of industry workers and the environment around them.

Occupational Toxicology: This deals with assessing the potential of adverse effects from chemicals in occupational environment and the recommendations of appropriate protective and precautionary measures.

Regulatory Toxicology: This deals with administrative functions concerned with the development and interpretation of mandatory toxicology testing programs and controlling the use, distribution, and availability of chemicals used commercially and therapeutically. For example, the Food and Drug Administration (FDA) regulates drugs, cosmetics, and food additives.

Regulation: Regulation is the control, by statute, of the manufacture, transportation, sale, or disposal of chemicals deemed to be toxic after testing procedures or according to criteria put forth in applicable laws.

Toxicodynamics: The study of biochemical and physiological effects of toxicants and their mechanism of action.

Toxicokinetics: The study of absorption, distribution, metabolism, and excretion of toxicants in the body.

Toxicovigilance: This deals with the process of identification, investigation, and evaluation of various toxic effects in the community with the aim of taking measures to reduce or control exposures involving the substances that produce these effects.

Toxinology: This deals with assessing the toxicity of substances of plant and animal origins and those produced by pathogenic bacteria/organisms.

Toxicoepidemiology: The study of quantitative analysis of toxicity incidences in organisms, factors affecting toxicity, and species involved, and the use of such knowledge for planning prevention and control strategies.

2.3 TOXICANT AND TYPES OF TOXICANTS

Poison: Poison is derived from the Latin *potus*, a drink that could harm or kill. It is any substance that when taken inwardly in a very small dose or applied in any kind of manner to a living body depraves the health or entirely destroys life. Although the word "toxicant" has essentially the same medical meaning, there are psychological and legal implications involved in the use of the word "poison" that makes manufacturers reluctant to apply it to chemicals, particularly those intended for widespread use in large quantities, unless they are required to do so by law. The term "toxicant" is more acceptable to both manufacturers and legislators.

Toxicant: Toxicant is synonym of poison; it is produced by living organisms in small quantities and is generally classified as biotoxin. These may be phytotoxins (produced by plants), mycotoxins (produced by fungi), zootoxins (produced by lower animals), and bacteriotoxins (produced by bacteria).

Endotoxins: These are found within bacterial cells.

Exotoxins: These are elaborated from bacterial cells.

Venom: A toxicant synthesized in a specialized gland and ejected by the process of biting or stinging. Venom is also a zootoxin, but it is transmitted by the process of biting or stinging.

Systemic Toxicant: A toxicant that affects the entire body or many organs rather than a specific site. For example, potassium cyanide is a systemic toxicant that affects virtually every cell and organ in the body by interfering with the cell's ability to utilize oxygen.

Organ Toxicant: A toxicant that affects only specific organs or tissues (may be called tissue toxicant) while not producing damage to the body as a whole. For example, benzene is a specific organ toxicant in that it is primarily toxic to the blood-forming tissues.

Pollutant: Any undesirable solid, liquid, or gaseous matter resulting from the discharge or admixture of noxious materials that contaminates the environment and contributes to pollution.

2.4 TOXICITY AND TOXIC EFFECTS

Toxic and toxicity are relative terms commonly used to compare one chemical with another.

Toxicity: The state of being poisonous or the capacity to cause injury in living organisms.

Toxicosis: The condition or disease state that results from exposure to a toxicant. The term "toxicosis" is often used interchangeably with the term "poisoning" or "intoxication."

Toxic Effects: Undesirable effects produced by a toxicant/drug that are detrimental to either survival or normal functioning of the individual.

Side Effects: Undesirable effects that result from the normal pharmacological actions of drugs. These results may not be detrimental or harmful to the individual.

Selective Toxicity: Toxicity produced by a chemical in one kind of living matter without harming another form of life, even though the two exist in intimate contact.

Safety: Means/implies practical certainty that injury will not result from use of a substance under specified conditions of quantity and manner of use.

Risk-to-Benefit Ratio: This implies that even a toxic agent may warrant use if its benefits for a significant number of people are much greater than the dangers,.

Risk: Expected frequency of occurrence of a harmful effect such as injury or loss arising from exposure to a chemical or physical agent under specified conditions.

Risk Assessment: A quantitative assessment of the probability of deleterious effects under given exposure conditions.

Hazard: The qualitative description of the adverse effect arising from a particular chemical or physical agent with no regard for dose or exposure. The term "hazard" is related to the risk, but it mainly expresses likelihood or probability of danger, irrespective of dose or exposure. Also a property or set of properties of the chemical substance that may cause an adverse health or ecological effect if there is exposure at a sufficient level.

Tolerance: A state or condition in which the size of the dose required for producing a toxic effect increases with repeated exposure. Also, a state of decreased responsiveness to the toxic effect of a chemical resulting from prior exposure to that compound or structurally related compound.

Acceptable Risk: The probability of suffering from disease or injury during exposure to a substance; it is considered to be small but acceptable to the individual.

Acceptable Exposure: Unintentional contact with a chemical or physical agent that results in harmful effects.

Margin of Exposure (MOE): The ratio of the no observed adverse effect level (NOAEL) for the critical effect to the theoretical, predicted, or estimated exposure dose or concentration.

Threshold Limit Values (TLV): The airborne concentration of a substance that represents conditions under which it is believed that nearly all workers may be repeatedly exposed without adverse effects. These values are expressed as time weight concentration for a 7- to 8-h work day for 40 weeks.

2.4.1 TOXICITY IN RELATION TO FREQUENCY AND DURATION OF EXPOSURE

Acute Toxicity: Toxic effects produced by a single dose or multiple doses during a 24-h period.

Subacute Toxicity: The study of repeated exposure to a toxicant and its effects for 30 days.

Subchronic Toxicity: The study of repeated exposure to a toxicant and its effects for 1 to 3 months.

Chronic Toxicity: The study of repeated exposure to a toxicant and its effects for more than 3 months.

2.4.2 TOXICITY IN RELATION TO TIME OF DEVELOPMENT AND DURATION OF INDUCED EFFECTS

Transient or Reversible or Temporary Toxicity: The toxicity or harmful effect that remains for a short duration of time (eg, narcosis-produced organic solvents).

Persistent or Permanent or Irreversible Toxicity: The toxicity or harmful effect that persists throughout the life span of the individual and is of a permanent nature (eg, scarring of skin produced by corrosives).

Immediate Toxicity: The toxicity that develops soon after a single exposure to a toxicant (eg, cyanide poisoning).

Delayed Toxicity: The toxicity or harmful effect that has a delayed onset of action (eg, peripheral neuropathy produced by some organophosphorus insecticides).

Cumulative Toxicity: Progressive toxicity or harmful effect produced by the summation of incremental injury resulting from successive exposures (eg, liver fibrosis produced by ethanol).

2.5 DOSE AND RELATED TERMS

Dose: The total or absolute quantity or amount of a substance applied or administered at one time to an individual to achieve the desired pharmacological or toxicological response.

Lethal Dose (LD): The lowest dose that causes death in any animal during the period of observation. Various percentages can be attached to the LD value to indicate doses required to kill 1% (LD_1), 50% (LD_{50}), or 99% (LD_{99}) of the test animals in the population.

Lethal Dose 50 (LD_{50}): Also known as median lethal dose (MLD). It is the dose of the toxicant that causes death of 50% of animals under defined conditions such as species, route of exposure, and duration of exposure. It is a commonly used measure of toxicity.

Lethal Concentration (LC): The lowest concentration of the compound in feed (or water in the case of fish) that causes death during the period of observation. It is expressed as milligrams of compound per kilogram of feed (or water).

Lethal Concentration-50 (LC_{50}): The concentration of the compound in feed (or water in the case of fish) that is lethal to 50% of the exposed population. It mainly expresses acute lethal toxicity.

No Observed Effect Level (NOEL): The highest dose level/concentration of a substance that, under defined conditions of exposure, causes no effect (alteration) on morphology, functional capacity, growth, development, or life span of the test animals.

No Observed Adverse Effect Level (NOAEL): The highest dose level/concentration of a substance that, under defined conditions of exposure, causes no observable/detectable effect (alteration) on morphology, functional capacity, growth, development, or life span of the test animals. NOAEL is a variant of NOEL that specifies that only the effect in question is adverse.

Lowest Observed Adverse Effect Level (LOAEL): The highest exposure level/dose level/concentration of a substance under defined conditions of exposure to an observable/detectable effect (alteration) on morphology, functional capacity, growth, development, or life span of the test animals observed.

Reference Dose/Reference Concentration (RfD/RfC): For noncancerous effects, oral intake (RfD) or inhalation reference concentration (RfC) of airborne materials is calculated using the NOAEL or LOAEL as a starting point. These values are developed from the experimentally determined NOAEL or LOAEL.

Maximum Allowable or Admissible/Acceptable Concentration (MAC): The regulatory value defining the upper limit of concentration of certain atmospheric contaminants allowed in the ambient air of the work place.

Maximum Residue Limit/Maximum Residue Level (MRL): The maximum amount of a pesticide or grog (mainly veterinary pharmaceutical) residue that is legally permitted or recognized as acceptable in or on food commodities and animal feeds. Although both terms have the same meaning, in practice the term "maximum residue limit" is used for the pesticide residue and the term "maximum residue level" is applicable for the drug residue.

Maximum Tolerated Dose (MTD): The highest dose/amount of a substance that causes toxic effects but no mortality in the test organism. In a chronic toxicity study, the MLD can cause limited toxic effects in the test organism, but it should not decrease the body weight more than 10% compared with the control group or produce overt toxicity (death of cells or organ dysfunction). The value is often denoted by LD_0.

Maximum Tolerated Concentration (MTC): The highest concentration of a substance in an environment medium that causes toxic symptoms but no mortality in the test organism.

Absolute Lethal Dose (LD_{100}): The lowest dose of substance that, under defined conditions, is lethal to 100% of exposed animals. The value is dependent on the number of organisms used in its assessment.

Absolute Lethal Concentration (LC_{100}): The lowest concentration of substance in an environment medium that, under defined conditions, is lethal to 100% of exposed organisms or species.

Acceptable Daily Intake (ADI): The estimated amount of substance in food or drinking water that can be ingested daily over a lifetime by humans without appreciable health risk. ADI is normally used for food additives (the term "tolerable daily intake" is used for contamination).

2.6 OTHER COMMON TERMS

Alternative Test: Alternative techniques that can provide the same level of information as current animal tests but use fewer animals, cause less suffering, or avoid the use of animals completely. Such methods, as they become available, must be considered whenever possible for hazard characterization and consequent classification and labeling for intrinsic hazards and chemical safety assessment.

Cheminformatics (also Known as Chemoinformatics, Chemioinformatics, and Chemical Informatics): Cheminformatics is the use of computer and informational techniques applied to a range of problems in the field of chemistry. These in silico techniques are used in, for example, pharmaceutical companies in the process of drug discovery.

Endpoint Study Record: International Uniform Chemical Information Database (IUCLID) format of the technical dossier used to report study summaries and robust study summaries of the information derived for the specific endpoint according to the REACH Regulation.

Endpoint: An observable or measurable inherent property/data point of a chemical substance. It can refer to a physical–chemical property like vapor pressure, or to degradability, or to a biological effect that a given substance has on human health or the environment (eg, carcinogenicity, irritation, aquatic toxicity).

In Vitro Test: Literally stands for "in glass" or "in tube"; refers to the test taking place outside of the body of an organism, usually involving isolated organs, tissues, cells, or biochemical systems.

In Vivo Test: A test conducted within a living organism.

In Silico: A phrase coined as an analogy to the familiar phrases in vivo and in vitro. It is an expression used to denote "performed on computer or via computer simulation" and means scientific experiments or research conducted or produced by means of computer modeling or computer simulation.

IUCLID Flag: An option used in the IUCLID software to indicate submitted data type (eg, experimental data) or their use for regulatory purposes (eg, confidentiality).

Prediction Model: A theoretical formula, algorithm, or program used to convert the experimental results obtained by using a test method into a prediction of the toxic property/effect of the chemical substance.

QSARs and SARs (Q(SAR)): Theoretical models that can be used to predict in a quantitative or qualitative manner the physicochemical, biological (eg, (eco)toxicological), and environmental fate properties of compounds from the knowledge of their chemical structure. A SAR is a qualitative relationship that relates a (sub-) structure to the presence or absence of a property or activity of interest. A QSAR is a mathematical model relating one or more quantitative parameters, which are derived from the chemical structure, to a quantitative measure of a property or activity.

Test (or Assay): An experimental system set-up to obtain information about the intrinsic properties or adverse effects of a chemical substance.

Validated Test: A test in which the performance characteristics, advantages, and limitations have been adequately determined for a specific purpose.

Validation: The process by which the reliability and relevance of a test method are evaluated for the purpose of supporting a specific use.

Vertebrate Animal: Animals that belong to the subphylum *Vertebrata*, which are chordates with backbones and spinal columns.

2.7 SOURCES OF POISONING

The exposure of humans and other organisms to toxicants may result from many activities such as intentional ingestion, occupational exposure, environmental exposure, and accidental and intentional (suicidal or homicidal) poisoning. The toxicity of a particular compound may vary with the portal of entry into the body, whether through the alimentary canal, the lungs, or the skin.

2.7.1 ACCIDENTAL POISONING

Accidental poisoning may occur when humans or animals ingest a toxicant accidentally or it is added unintentionally to food or through feed, fodder, or drinking water. Such toxicants come from either natural sources or human-made sources. Natural sources include ingestion of toxic plants, biting or stinging by poisonous reptiles, ingestion of food contaminated with toxins, water contaminated with minerals, and others. Human-made sources include therapeutic agents, household products, agrochemicals, and others.

2.7.2 MALICIOUS POISONING

Malicious poisoning is the unlawful or criminal killing of a human or animal by administering certain toxic/poisonous agents. An incidence of such poisoning is more prevalent in humans and less so in animals.

2.7.3 OCCUPATIONAL EXPOSURE

Occupation exposure to workers is very common because humans live in a chemical environment. Estimates indicate that approximately 68,000 to 101,000 chemicals are in common use. Industrialization and creation of large urban centers have led to the contamination of air, water, and soil. Industrial workers are exposed to these chemicals during the synthesis, manufacture, or packaging of these substances or through their use in the occupational setting. The major emphasis of occupational toxicology is to identify the agent of concern, define the conditions leading to their safe use, and prevent absorption of harmful amounts. Guidelines have been issued to establish safe ambient air concentrations for many chemicals found in the workplace. For toxicological implications of chronic exposure to various chemicals, the reader may refer to other chapters about toxic agents in this book.

2.8 DURATION AND FREQUENCY OF EXPOSURE

The exposure of experimental animals to chemicals can be divided into four categories: acute, sub-acute, sub-chronic, and chronic.

Acute exposure is defined as exposure to a chemical for less than 24 h. Examples of exposure routes are: intraperitoneal (IP), intravenous (IV), and subcutaneous (SC) injection; per os (oral intubation); and dermal application. The exposure usually refers to a single administration; repeated exposures may be given within a 24-h period for some slightly toxic or practically nontoxic chemicals. Acute exposure by inhalation refers to continuous exposure for less than 24 h, most frequently for 4 h.

Repeated exposure is divided into three categories: sub-acute, sub-chronic, and chronic.

1. *Sub-acute exposure* refers to repeated exposure to a chemical for 1 month or less.
2. *Sub-chronic exposure* refers to repeated exposure to a chemical for 1 to 3 months.
3. *Chronic exposure* refers to repeated exposure to a chemical for more than 3 months (usually this refers to studies with at least 1 year of repeated dosing).

These three categories of repeated exposure can be by any route, but most often they occur by the oral route, with the chemical added directly to the diet. In human exposure situations, the frequency and duration of exposure are usually not as clearly defined as in controlled animal studies. However, almost the same terms are used to describe general exposure situations. Thus, workplace or environmental exposures may be described as *acute* (occurring from a single incident or episode), *sub-chronic* (occurring repeatedly over several weeks or months), or *chronic* (occurring repeatedly for many months or years).

CHAPTER

3 Classification of poisons/toxicants

CHAPTER OUTLINE

3.1 INTRODUCTION

Toxic agents are classified in number of ways depending on the interests and needs of the classifier. There is no single classification applicable for the entire spectrum of toxic agents; therefore, combinations of classification systems based on several factors may provide the best rating system. Classifications of poisons may take into account both the chemical and biological properties of the agent; however, exposure characteristics are also useful in toxicology. Classification based on sources of toxicants (plant toxins, animal toxicants, mineral toxicants, synthetic toxicants), physical state of toxicants (gaseous toxicants, liquid toxicants, solid toxicants, dust toxicants), target organ/system (neurotoxicants, hepatotoxicants, nephrotoxicants, pulmotoxicants, hematotoxicants, dermatotoxicants), chemical nature/structure of toxicants (metals, nonmetals, acids, and alkalies), organic toxicants (carbon compounds other than oxides of carbon, the carbonates, and metallic carbides and cyanides), analytical behavior of toxicants (volatile toxicants, extractive toxicants, metals, and metalloids), type of toxicity (acute, subacute, chronic, etc.), toxic effects (carcinogens, mutagens, teratogens, clastogens), usage (insecticides, fungicides, herbicides, rodenticides, food additives, etc.), mechanism of action, and environmental and public health considerations.

3.2 CLASSIFICATION OF POISONS

According to the main symptoms produced, poisons are basically classified into four groups, namely, corrosive poisons, irritant poisons, systemic poisons, and other poisons. The details are summarized in Tables 3.1–3.4.

Fundamentals of Toxicology. DOI: http://dx.doi.org/10.1016/B978-0-12-805426-0.00003-2

To help physicians and to provide them with some idea regarding the hazardous nature of various poisons in humans, a "toxicity rating" system has been created for common poisons. The higher the toxicity rating for a particular substance (over a range of 1–6), the greater its potency. The toxicity rating based on toxic potential of substances (super toxic, extremely toxic, very toxic, moderately toxic, slightly toxic, and practically nontoxic) is summarized in Table 3.5.

Table 3.1 Corrosive Poisons (Caustics)

Strong Acids		Strong Alkalies	
Inorganic or Mineral Acids	**Organic Acids**	**Hydrates of**	**Carbonates of**
Sulphuric acid	Carbolic acid	Sodium	Potassium
Nitric acid	Oxalic acid	Sodium	Potassium
	Hydrochloric acid		

Table 3.2 Irritant Poisons

Inorganic	Organic	Mechanical
Nonmetallic: phosphorus, halogens *Metallic*: arsenic, mercury, lead, copper, etc.	*Vegetable*: Abrus, castor, croton, calatropia, ergot, etc. *Animal*: snake or insect bites and stings	Diamond dust, glass powder, hair, nails, pins, etc.

Table 3.3 Systemic Poisons

Central Nervous System (Neurotoxins)	Cardiovascular	Lungs (Asphyxiants)
Central Soniferous • Opium • Pethidine *Inebriants* • Alcohols, anesthetics • Sedative hypnotics • Insecticides (hydrocarbons) • Benzodiazepines, etc. *Delirients* • Datura • Cannabis • Cocaine, etc. *Spinal* Strychnine, gelsemium, etc. *Peripheral* Curare, conium, etc.	Oleanders, aconite, nicotine	Carbon monoxide, carbon dioxide, irrespirable gas, cyanogens gas, Amol cyanides

Table 3.4 Miscellaneous Poisons

Domestic poisons	Insecticides (aluminum phosphide, rat poison), kerosene, diesel, petrol, cleaning agents, soaps, detergents, disinfectants, cosmetics, etc.
Therapeutic substance	Salicylates, paracetamol, antidepressants, sedatives, antipsychotics, insulin, etc.
Food poisons	Bacterial, viral, mushrooms, chemicals, etc.
Drugs of dependence	Alcohol, tobacco, hypnotics, hallucinogens, stimulants, organic solvents, etc.

Table 3.5 Toxicity Rating

	Probable Lethal Dose (Human)	
Toxicity Rating or Class	**General Dose, mg/kg**	**For a 70-kg Man**
6 (super toxic)	<5 mg/kg	A few drops
5 (extremely toxic)	5–50 mg/kg	A pinch to 1 teaspoon
4 (very toxic)	51–500 mg/kg	1 teaspoon to 2 tablespoons
3 (moderately toxic)	501 mg/kg to 5 g/kg	1 ounce to 1 pint (1 pound)
2 (slightly toxic)	5.1 g/kg to 15 g/kg	1 pint to 1 quart (2 pounds)
1 (practically nontoxic)	>15 g/kg	More than 2 pounds

3.3 ACTIONS OF POISONS

Poisons usually act in three ways: locally, remotely, and both locally and remotely.

- *Locally Acting*: The chemicals act only at the site of application, such as skin/mucosa (eg, corrosive poisons).
- *Remotely Acting*: These act only after being absorbed into the circulatory system (eg, narcotic poisons, cardiac poisons, etc.).
- *Both Locally and Remotely Acting*: These act by local and remote actions (eg, carbolic acid, etc.).

CHAPTER

Factors affecting toxicity

4

CHAPTER OUTLINE

4.1 INTRODUCTION

It is well known that the sensitivity to the adverse effects of xenobiotics is not the same for all species. For example, unlike most mammals, rabbits may ingest large amounts of belladonna (*Atropa belladonna*), an extremely toxic chemical. It is also well known that the exposure of a population to a given amount of a toxicant may not affect each individual to a similar extent because of the occurrence of several factors capable of modulating the overall toxic response. Age is also an important determinant of chemical toxicity for most compounds. Toxicity is generally higher in younger individuals for a number of reasons, including, among others, a limited ability to biotransform and excrete xenobiotics. Thus, several factors, both of environmental origin as well as pertaining to individuals or mediated by the xenobiotic itself, may influence the response to foreign compounds.

4.2 FACTORS AFFECTING TOXICITY

These factors capable of modulating chemical toxicity can be grouped as:

1. Host factors (factors related to subject)
2. Factors related to toxicant or associated with xenobiotics
3. Environmental conditions

Thus, there could be individual or nonindividual factors that can affect the response of any drug or chemical.

Fundamentals of Toxicology. DOI: http://dx.doi.org/10.1016/B978-0-12-805426-0.00004-4

4.2.1 HOST FACTORS

Size Size or weight of an individual is an important variable that determines the dose of a chemical agent required to elicit a given response. If the same amount of a chemical is given to individuals of different sizes, then the concentration of the chemical attained in the tissues will be different and, hence, the effect induced will vary. Large individuals can tolerate a larger dose than individuals of small size. For this reason, the dosage or the amount of a chemical to be given or the amount of chemical allowed as acceptable daily intake (ADI) is expressed as per unit of body weight. The metabolism and activity are proportional to the surface area of the body and, accordingly, this function has been used for fixing tolerance limits and for determining the ADI for various chemical agents.

Age Young animals or human infants are uniquely susceptible to chemicals that are relatively safer during a later period of life. The difference in response during early life is a consequence of the relative inefficiency of various metabolic and excretory pathways, the greater susceptibility of certain tissues, immaturity of the blood–brain barrier, and other factors. It is well known that a number of enzyme systems are poorly developed at birth. This deficiency is primarily quantitative, with the processes for biotransformation or excretion of the chemical agent being present but functioning at a level significantly below that of the adult. The oxidative pathways concerned with metabolism of a variety of chemical agents operate in the newborn at levels well below those of the adults. For example, deficiency of glucuronyl transferase activity results in enhanced toxicity of chemicals that are dependent on this route of detoxification and contributes to the accumulation of unbound bilirubin, which may lead to jaundice. Immaturity of kidney, brain, or other organs may also render them more sensitive to drugs or chemicals. Immaturity of the blood–brain barrier may allow easier access of the chemical agent of the central nervous system (CNS) than in the adult.

Species and strains Species variation can greatly influence the toxicity of a specific compound. The relative toxicity of some chemicals, such as endosulfan, when tested in several species varied markedly. Often, differences in toxicity are due to different types of biotransformation, which can take place in various tissues. The compound administered to one species may be rapidly metabolized to a nontoxic compound or, at times, to a more toxic compound; in a second species, the same compound may be metabolized at a very slow rate or, in fact, may be metabolized by another mechanism producing a different metabolite.

Differences in the strain of animals also induce a variation in response of chemical agents, and such differences have been detected in acute toxicity measurement of various inbred strains of mice. Because humans are a remarkably heterogeneous species, the rate of metabolism of any compound may differ greatly from person to person.

Sex The sex of an animal often has an influence on the toxicity of a chemical agent. Major differences are shown to be under direct endocrine influence. The nephrotoxic effect of chloroform in the male mouse can be reduced by estrogen treatment and castration; androgen treatment in the female mouse induces susceptibility to this effect. In such instances, the effect of sex hormones on the enzymatic biotransformation of a compound might be responsible for the sex differences. Females generally require a lower dosage than males because of their smaller size. Because variation in toxicity due to sex is well known, the chemical agents or drugs must be used with special care during pregnancy because they could lead to teratogenic effects in females. During lactation, it is important to remember that some chemicals or drugs may be excreted in milk and may even act on the offspring. Thus, it is desirable to measure acute toxicity in both male and female animals of any species.

Feed and feeding The composition of the feed or food can affect the results of toxicity tests. High-fat diets can sensitize animals to the hepatotoxic effects of chloroform, whereas high-carbohydrate and high-protein diets provide protection from these effects. It may be of significance to mention that the activity of hepatic drug-metabolizing enzyme systems decreases in mice fed a low-protein diet, and vitamin C deficiency has been shown to affect the rate of drug metabolism in guinea pigs. Altered reactions have been reported in acute toxicity in animals fed synthetic diets. Even some food ingredients might induce a toxic reaction during a drug treatment. For example, sympathomimetic effects due to the interaction of monoamine oxidase inhibitors and cheese with a high tyramine content have been demonstrated. These findings indicate that it is necessary to provide a standard and nutritionally adequate diet in toxicity studies. However, the study of toxicity in animals with some nutritional deficiency (eg, protein) is of considerable interest. For example, decrease in absorption of the compounds in animals feed prior to intubation is frequently encountered in oral toxicity tests. Therefore, to assume more uniform absorption, it is customary to withhold the feed for 16–18 h prior to intubation. However, starvation-induced catabolic effects may also influence the results of toxicity. For practical reasons, overnight starvation is a common practice. Water is offered ad libitum before and after dosage.

Changes in the internal environment Several physiological factors, such as physical activity, stress conditions, hormonal state of animals, and degenerative changes in internal organs, are known to influence the toxicity of any compound; therefore, toxicity tests are performed with healthy animals. Changes in metabolism or body composition during pregnancy and lactation, as well as after major surgery, could influence toxicological responses.

Alteration of chemical toxicity induced by a compound given prior to the one undergoing investigation is of great importance. For example, some compounds may induce increased synthesis of liver microsomal enzymes and influence the metabolism of another. Inhibition of drug or chemical agent metabolism, displacement of protein binding of a chemical, or inhibition of its renal clearance can also be accomplished by chemical agents.

Pathologic conditions often modify the effect of chemical agents to a very considerable extent because animals or humans will respond in different ways to the same chemical when they are healthy as opposed to when they are ill. Any one of these factors will greatly enhance chemical or drug toxicity.

Habitually used drugs The habitual use of certain psychoactive drugs by humans is known to augment or decrease toxic reactions to drugs in humans. The widespread use of caffeine as tea, coffee, and caffeine-containing soft drinks, alcohol, and nicotine are commonly abused drugs for social purposes. The habitual, and particularly excessive, use of these chemicals could affect the sensitivity of humans to toxic doses of drugs and other chemicals.

Idiosyncratic reaction/toxicity Occasionally, toxicity peculiar to an individual or that appears in a few persons but not in the general population has been observed. The incidence of idiosyncratic toxicity is low, varying from less than 1 person in 100,000 to as high as 1 in 10. Idiosyncratic drug reactions often occur after sensitization followed by re-exposure to a drug. A delay of 3 to 4 weeks after a 1- to 2-week course of medication can be seen for some drugs (eg, amoxicillin-clavulanic acid) before clinical signs become evident, but onset is expedited with rechallenge. Various drugs are believed to cause immune-mediated idiosyncratic reactions in humans, including halothane, diclofenac, phenytoin, and sulfonamides. Skin reactions to drugs or chemicals taken systemically (reactions such as urticaria and angioneurotic edema, bronchial asthma, and anaphylactic shock) have been commonly observed.

Patients with a deficiency of glucose-6-phosphate dehydrogenase, for example, develop hemolysis after ingesting certain drugs or foods. Some idiosyncratic drug reactions can be seen after very long latency (up to 12 months) but are usually not associated with features of hypersensitivity and have been variable in response to a rechallenge. These are classified as nonimmune-mediated idiosyncratic reactions. Examples of drugs that are known to cause this type of idiosyncratic reaction include troglitazone, valproate, amiodarone, ketoconazole, disulfiram, and isoniazid. However, some involvement of allergic mechanism cannot be ruled out.

4.2.2 FACTORS RELATED TO THE TOXICANT OR ASSOCIATED WITH XENOBIOTICS

Physical state and chemical properties of the toxicant The physical state and chemical properties of the toxicant such as: (1) solubility in water; (2) solubility in vegetable oils; (3) the suspending medium; (4) the chemical stability of the chemical agent; (5) the particle size; (6) rates of disintegration of formulations of chemicals; (7) the crystal form; and (8) the grittiness of inert substances given in bulk amounts.

For example, fine particles are more readily absorbed than coarse ones (in the case of poisons bearing irritating properties, eg, α-naphthylthiourea, zinc phosphide). Small particles come into contact with a wider surface of the gastric mucosa and therefore may be more likely to elicit protective vomiting. Some chemicals such as trichlorphon, which is sold as a wettable powder to control external parasites, may be easily converted in alkaline solutions to dichlorvos, which has an eightfold lower oral LD_{50} in rats compared to the parent compound.

Solvents and other substances included in commercial preparations may also affect the overall toxicity of the active principle(s). Nonpolar solvents may considerably increase the absorption rate of lipophilic poisons, especially when considering exposure by the dermal route.

Routes and rate of administration Generally, toxicity is the highest by the route that carries the compound to the blood stream most rapidly. For most xenobiotics, parenteral routes of exposure entail more prompt and complete bioavailability than the oral route, often resulting in a lower LD_{50}. The intravenous toxic dose is greatly influenced by the rate of injection. The gastrointestinal absorption of a compound varies widely. The differences between oral and parenteral LD_{50} give some indication regarding the extent of absorption of a compound. In addition, orally ingested poisons may undergo first-pass metabolism that, in certain cases, may lead to almost complete detoxification. As an example, pyrethrum-based insecticides are practically nontoxic in mammalian species, in which they are extensively hydrolyzed in the gut, but not in fish, in which a significant amount of molecules may enter the body through the gills.

Previous or coincident exposure to other chemicals (drug–drug Interactions) A variety of chemicals (drugs, plant toxins, pesticides, environmental pollutants) are capable of increasing (enzyme inducers) or decreasing (enzyme inhibitors) the expression and activity of hepatic and extrahepatic phase I and phase II enzyme systems participating in the biotransformation reactions, thereby modulating the toxicity of several xenobiotics. Thus, administration of two or more chemicals of different structures when administered simultaneously may lead to an additive effect, summation, negative summation, antagonism, or potentiation. If the agents act on the same organ or tissue and the effect produced is the algebraic sum of their independent actions, then it is called an additive effect.

If the compound leads to enzyme induction, then this phenomenon takes place generally slowly because it requires prolonged exposure to the inducing molecule(s). For a given toxicant, the modulation of the biotransformation capacity mentioned may have different clinically relevant outcomes according to the nature of the toxicant under consideration and the nature of its resulting metabolite(s). In the case of enzyme induction, a decrease in the overall toxicity is expected if the parent compound itself is responsible for the toxic action(s); however, the opposite holds true whether one or more (re)active metabolites arising from biotransformation reactions mediates the toxic damage.

On the contrary, enzyme inhibition is expected to entail beneficial effects in poisonings from toxicants that necessitate a metabolic activation; in certain cases, inhibitors may be used for therapeutic purposes. Cimetidine is recommended to treat acetaminophen toxicosis in dogs and cats because of its inhibitory effects on CYP-mediated generation of the reactive metabolite NAPQI, which is responsible for severe liver injury occurring in poisoned animals.

Enzyme inhibition may enhance the toxic potency of chemicals acting per se (ie, not requiring a metabolic activation) and provide a rationale for explaining many drug–drug interactions.

Drug–drug interactions may also occur in the bloodstream. Anticoagulant rodenticides like warfarin, bromadiolone, or brodifacoum are characterized by relatively long plasma half-lives due to a high degree of plasma protein-binding.

Finally, the co-administration of certain drugs may also modulate the toxicity of several poisons by acting at the receptor level. For instance, drugs that have neuromuscular blocking properties that are elicited through their action on nicotinic receptors (eg, d-tubocurarine or succinylcholine) may enhance the toxicity of organophosphates or carbamates, whereas the reverse holds true in the case of exposure to parasympatholytic agents like atropine, which is widely used as an antagonist in clinical practice.

Tolerance It is well known that the toxic reaction of an animal to a given dose of a drug may decrease, remain unchanged, or increase on subsequent administration of that dose. A decrease in toxic response is usually called tolerance, and an increase is called hypersusceptibility. Enzyme induction, or the increased activity of enzymes concerned with detoxification and elimination of a drug, is a common mechanism for the development of tolerance to a drug on repeated administration.

A decrease in the sensitivity of the end-organs to the toxic effects of the drug is also known to cause tolerance. Chloropromazin, for example, decreases the CNS of normal albino rats and lessens their locomotor activity. On repeated administration of chlorpromazine, there occurs an increase in excitatory feedback to the centers depressed by chlorpromazine with a reluctant decrease in their sensitivity to depression by the drug. On abrupt withdrawal of the drug, excitatory feedback is no longer balanced by the depressant action of the drug and a marked increase in activity of the brain follows, with insomnia and augmented locomotor activity.

4.2.3 ENVIRONMENTAL CONDITIONS

The environment can affect the toxic response to chemicals given to animals or humans. There are three basic factors in the environment of laboratory animals used in toxicity testing:

1. The presence of other species of animals, usually humans. Laboratory animals develop an attitude, maybe hostility, indifference, or affection, depending largely on the operator in the animal. The attitude of the animal can influence the toxic response to drugs.
2. The presence of other animals of the same species. The presence of another male or female of the same species can affect a toxic reaction to certain chemicals, probably due to aggression or fear.
3. *Physical environment*. The physical environment under which a toxicity test is performed causes considerable significance in the toxic response (eg, light,

temperature, relative humidity, etc.). Similarly, temperature can influence the LD_{50} of several chemicals in rats (change in LD_{50} values at 37°C and 26°C). A warm, humid environment is known to enhance dermal absorption as well as affect toxicity in certain inhalation toxicity studies. Even the light and dark cycles of the day, number of animals in the cage, construction of the cage, and seasonal variations are reported to influence the toxicity. Because it is rarely possible to study the effects of all variations in environmental conditions, it is important to state under what conditions an experiment was performed so that one can explain the reason for the variation when duplicating the experiment and getting divergent results.

For example, high ambient temperatures are reported to enhance the toxicity of chlorophenols and nitrophenols that cause increased production of heat by uncoupling mitochondrial oxidative phosphorylation. Conversely, cold temperatures are predisposing factors for α-chloralose, a rodenticide/avicide formerly used as an anesthetic agent that may induce life-threatening hypothermia, especially in cats, by acting on hypothalamic thermoreceptors.

Thus, the exposure to poisons may elicit different outcomes according to a number of factors. In most cases, the variation in the toxic response is based on the different expressions of enzymes or proteins involved in the kinetics of poisons, which may vary according to diet, species, breed, and physiopathological factors, or the previous or concomitant exposure to several foreign compounds. Although until recently such events could not be explained, the current unprecedented development of molecular techniques has made it possible to gain insight into many of the mechanisms underlying most of the differences in the response to foreign compounds.

CHAPTER

Natural laws concerning toxicology

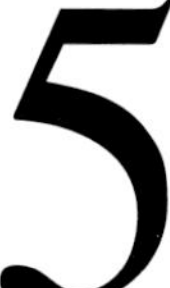

CHAPTER OUTLINE

5.1 INTRODUCTION

The major routes (pathways) by which toxic agents gain access to the body are the GI tract (ingestion), lungs (inhalation), skin (topical, percutaneous, or dermal), and other parenteral routes (other than intestinal canal). Toxic agents generally produce the greatest effect and the most rapid response when administered directly into the bloodstream (intravenous (IV) route). An approximate descending order of effectiveness for the other routes is inhalation, intraperitoneal (IP), subcutaneous (SC), intramuscular (IM), intradermal, oral (per os), dermal, and added directly to the diet. In human exposure situations, the frequency and duration of exposure are usually not as clearly defined as in controlled animal studies, but many of the same terms are used to describe general exposure situations. Thus, work place or environmental exposures may be described as acute (occurring from a single incident or episode), subchronic (occurring repeatedly over several weeks or months), or chronic (occurring repeatedly for many months or years).

Fundamentals of Toxicology. DOI: http://dx.doi.org/10.1016/B978-0-12-805426-0.00005-6

Generally, toxicity is the highest by the route that carries the compound to the blood stream most rapidly. However, a compound could be more toxic orally than parenterally if an active product is formed in the GI tract. The GI absorption of a compound varies widely. The difference between the oral and parenteral lethal dose-50 (LD_{50}) gives some indication regarding the extent of absorption of a compound. The IV toxic dose is greatly influenced by the rate of injection. These variables should be kept in mind, especially when the estimation of lethal dose is attempted in any species of animals.

5.2 TOLERANCE

The toxic reaction of an animal to a given dose of a drug may decrease, remain unchanged, or increase after subsequent daily administration of that dose. A decrease in toxic response is usually called tolerance, and an increase is called hypersusceptibility. Enzyme induction, or the increased activity of the enzymes concerned with detoxification and elimination of the compound, is a common mechanism for the development of tolerance to a drug/toxicant after repeated administration.

A decrease in the sensitivity of the end-organs to the toxic effects of the drug is also known to cause tolerance. Chlorpromazine, for example, after repeated administration decreases the central nervous system (CNS) of normal albino rats and lessens their locomotor activity. After abrupt withdrawal of the drug, the excitatory feedback is no longer balanced by the depressant action of the drug. This is followed by a marked increase in the activity of the brain with insomnia and an increase in locomotor activity.

5.3 DOSE

Most commonly, the term "dose" is used to specify the amount of chemical administered, which is usually expressed per unit of body weight. To study the effect of a drug or other chemical in an animal, that animal has to be dosed. Dosing is the act of introducing a drug or chemical into a living system. As has been explained previously, there are several factors (including the handling of animals) and methods used in these experiments (influencing the outcome of response or toxicity) that are all very important. The purpose of this chapter is not to highlight the methods used in toxicology; however, using the rat as an example, some sketch diagrams for oral or parenteral administration of drugs or chemicals are shown in Fig. 5.1A–H.

As mentioned previously, toxicity is a relative event that depends not only on the toxic properties of the chemical and the dose administered but also on individual and interspecies variation in the metabolic processing of the chemical. The first recognition of the relationship between the dose of a compound and the response obtained has been attributed to Paracelsus. It is noteworthy that his

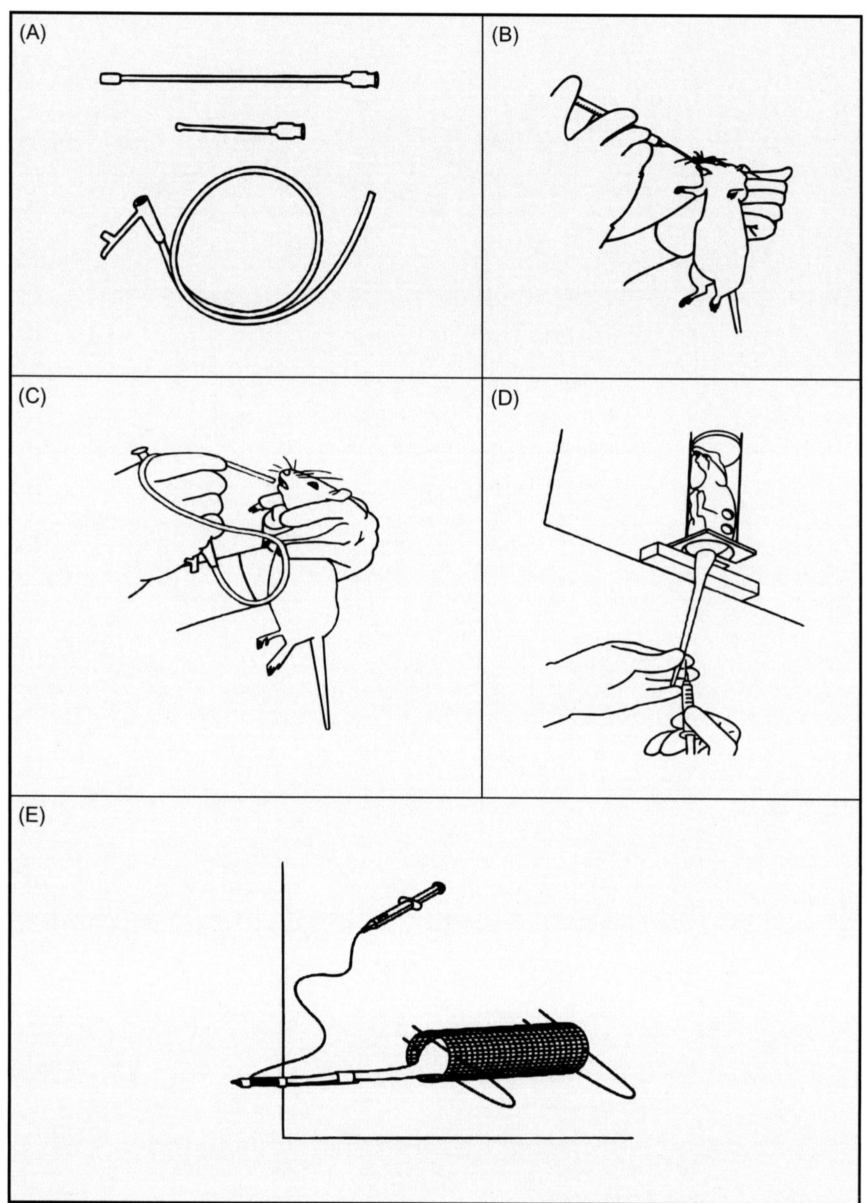

FIGURE 5.1

Sketches (A) to (H) show different methods used during administration of any drug/or chemical in rats. (A) Gavage capsule needle, size 8-French infant feeding needle, and gavage needle. (B) Gavage dosing with ball-tipped needle. Note the method of restraint. (C) Dosing with infant feeding dose. Alternate method of restraint. (D) Tail vein injection. (E) Tail vein infusion. The tail vein has been stabilized with a splinter. (F) Intraperitoneal injection technique. (G) Intramuscular injection technique. (H) Subcutaneous injection technique.

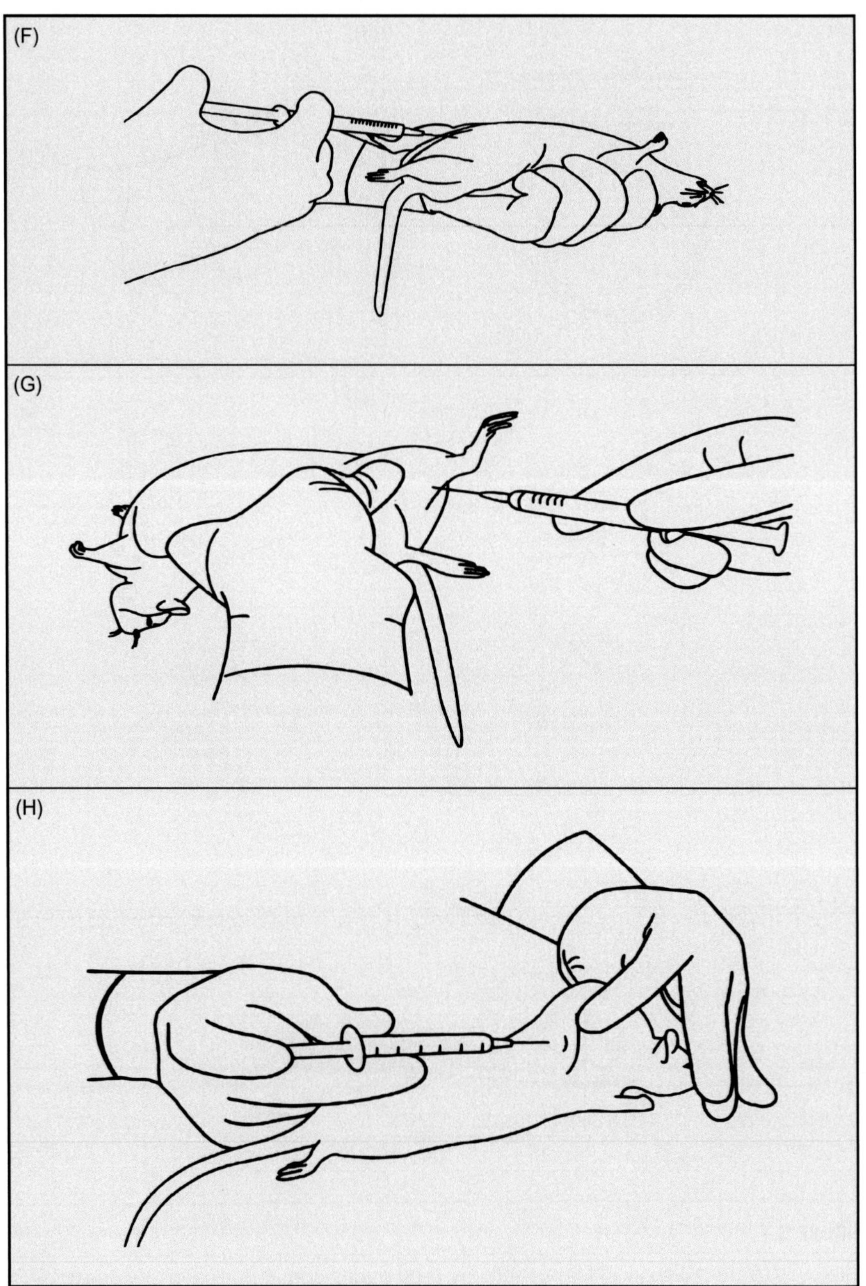

FIGURE 5.1

(Continued)

statement includes not only that all substances can be toxic at some dose but also that "the right dose differentiates a poison from a remedy," a concept that is the basis for pharmaceutical therapy (ie, a typical dose–response curve in which the percentage of organisms or systems responding to a chemical is plotted against the dose). For many chemicals there will be a dose below which no effect or response is observed. This is known as the threshold dose. This concept is of significance because it implies that a no observed effect level (NOEL) can be determined and that this value can be used to determine the safe intake for food additives and contaminants such as pesticides (but not chemical carcinogens).

5.4 TIME ACTION CURVES

The relationship between dose and response is usually established when the chemical/drug effect at a particular dose has reached a maximum or a steady level. Naturally, the chemical effects do not develop instantaneously or continue indefinitely; they change with time. Thus, the magnitude of a chemical effect at any given moment is a function not only of the dose but also of the amount of time elapsed since the chemical made contact with the reactive tissues. This curve represents several important features. There are three distinct phases and a fourth phase that may be present or pronounced with some chemicals but absent with others (Fig. 5.2); these include:

- Time of onset of action (*T*a)
- Time to peak effect (*T*b)
- Duration of action (*T*c)
- Residual effects (*T*d)

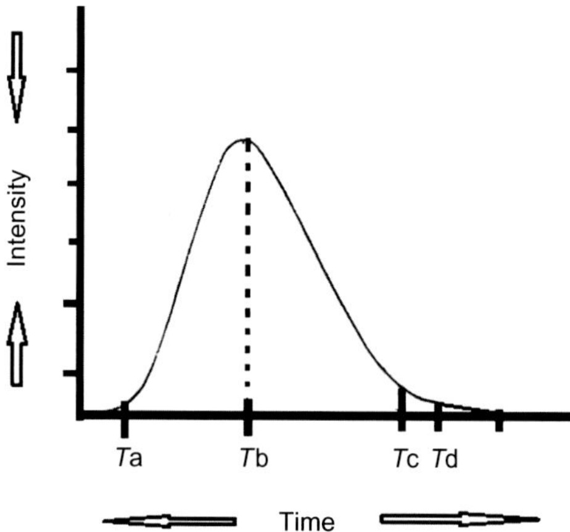

FIGURE 5.2

Hypothetical curve showing time–effect relationship of a toxicant. *T*a, latency time; *T*b, peak time; *T*c, persistence time; *T*d, residual effect.

Phase I: Time of onset of action (*T*a). Following the administration of a chemical agent to a system, there is a delay in time before the first signs of chemical effects are manifested. The lag in onset is of finite time, but for some chemicals the delay may be so short that it gives the appearance of an instantaneous action. There are various reasons responsible for the chemical effect to reach an observable level.

Phase II: Time to peak effect (*T*b). The maximum response will occur when the most resistant cell has been affected to its maximum or when the chemical has reached the most inaccessible cells of the responsive tissue.

Phase III: Duration of action (*T*c). The duration of action extends from the moment of onset of perceptible effects to the time when an action can no longer be measured. It will depend on the rate at which it is metabolized, altered, or otherwise inactivated or removed from the body.

Phase IV: Residual effects (*T*d). Even after its primary actions are terminated, many chemicals are known to exert a residual action. It is not always possible to determine whether the residual effect is caused by the persistence of minute quantities of the chemical or by persistence of subliminal effects.

5.5 DOSE–RESPONSE RELATIONSHIP

"Effect" and "response" are often used interchangeably to denote a biological change, either in an individual or in a population, associated with an exposure or dose. However, some toxicologists have found it useful to differentiate between an effect and a response by applying the term "effect" to a biological change and the term "response" to the proportion of a population that demonstrates a defined effect.

From a practical perspective, there are two types of dose–response relationships:

1. The individual dose–response relationship, which describes the response of an *individual* organism to varying doses of a chemical, often referred to as a "graded" response because the measured effect is continuous over a range of doses.
2. A quantal dose–response relationship, which characterizes the distribution of individual responses to different doses in a *population* of individual organisms. Thus, the dose–response relationship has two broad types:
   a. graded or gradual dose–response relationship
   b. quantal or all-or-none dose–response relationship

5.5.1 GRADED OR GRADUAL DOSE–RESPONSE RELATIONSHIP

The graded or gradual response involves a continuous change in the effect with changing doses. This type of relationship is useful for measuring the incremental responses of a compound and can be seen in an individual organism as,

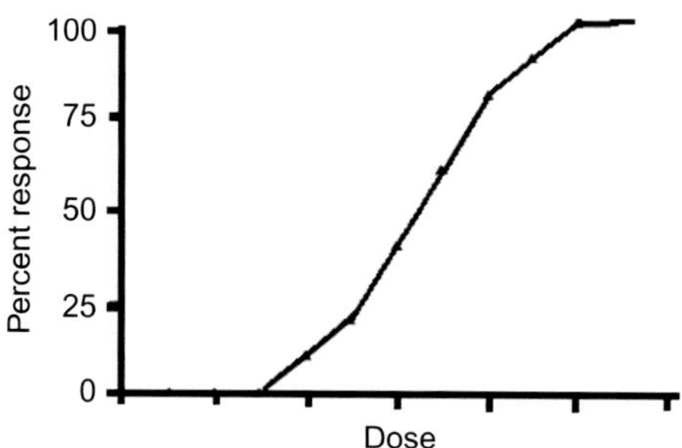

FIGURE 5.3

A typical dose–response curve in which the percentage of organisms or systems responding to a chemical is plotted against the dose.

for example, the contraction of the small intestine produced by carbachol, convulsions produced by strychnine, and inhibition of cholinesterase (ChE) produced by organophosphorus (OP) insecticides. This type of relationship is useful for studying efficiency of therapeutic drugs or toxic symptoms produced by a toxicant. A typical dose–response curve in which the percentage of organisms or systems responding to a chemical is plotted against the dose is shown in Fig. 5.3.

The graded dose–response relationship is based on the following presumptions:

1. The pharmacological/toxicological effect is a result of the known drug/toxicant.
2. There is a molecular or receptor site(s) with which the drug/toxicant interacts to produce the response.
3. The production of a response and the degree of response are related to the concentration of the drug/toxicant at the molecular or receptor site.
4. The concentration of the drug/toxicant at the molecular or receptor site, in turn, is related to the administered dose of the agent.
5. The effect of drug/toxicant is proportional to the fractions of molecular or receptor site occupied by the agent; therefore by increasing or decreasing the dose, the response also increases or decreases, respectively. The maximal effect occurs when the drug/toxicant occupies all molecular or receptor sites.

The logarithmic transformation of dose is often used for the dose–response relationship because:

1. It permits display of a wide range of doses on a single graph.
2. It facilitates visual and mathematical comparisons between the dose–response curve for different agents or for different responses to a single agent.
3. Log–dose plots usually provide a more linear representation of data.

5.5.2 QUANTAL OR ALL-OR-NONE DOSE–RESPONSE RELATIONSHIP

A quantal dose–response relationship is one involving an all-or-none response; for example, on increasing the dose of a compound, the response is either produced or not produced. This relationship is seen with certain responses that follow the all-or-none phenomenon and cannot be graded (eg, death). In toxicology, the quantal dose–response relationship is extensively used for the calculation of the lethal dose because in it we observe only mortality. The quantal dose–response relationship is always seen in a population because the assumption is made that the individual responds to the maximal possible or not at all. The graph of a quantal dose–response relationship does not show the intensity of effect, but rather the frequency with which any dose produces the all-or-none phenomenon. A widely used statistical approach for estimating the response of a population to toxic exposure is the "effective dose" (ED) or "lethal dose" (LD). Generally, the mid-point, or 50%, response level is used, giving rise to the effective dose-50 (ED_{50}) or LD_{50} value. However, any response level, such as an ED_1, ED_{10}, or ED_{30} or lethal dose-1 (LD_1), LD_{10}, or LD_{30}, could be chosen. A graphical representation of an approximate ED_{50} is shown in Figs. 5.4 and 5.5. Please note that these responses may be mortality (LD) or ED.

In quantal dose–response, the log–dose response curve is sigmoid in character. The sigmoid curve has a relatively linear portion between 16% and 84% and is used to determine the slope of the curve. A small portion of the population at the left and right sides of the curve responds to low and high doses and constitutes hyper-reactive (hypersensitive) and hyporeactive (hyposensitive) groups respectively. If a compound produces its effect at a very low dosage, then the individual is said to be hyper-reactive or hypersensitive; if the same effect is produced by the compound at unusually large doses, then the individual is said to be hyporeactive or hyposensitive.

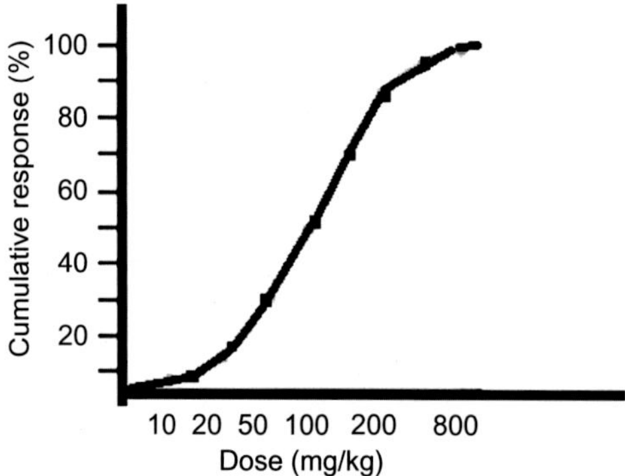

FIGURE 5.4

Typical sigmoid S-shaped curve showing quantal dose–response relationship. The response may be effective dose or morality.

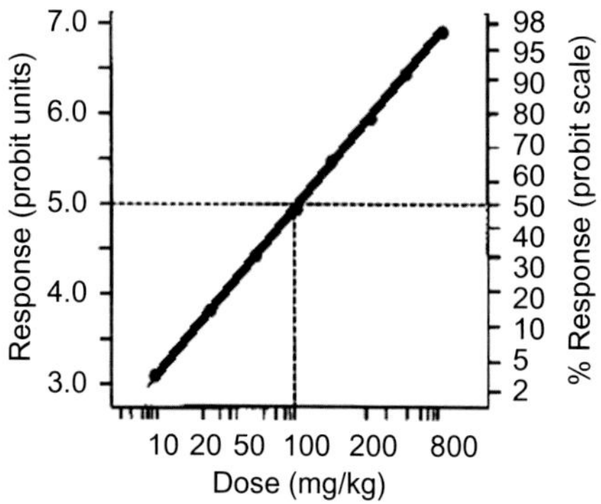

FIGURE 5.5

Quantal dose–response relationship showing linear transformation of dose–response data by log-probit plot. Percentage response may be effective dose or morality.

LD_{50}: Also called median lethal dose (MLD), is the dose that is lethal to 50% of animals exposed to a given toxicant under defined conditions. The LD_{50} value is a common way of expressing acute toxicity and may not pertain to the severity of clinical signs observed in the characteristic changes caused by the toxicant but depend only on the lethality produced by the toxicant. Although recently some toxicological organizations and government regulatory agencies have greatly reduced reliance on the LD_{50} (to reduce the number of animals needed for study), it is still considered an important index to assess the toxicity of chemicals.

5.6 STATISTICAL CONCEPT OF TOXICITY

The calculation of the LD_{50} value is a statistical estimate of the dose necessary to kill 50% of a very large population of the test species. Experimentally, this is achieved by administering a chemical at graded doses to a group of animals and then observing the resultant mortalities in a set time period (usually 1–2 weeks). Generally, rats and mice are the species of choice, but other species such as rabbits, guinea pigs, and hamsters may be used.

The LD_{50} value is obtained by plotting the percentage of individuals succumbing to a given dose of lethal chemical as ordinate against the dose of the compound used as abscissa. In this way, one obtains as S-shaped curve as shown Fig. 5.4. The shape of the curve indicates the degree of variation. The LD_{50} is obtained from the curve by drawing a horizontal line from the 50% mortality point on the ordinate where it intersects the curve. At the point of intersection the vertical line is drawn, and this line intersects at the LD_{50} point. This dose is designated as LD_{50}. The same data from the sigmoid curve or a bell-shaped curve will form a straight line when transformed into probit units (Fig. 5.5). These values are statistically obtained and represent the best estimation of the dose required to kill 50% of the animals. The information with respect to the lethal dose for 95% or for 5% of the animals can also be derived by a similar procedure. The estimation is always accompanied by some error of the value, such as probability range of the value. The limits of the probability range are arbitrarily selected by the experimenter to indicate that similar results would be obtained in 90 or 95 of 100 tests performed in a manner identical to that described. Several methods have been described for making such estimations. The standard procedures are described in the literature. The description of detailed procedures is beyond the scope of this chapter. Similarly, the LD_1 and LD_{99} can be easily estimated from the equations used to estimate the LD_{50}.

Biological similarities in values of the LD_{50} suggest that toxicity in humans will be similar to that found in animals. If the same LD_{50} is found in a wide variety of animal species, then the toxic reaction in humans is more likely to be similar to that in animals than if there is variation between biologically different species.

Suppose that a compound is administered to a uniform population of biologic specimens. The typical line at LD_{50} is drawn to intersect the curve at 50 on the ordinate. The point of intersection on this line with the abscissa gives the dose that is lethal for 50% of the test animals.

The evaluation of the LD_{50} in several animal species is a fair guide to the acute lethal toxicity of the same compound in humans. One such scheme utilizes ranges of doses with descriptive terms for toxicity. LD_{50} values are also useful for making an objective comparison of inherent toxicity of different compounds. Some compounds are so toxic that exposure to a few drops will result in toxicity. On the contrary, other compounds are relatively harmless and may be ingested without any harm. A general guideline for the probable lethal oral dose for a human is summarized in Chapter 3, Classification of Poisons/Toxicants (Table 3.5).

5.7 VARIABLES OF DOSE–RESPONSE CURVE

Irrespective of the shape (linear, sigmoid, hyperbolic), the dose–response curve has four characteristic variables: efficacy, potency, slope, and biological variations. These terms may be defined as follows.

Efficacy: The maximal effect or response produced by an agent is called its maximal efficacy or efficacy.

Potency: Potency is a comparative measure that refers to the different doses of two agents needed to produce the same effect.

Slope: The slope of a dose–response curve gives the relationship between the receptor/target site and the agent.

Biological Variations: Variation or variance can be defined as the appearance of differences in the magnitude of response among individuals in the same population given the same dose of a compound.

5.8 FREQUENTLY USED TERMS FOR SAFETY EVALUATION OF DRUGS

The margin of safety of a compound is determined from the results of two studies, such as an ED study and an LD study. A ratio between selected ED and LD values is then used to express the margin of safety. The larger the ratio, the greater is the margin of safety.

Therapeutic Index (TI): TI may be defined as the ratio of the LD_{50} and the ED_{50}.

$$TI = LD_{50}/ED_{50}$$

where LD_{50} is the dose that is lethal for 50% of the population and ED_{50} is the dose that is effective for 50% of the population.

The TI measure is commonly used for evaluating the safety and usefulness of therapeutic agents. The higher the index, the safer is the drug.

Therapeutic Ratio (TR): The TR may be defined as the ratio of the lethal dose-25 (LD_{25}) and the effective dose-75 (ED_{75}).

$$TR = LD_{25}/ED_{75}$$

where LD_{25} is the dose that is lethal for 25% of the population and ED_{75} is the dose that is effective for 75% of the population.

TR is considered a better index of safety of a compound because it also includes the steepness of curve. In toxicity cases, a flatter curve is considered more toxic, or hyper-reactive groups are at a much greater risk than the hyporeactive or normal group. Shallower curves usually have low therapeutic ratios.

Standard Safety Margin (SEM): SEM may be defined as the ratio of the LD_1 and the effective dose-99 (ED_{99}).

$$SEM = LD_1/ED_{99}$$

where LD_1 is the dose that is lethal for 1% of the population and ED_{99} is the dose that is effective for 99% of the population.

The SEM is a more conservative estimate than the TI because values are derived from extremes of the respective dose–response curves.

Chronicity Factor: Chronicity factor is the ratio of the acute LD_{50} (one dose) to chronic LD_{50} doses.

$$\text{Chronicity factor} = \text{acute } LD_{50}/\text{chronic } LD_{50}$$

The chronicity factor is used to assess the cumulative action of a toxicant. Compounds with cumulative effects have a higher chronicity factor.

Risk Ratio: The ratio between the inherent toxicity and the exposure level gives the risk ratio. Risk ratio indicates the risk of a compound. Substances of higher inherent toxicity may pose little risk because access of exposure of individuals to such agents is limited. Compounds of low toxicity may be dangerous if used extensively.

5.9 INTERACTION WITH RECEPTORS

Many toxicants/xenobiotics exert their effects by interacting with specific receptors in the body. This xenobiotic–receptor interaction leads to a change in the macromolecule, which in turn triggers a sequence of events resulting in a response of the tissue or organ. The intensity of the response produced by a toxicant/xenobiotic depends on its intrinsic activity, which in turn depends on the chemical structure of the compound.

Affinity: Affinity is the ability of a xenobiotic to combine with its receptors. A ligand of low affinity requires a higher concentration to produce the same effect as a ligand of high affinity. Agonists, partial agonists, antagonists, and inverse agonists have the same or similar affinity for the receptor.

Intrinsic Activity: A proportionately constant ability of the agonist to activate the receptor as compared to the maximally active compound in the series being studied. It is the maximum of unity for a full agonist and the minimum or zero for the antagonist.

5.10 TYPES OF XENOBIOTICS

Agonist: Agonist (full agonist) is an agent that interacts with a specific cellular constituent (ie, receptor) and elicits an observable positive response.

Partial Agonist (PA): PA is an agent that acts on the same receptor as other agonists in a group of endogenous ligands or xenobiotics but, regardless of its dose, it cannot produce the same maximal biological response as a full agonist.

Antagonist: Antagonist is an agent that interacts with the receptor or any other part of the effector mechanism to inhibit the action of an agonist. Antagonist has no activity of its own.

Inverse Agonist: Inverse agonist is a compound that interacts with the same part as the agonist, but it produces a response just opposite to that of the agonist.

5.11 XENOBIOTIC/DRUG INTERACTION

When two or more xenobiotics are used together, the pharmacological/toxicological response is not necessarily the same of two agents used individually because one agent may interfere with the action of another agent. This is called xenobiotic/drug interaction.

Addition/Additive Effect: When the combined effect of two compounds given together is equal in magnitude to the sum of the effects of each compound given alone, the interaction is called addition and the effect produced is called the additive effect.

Potentiation/Potentiative Effect: When one compound has no effect of its own increases the effect of another compound, the interaction is called potentiation and the effect produced is called the potentiative effect.

Synergism/Synergistic Effect: When the combined effect of two compounds given together is greater in magnitude than the sum of the effects of each compound given alone, the interaction is called synergism and the effect produced is called the synergistic effect.

Antagonism/Antagonistic Effect: When the combined effect of two compounds given together is lesser in magnitude than the sum of the effects of each compound given alone, or when one compound with no effect of its own decreases or inhibits the effect of the other compound, the interaction is called antagonism and the effect produced is called the antagonistic effect.

5.12 NATURE AND EXTENT OF TOXICITY TESTING

The nature and extent of toxicity vary depending on the origin of toxic substances. They may be natural in origin or artificial or synthetic. The majority of toxicants/chemicals stem from an industrial or commercial pool of synthetic chemicals. The toxic effects of chemical may be physiological, biochemical, or pathological in nature. The changes produced by these agents can be complex and damaging not only to one organ or tissue but also to different cells. As has been discussed previously, a broad distinction is often made between corrosives, irritants, narcotics, and others. In brief, chemical agents may act locally by irritating the tissue with which they come in contact, resulting in severe tissue destruction (eg, caustic alkalis and mineral acids), or they may act systematically, being absorbed into the blood stream and carried to the site of action. For detailed classification of chemicals, the reader is referred to Chapter 3, Classification of Poisons/Toxicants.

It has become customary to classify toxicity as one of three types: acute, subacute, or chronic toxicity. Some chemicals are capable of producing all three types of toxicities. Development and reproduction toxicity, carcinogenicity, genotoxicity, and other special types of toxicity are often treated as separate groups because of their unique aspects of toxic action. Therefore, these aspects of toxicity are discussed separately in subsequent chapters.

CHAPTER

Hazard and risk assessment

6

CHAPTER OUTLINE

6.1 INTRODUCTION

We often perform toxicological research to understand the mechanisms and associated health risks following exposure to hazardous agents. The problem of understanding the hazards and risks associated with unintentional or coincidental exposures to chemicals is a complex one, with multiple uncertainties. Therefore, risk assessment (RA) is a systematic scientific characterization of potential *adverse health effects* following exposure to these hazardous agents. The RA activities are designed to *identify*, *describe*, and *measure qualities and quantities* from these toxicological studies, which are often conducted with homogeneous animal models at doses and exposure durations not encountered in a more heterogeneous human population.

Thus, the assessment of risks to human health involves the scientific examination and evaluation of information in four areas: the hazardous nature of agents in the environment; the degree of human exposure to such agents; the response of people's health to exposure; and risk management. The product of a RA is information about the likelihood of health degradation following an exposure to hazardous agents.

Risk Assessment (RA): RA can be defined as the systematic scientific evaluation of potential adverse health effects resulting from human exposures to hazardous agents or situations.

Risk is defined as the probability of an adverse outcome based on the exposure and potency of the hazardous agent(s).

Fundamentals of Toxicology. DOI: http://dx.doi.org/10.1016/B978-0-12-805426-0.00006-8

RA requires an integration of both qualitative and quantitative scientific information. For example, qualitative information about the overall evidence and nature of the endpoints and hazards are integrated with quantitative assessments of the exposures, host susceptibility factors, and the magnitude of the hazard. A description of the uncertainties and variability in the estimates is a significant part of risk characterization and an essential component of RA.

6.2 RISK ASSESSMENT APPROACH

Over the past several years, regulatory agencies in the United States have developed a systematic scientific and administrative framework for RA. Major regulatory agencies for the control and use of toxic chemicals and RA in the United States are summarized in Table 6.1.

The functional elements for RA are well defined and widely accepted. The factors and elements are important in the evaluation and have been established by various regulatory agencies, including those in the United States. Therefore, for risk analysis, the models used in RA may involve considerations such as those provided in Table 6.2.

Table 6.1 Major Regulatory Agencies for Control and Use of Toxic Chemicals and Risk Assessment in the United States

EPA: Air Pollutants Clean Air Act 1970
Water pollutants: Federal Water Pollution Control Act 1948
Drinking water: Safe Drinking Water Act 1974
Pesticides, Fungicides, Insecticides & Rodenticides Act (FIFRA) 1947
Food Quality Protection Act (FQPA) 1996
Ocean dumping: Marine Protection, Research, and Sanctuaries Act (MPRSA) and Ocean Dumping Act (1972)
Toxic chemicals: Toxic Substances Control Act (TSCA) 1976
Hazardous wastes: Resource Conservation and Recovery Act (RCRA) 1976
Abandoned Hazardous Wastes Superfund (CERCLA) 1980
CEQ environmental impacts: National Environmental Policy Act (NEPA) 1969
OSHA: Workplace Occupational Safety and Health (OSH) Act 1970
Foods, drugs, and cosmetics (FDA): Food and Drugs Act 1906
Food, Drugs, and Cosmetics Act (FDC) 1938
FDA Modernization Act 1997
CPSC dangerous consumer products: Consumer Product Safety Act (CPSA) 1972
Transport of hazardous materials (DOT): Hazardous Materials Transportation Act (HMTA) 1975

EPA, *Environmental Protection Agency;* CEQ, *Council for Environmental Quality (now Office of Environmental Policy);* OSHA, *Occupational Safety and Health Administration;* FDA, *Food and Drug Administration;* CPSC, *Consumer Product Safety Commission;* DOT, *Department of Transportation.*

Table 6.2 Data Required for Preliminary Evaluation of Risk Assessment in Human Health

Data Required	Quality Data
Physiochemical processes	Observed effects on humans
Toxicity	Derived from animal studies
Release/transport/uptake	Applicable to expected dosage
Chemical–physical interaction	Most current to support specific conclusions

Physiochemical processes include the following:

1. Human reactions to hazard exposure
2. Population demographics
3. Animal or human similarity or dissimilarity
4. Industrial control pollution methods

6.2.1 PRELIMINARY EVALUATION

Chemicals are normally classified as hazardous or toxic based on the results of animal studies that are then extrapolated to humans. Toxicity may be established without such observations based on experience with similar chemicals/or materials.

6.2.2 TOXICITY ASSESSMENT

The main evidence used in an assessment of toxicity comes from two sources:

1. Human studies (epidemiological studies)
2. Animal studies

Some supporting information may be obtained from clinical and in vitro studies.

Thus, the risk approach identifies the following four major elements of RA. The information developed in the RA process is utilized in risk management, and decisions are made regarding the need for and the degree of steps to be taken to control exposures to the chemical of concern (Fig. 6.1).

1. Hazard identification
   a. Epidemiology
   b. Animal studies
   c. Short-term assays
   d. Structure–activity relationship
2. Exposure assessment
   a. Identification of exposed populations
   b. Identification of routes of exposure
   c. Identification of degree of exposure

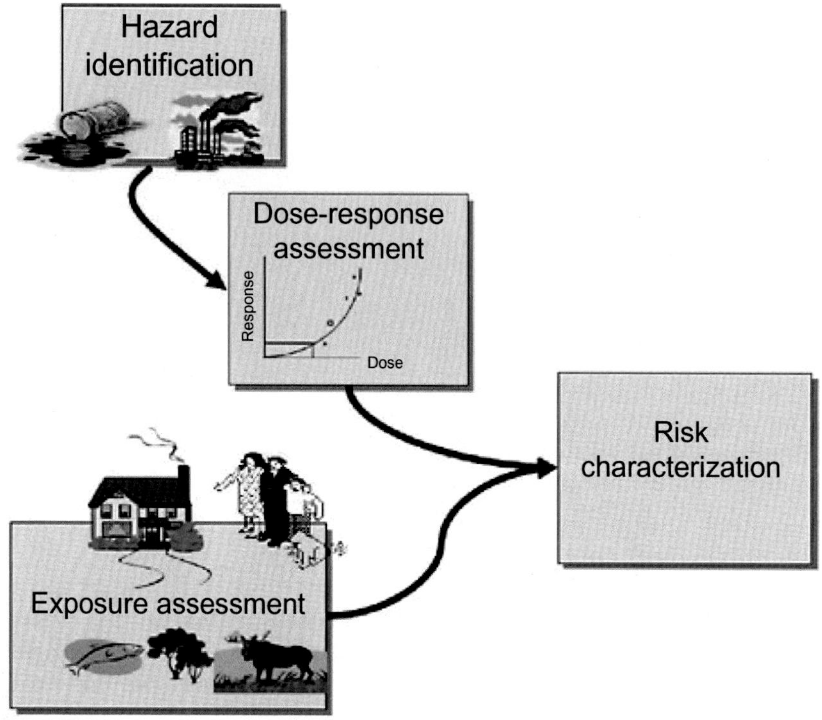

FIGURE 6.1

The four major elements of risk assessment. The information developed in the risk assessment process is utilized in risk management, whereby decisions are made based on the need for and degree of the steps that should be taken to control exposures of chemicals of concern.

Source: NRC, 2007. Models in Environmental Regulatory Decision Making. The National Academies Press, Wasington, DC. Available at: http://www.nap.edu/read/11972/chapter/4.

3. Dose–response assessment
   a. Quantitative toxicity information collected
   b. Dose–response relationship established
   c. Extrapolation of animal data to humans
4. Risk characterization
   a. Estimation of the potential for adverse health effects to occur
   b. Evaluation of uncertainty
   c. Summarization of risk information

In principle, carefully performed epidemiological studies can provide very convincing evidence about a possible relationship between a toxicant and a disease. Because animals are not humans, care must be taken in extending such results to human conditions. When possible, multiple species should be involved in animal tests to minimize the effects of interspecies differences.

The data obtained from various experiments are separated into those that do not increase the likelihood of cancer and those that do. For noncancer-related end points, the concept of no observed adverse effect level (NOAEL) is applied.

As described in previous chapter, approaches for characterizing dose–response relationships include identification of effect levels such as LD_{50} (dose producing 50% lethality), LC_{50} (concentration producing 50% lethality), ED_{10} (dose producing 10% response), and NOAELs. NOAELs have traditionally served as the basis for RA calculations, such as reference doses or acceptable daily intake (ADI) values. Reference doses (RfDs) or concentrations (RfCs) are estimates of daily exposure to an agent that is assumed to be without an adverse health impact in humans. The ADIs are used by WHO for pesticides and food additives to define "the daily intake of chemical, which during an entire lifetime appears to be without appreciable risk on the basis of all known facts at that time." Reference doses and ADI values typically are calculated from NOAEL values by dividing by uncertainty factor (UF) and/or modifying factors (MF). Tolerable daily intake (TDI) can be used to describe the intake of chemicals that are not "acceptable" but are "tolerable" because they are below levels thought to cause adverse health effects. These are calculated in a manner similar to that for ADI. In principle, dividing by the uncertainty factors allows for interspecies (animal-to-human) and intraspecies (human-to-human) variability with default values of 10 each. An additional uncertainty factor is used to account for experimental inadequacies, for example, to extrapolate from studies with short exposure to a situation more relevant for chronic study or to account for inadequate numbers of animals or other experimental limitations. If only a LOAEL value is available, then an additional 10-fold factor is commonly used to arrive at a value more comparable to a NOAEL value. Traditionally, a safety factor of 100 is used for RfD calculations to extrapolate from a well-conducted animal bioassay (10-fold factor, animal-to-human) and to account for human variability in response (10-fold factor, human-to-human variability).

An assumption is made that exposure below a certain level, the NOAEL, will have no adverse health consequences. An acceptable reference dose, RfD, is then established by:

$$\mathrm{RfD} = \mathrm{NOAEL}/(\mathrm{UF} \times \mathrm{MF})$$

$$\mathrm{ADI} = \mathrm{NOAEL}/(\mathrm{UF} \times \mathrm{MF})$$

where the uncertainty factor (UF) is typically equal to 100 and MF is the modifying factor.

For cancer end points, the only strictly safe exposure level is at zero dose, although for very small doses the risk is extremely low and is not considered significant.

6.2.3 EXPOSURE ASSESSMENT

Estimation of exposure begins with the detailed description of the toxic agent. In circumstances where exposure has already occurred, it is easy to obtain sufficient information to make an assessment of the exposure. Due to lifestyle changes in the population, long-term modeling becomes difficult. However, it helps the expert to estimate the dose input for a human subject.

Therefore, the primary objectives of the exposure assessment are to determine the source, type, magnitude, and duration of contact with the chemical of interest. Risk Commission frameworks for risk assessment and risk management provide a consistent framework-based approach for evaluating risks and taking action to reduce risks. The objectives of risk assessments vary with issues, risk management needs, and statutory requirements. Hence, toxicology, epidemiology, exposure assessment, and clinical observations can be linked with biomarkers, cross-species investigations of mechanisms of effects, and systematic approaches to risk assessment, risk communication, and risk management. Conceptually, calculations are designed to represent a "plausible estimate" of the exposure of individuals in the upper 90th percentile of the exposure distribution. Upper-bound estimations would be "bounding calculations" designed to represent exposures at levels that exceed the exposures experienced by all individuals in the exposure distribution and are calculated by assuming limits for all exposure variables. For example, risk calculations of arsenic (As) exposure via a soil ingestion route is calculated using point estimates, and a lifetime average daily dose (LADD) is calculated as follows:

$$\text{LADD} = \frac{\begin{array}{c}\text{Concentration of toxicant in exposure media} \times \text{Contact rate} \times \\ \text{Contact fraction} \times \text{Exposure duration}\end{array}}{\text{(Body weight) (Lifetime)}}$$

Many exposures are now estimated using exposure factor probability distributions rather than single-point estimates for the factors within the LADD equation. In general, estimates for cancer risk use average exposure over a lifetime (see previous LADD example). In a few cases, short-term exposure limits (STELs) (eg, ethylene oxide) and characterization of brief but high levels of exposure are required. In these cases, exposures are not averaged over the lifetime and the effects of high, short-term doses are estimated. With developmental toxicity, a single exposure can be sufficient to produce an adverse developmental effect; therefore, daily doses are used rather than lifetime weighted averages.

There is a great concern about involuntary exposures (especially in the food supply, drinking water, and air) and unfamiliar hazards, such as radioactive waste, electromagnetic fields, asbestos insulation, and genetically modified crops and foods.

In brief, the hazard and RA is based on four components: hazard identification, research, risk assessment, and risk management. The approach is based on uncertainty and the use of various mathematical models while keeping in mind the public health concern and the economic, social, and political contexts for risk management options. Such decisions are made by a risk management group. The details of the models used and the recent approach of the "benchmark dose" are beyond the scope of this chapter.

6.3 CONCLUSION

As scientists, we must clearly communicate the uncertainty associated with our extrapolations; otherwise, we are being dishonest. Our most vigorous efforts must be focused on those activities that best allow us to address these problems. These studies should include designing better studies from the perspective of RA, that is, they should cover a broader range of doses with a focus on the molecular and cellular mechanisms. Advances in toxicology are certain to improve the quality of risk assessments, to find substitute data for assumptions, and to help describe the models with more credibility.

UNIT II

CHAPTER

Absorption, distribution, and excretion of toxicants 7

CHAPTER OUTLINE

7.1 INTRODUCTION

The disposition of a chemical or *xenobiotic* is defined as the composite actions of its *absorption*, *distribution*, *biotransformation*, and *elimination*. This chapter focuses on the contribution of absorption, distribution, and elimination to

Fundamentals of Toxicology. DOI: http://dx.doi.org/10.1016/B978-0-12-805426-0.00007-X

xenobiotic toxicity. Toxicants exert their effect only when they interact with specific receptor sites, which may be located in distant organs. To reach the target site, the toxicant must be absorbed effectively into the blood stream, distributed efficiently to the site of action, and subsequently metabolized and excreted from the body. The processes of absorption and distribution are responsible for placement or deployment of these toxicants in the body, and metabolism and excretion are responsible for elimination of the toxicants from the body. Because all these processes involve passage across biological membranes, we begin with a discussion of this important and ubiquitous barrier.

7.2 TRANSLOCATION OF XENOBIOTICS ACROSS MEMBRANES

Translocations may take place either by simple diffusion or filtration or through specialized transport, which may be active, facilitated, or pinocytosis. The primary routes of exposure for toxic substances are oral, respiratory, and dermal. The gastrointestinal (GI), respiratory, and dermal systems are lined with epithelia that present significant barriers to the entry of foreign substances due to tight junctions between their cells or continuous lipid layers in the case of skin. The membranes of cells that form viable epithelial barriers are traversed by transporter proteins that either actively exclude xenobiotics or facilitate the movement of specific substrates across the barrier. The onset, duration, and intensity of a substance's toxic effects are therefore dependent on the toxicant's ability to permeate lipid cell membranes directly and its interactions with transporter proteins. Dermal penetration is unique in the sense that the outer epithelial cellular layers (corneocytes) are nonviable and do not contain transporter proteins. Absorption, in this case, is therefore dependent on the ability of toxicants to penetrate the intercellular lipid matrix found between corneocytes.

Toxicants usually pass through a number of cells, such as the stratified epithelium of the skin, the thin cell layers of the lungs or the GI tract, capillary endothelium, and ultimately the cells of the target organ. The plasma membranes surrounding all these cells are remarkably similar.

7.2.1 MEMBRANE PERMEABILITY

As stated previously, there are several barriers through which a chemical substance may pass before achieving a sufficient concentration of cells producing the characteristic action. There is a succession of membranes of three main types: (1) those like the skin, composed of several types of layers of cells; (2) those composed of a single layer of cells, such as the intestinal epithelium; and (3) those less than one cell in thickness, such as the membrane of a single cell. Biological cells have a fundamental structure, the cell membrane (or, as it is often called, the plasma membrane). The thickness of the membranes is approximately 100 Å. The pores in various biological membranes vary from 4 to 40 Å. The lipid layer of the cell membrane is readily penetrated by lipid-soluble substances. Current concepts indicate that the cell membrane is a biomolecular layer of lipid molecules coated on each side with a protein layer. The structure of the plasma membranes thus suggest that the important physio-chemical properties of any xenobiotic that influence its passage across the membrane are its size, shape, degree of ionization, and lipid solubility of the ionized and nonionized forms.

7.2.2 MECHANISM OF CHEMICAL TRANSFER

The mechanism by which a chemical agent may pass through a membrane has been summarized in Table 7.1. In general, it can be divided into two types: (1) passive transfer, in which the membrane is inert, and (2) specialized transport, in which the membrane has an active part in the transfer of chemical agents through the membranes. There is yet another mechanism known as pinocytosis.

7.2.3 PROCESSES OF TRANSPORT

Processes of the transport of toxicants across membranes are discussed here.

7.2.3.1 Passive transport

Passive Diffusion: Most toxicants cross membranes by simple diffusion (chemicals traverse from regions of higher concentration to regions of lower concentration) without any energy expenditure. Small hydrophilic molecules

Table 7.1 Transfer of Molecules Across Biological Membranes

Transfer Process	Mechanism	Substrate Specificity
Passive diffusion	Diffusion through lipoidal membrane down to a concentration gradient	None, most foreign compounds
Filtration	Diffusion through aqueous pores in the membrane down to concentration gradient	Hydrophilic molecules and ions of the molecular weight (eg, water, urea)
Facilitated diffusion	Carrier transport through membrane down to a concentration gradient; saturated by excess substrate	Narrow, mainly for molecules concerned with the process of intermediary metabolism (eg, sugars and amino acids)
Active transport	Carrier transport through membrane against a concentration gradient requires metabolic energy; saturated by excess substrate	Narrow, mainly for molecules concerned with the process of intermediary metabolism (eg, sugars and amino acids)
Pinocytosis	Invaginations of the membrane absorb extracellular material	Uncertain

(up to approximately 600 Da) permeate membranes through aqueous pores in a process termed paracellular diffusion, whereas hydrophobic molecules diffuse across the lipid domain of membranes (transcellular diffusion). The smaller a hydrophilic molecule is, the more readily it traverses membranes by simple diffusion through aqueous pores. Consequently, a small, water-soluble compound such as ethanol is rapidly absorbed into the blood from the GI tract and is distributed just as rapidly throughout the body by simple diffusion from blood into all tissues. However, after a steady state is attained, the concentration of the chemical is the same on both sides of the membrane. Both nonpolar and polar substances that posses sufficient lipid solubility diffuse through the membrane in this manner.

Many chemicals of toxicological interest exist in solution in ionized and nonionized forms. The ionized form is often unable to penetrate the cell membrane because of its low lipid solubility; however, in contrast, the unionized (undissociated) agents penetrate biological membranes by diffusion because they are usually much more lipid-soluble than the ionized form. Diffusion is dependent on the lipid solubility of the nonionized form of the compound.

The majority of chemicals to which most of the population is exposed are organic acids or bases. Their absorption is dependent on their dissociation constant (the dissociation constant is the fraction of the compound present in the ionized form). Weak acids and weak bases are only partly ionized (dissociated) in water; strong acids and strong bases are completely ionized. The dissociation constant is expressed for both acids and bases as a pKa, which is simply the negative logarithm of the acidic dissociation constant. It may seem confusing to express the dissociation of both acids and bases as acid dissociation constants, but everything is relative and the use of pKa values makes it easy to make calculations.

An acid with a low pKa is a strong acid, and one with a high pKa is a weak acid. Conversely, a base with a low pKa is a weak base, and one with a high pKa is a strong base. The weak acids are absorbed readily from the stomach because they all are almost completely nonionized at the gastric pH. Weak bases are not absorbed well; indeed, they would tend to accumulate within the stomach at the expense of the chemical agent in the blood stream. Naturally, in the more alkaline intestine, bases would be absorbed better and acids would be absorbed more poorly.

The concentration of a chemical that is in an ionized form or a nonionized form depends on both pKa of the chemical and the pH of the solution in which it is dissolved. The relationship may be derived by mathematical transformation with the Henderson Hasselbalch equation:

For weak acidic compound:

$$\mathrm{pKa} - \mathrm{pH} = \log \frac{\text{Concentration of unionized compound}}{\text{Concentration of ionized compound}}$$

$$\%\ \text{ionized compound} = \frac{100}{1 + \text{antilog}\ (\mathrm{pKa} - \mathrm{pH})}$$

For weak basic compound:

$$\mathrm{pH} - \mathrm{pKa} = \log \frac{\text{Concentration of unionized compound}}{\text{Concentration of ionized compound}}$$

$$\%\ \text{ionized compound} = \frac{100}{1 + \text{antilog}\ (\mathrm{pH} - \mathrm{pKa})}$$

It is therefore assumed that the gastric mucosal wall acts as a simple lipoid barrier that is permeable only in the lipid-soluble, nondissociated form of the acid. Thus, in plasma, the ratio of the nonionized drug to the ionized drug is 1:1000; in gastric juice, the ratio is 1:0.001. Therefore, the total concentration ratio between the plasma and the gastric sides of the barrier is 1000:1. For a weak base with a pKa of 4.4, the ratio is reversed.

Filtration: When water flows in bulk across a porous membrane, any solute small enough to pass through the pores flows with it. Passage through these channels is called *filtration* and involves the bulk flow of water caused by hydrostatic or osmotic force (examples include hydrophilic molecules and ions with molecular weight such as water and urea).

7.2.3.2 Specialized active transport

There are numerous compounds whose movement across membranes cannot be explained by simple diffusion or filtration. Some compounds are too large to pass through aqueous pores or are too insoluble in lipids to diffuse across the lipid domains of membranes. Nevertheless, they are often transported very rapidly across membranes, even against concentration gradients. To explain these phenomena, specialized transport systems have been identified. These systems are responsible for the transport (both influx and efflux) across cell membranes of many nutrients, such as sugars, amino acids, pyrimidines, and others.

At least two types of carrier transporters exist for the transport of several foreign molecules in the body.

Active Transport: The active transport process has the following properties: (1) the movement of chemicals against electrochemical or concentration gradients; (2) the system can be saturated; (3) competitive inhibition can occur among substrates among compounds that are carried by the same transporter; (4) the system has a characteristic of selectivity (ie, a compound must have a certain basic chemical structure to be transported by the system); and (5) the system requires expenditure of energy, so that metabolic inhibitors block the transport process.

In this process, substances are actively transported across cell membranes and are presumed to pass into the cells that form a complex with the membrane-bound macromolecular carrier on one side of the membrane. The complex subsequently traverses to the other side of the membrane, where the substance is released. Afterward, the carrier returns to the original surface to repeat the transport cycle.

Facilitated Diffusion: Facilitated diffusion applies to carrier-mediated transport that exhibits the properties of active transport, except that the substrate is not moved against an electrochemical or concentration gradient and the transport process does not require the input of energy.

7.2.3.3 Additional transport processes

Other forms of specialized transport have been proposed, but their overall importance is not as well established as that of active transport and facilitated diffusion. Phagocytosis and pinocytosis are proposed mechanisms for cell membranes by which cells engulf small drops of external medium (particles). This type of transfer has been shown to be important for the removal of particulate matter from the alveoli by phagocytes and from blood by the reticuloendothelial system of the liver and spleen.

7.3 ABSORPTION

Absorption is defined as the process of movement of an unchanged compound from its site of administration or exposure to the blood stream. Most hazardous substances must gain access to the systemic circulation to exert their toxic effects through interaction with one or more internal organs, except those that cause a local reaction at the site of exposure. During absorption, toxic substances gain entrance to the body from the external environment by crossing cellular barriers. The schematic representation of various steps involved during absorption distribution and excretion and the possible toxicokinetic fate of a chemical after exposure by inhalation, dermal contact, and ingestion are presented in Fig. 7.1. Many factors influence absorption of xenobiotics. The absorption of xenobiotics is dependent on the solubility of the chemicals, the concentration of chemicals, the circulation, the site of absorption, the area of absorbing surface, and the route of administration. The possible routes by which xenobiotics enter the body are the GI tract, skin, and lungs. However, there are many parenteral routes that are often used in experimental studies of toxic agents. The commonest among them are intraperitoneal (IP), subcutaneous (SC), and intravenous (IV).

7.3.1 GASTROINTESTINAL ABSORPTION

The oral route is an important means by which xenobiotics enter the body system either directly or indirectly as environmental contaminants. Because absorption takes place along the whole length of the chemical properties of each xenobiotic, this determines whether it will be absorbed in the strongly acidic stomach or in the nearly neutral intestine.

As discussed previously, the principles governing the absorption of chemicals from the GI tract are the same as for the passage of chemicals across the biological

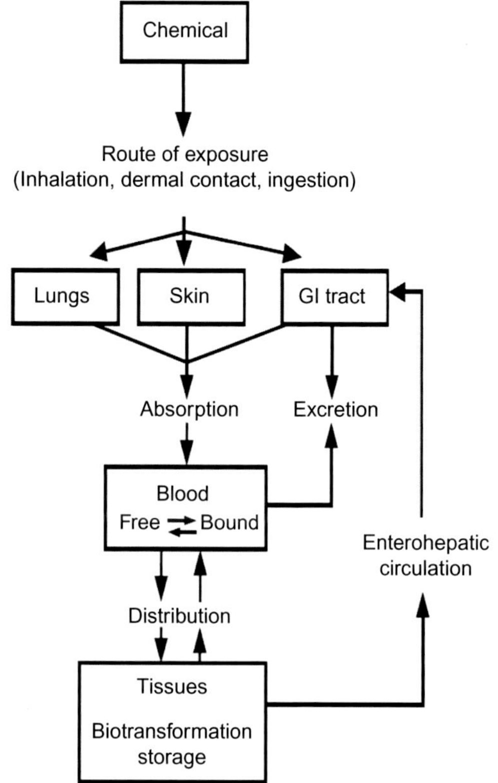

FIGURE 7.1

Schematic representation of absorption, distribution, and excretion. Possible toxicokinetic fate of a chemical after exposure by inhalation, dermal contact, and ingestion.

membranes. Some drugs such as nitroglycerin are better absorbed from a sublingual route of administration, and this route of absorption is important in medical practice. Most of the chemicals are absorbed through the GI tract by the nonionic diffusion across the lipid layer of the GI epithelial membrane. Certain inorganic and organic ions, sugars, amino acids, and pyrimidines are transported by specialized active processes. The chemicals that are weak acids are predominantly ionized at gastric juice pH, poorly absorbed through gastric mucosa, and are absorbed mainly through the intestinal mucosa. If the gastric contents are made alkaline, then acid compounds become more ionized and are less well absorbed. Conversely, basic compounds become less ionized and are better absorbed. In an intestine where the pH is approximately 5.3, the bases are more readily absorbed and weak acids are less readily absorbed than in the stomach.

The presence of food can impair the absorption of chemicals; for example, prolonged fasting has been shown to diminish the absorption of several chemicals, possibly by deleterious effects on the epithelium of the intestinal wall. Absorption from the GI tract may also be restricted or decreased if the chemical is unstable in GI fluid, or if it becomes bound to food or other GI contents. The chemicals may be altered by the action of acids, enzymes, or intestinal flora to form a new chemical or compound that may differ in toxicity from the parent compound. For example, snake venom is relatively nontoxic when given orally than when administered via the IV route because it is broken down by the digestive enzymes of the GI tract.

7.3.2 SKIN ABSORPTION

Skin is the most common tissue to come in contact with many chemicals. Fortunately, the skin restricts the diffusion and evaporation of water, except at the sweat glands. The epidermis, although only approximately 0.2 mm thick, largely limits absorption. The outer horny layer (stratum corneum) consists of a continuous sheet of flattened cells densely packed with keratin and constitutes a barrier to the penetration of water-soluble substances. However, some chemicals can be absorbed through the skin in sufficient quantities to produce systemic effects. For example, carbon tetrachloride and other organic solvents penetrate the skin in this way and can cause serious toxic effects. Pesticides (parathion, malathion) and nicotine insecticides have caused deaths in agricultural workers as a result of percutaneous absorption. Chlorovinylarsine dichloride (Lewisite), a mustard gas, is readily absorbed through contact with the skin.

The rate and degree of penetration of xenobiotics through the skin can vary in different areas of the body. Because the stratum corneum plays a critical role in determining the cutaneous permeability, abrasion or removal of this layer causes an abrupt increase in the permeability of the epidermis for all kinds of molecules, whether large, small, lipid-soluble, or water-soluble.

Chemicals penetrate through the epidermis, which is a rate-limiting factor. The rates are determined largely by their lipid/water partition coefficients, water-soluble ions, and polar molecules being virtually excluded. Even substances that are very lipid-soluble penetrate slowly in comparison with their rates of penetration of other thinner cell membranes. The underlying dermis, which consists of loosely arranged connective tissue and is vascularized, is freely permeable. In this respect, species differences are very important because many chemicals are poorly absorbed through the skin of a mammal but pass readily through the chitinous skeleton of the insects. For example, DDT is much less toxic to mammals than to insects when applied to the skin. Several injurious chemicals such as acids, alkalis, or mustard gases can injure the barrier cells, thereby increasing permeability. Dimethylsulfoxide can also facilitate the penetration of toxicants through the skin. This liquid is miscible with water and with many organic solvents, and is capable of increasing the penetration of ionized chemicals into the deeper layers of the skin. Such chemicals may be of practical use in medical practice,

(4) cellular fluids. The nonionized lipid/soluble fractions penetrate most readily. The rate of penetration of a chemical is not really a factor limiting chemical activity because equilibration in most tissues takes place quite rapidly. However, there are some exceptions; for example, bone and adipose tissues are rather poorly supplied with blood and, as such, longer time is required to achieve equilibration in these tissues. In addition, some chemicals may accumulate in various areas as a result of binding or due to their affinity for fat. The accumulation may be at the site of action of the chemical or some other location. In the latter situation, the accumulation may serve as a storage depot for the chemical. In this case, the chemical in the storage depot may be inactive, but the chemical in the storage depot is in equilibrium with free chemicals, thus helping to maintain the effective concentration of the chemical at the site of action. However, uneven distribution through the body may occur due to affinity for specific environments, such as fat for highly lipophilic compounds or bone for compounds that bind to Ca^{2+}. This can lead to extremely low concentrations in the blood plasma and accumulation with prolonged storage of the compound at the depot sites.

7.4.1 TISSUE PERMEABILITY BARRIERS

The biological complexity and specialization depend on the existence of permeability barriers across which concentration gradients can be established and maintained. Thus, in most tissues, including testes, cellular organization precludes continuous membrane barriers and raises the possibility of diffusion around membranes through extracellular spaces. In endothelia and epithelia, the extracellular diffusion occurs through narrow intercellular clefts between membranes of adjacent cells. This specialized intercellular cleft is known as the tight junction or zona occludents.

In permeability barriers, the effective tight junction occurs at the level of capillary endothelium (eg, brain, placenta, and thymus barriers). These barriers are called blood–organ barriers. In blood–bile barriers, the blood has direct access to the membranes of the hepatocytes. Tight junctions formed by adjacent hepatocytes constitute the physical barrier immediately interposed between blood and bile. Some of the so-called blood–organ barriers do not directly involve the blood. For example, in the blood–urine barrier, tight junction occurs near the luminal surface of bladder epithelial cells; in the blood–testes barrier, tight junction occurs within the seminiferous tubules. Thus, the blood–testes barrier resembles the blood–urine barrier more than the blood–brain barrier, with which it is often compared. A few important barriers are discussed here.

Blood–Brain Barrier: The blood–brain barrier is located between the plasma and extracellular space of the brain either at the capillary endothelial cells or at the glial field that surrounds the brain capillaries. The blood–cerebrospinal fluid barrier is located at the choroids plexus. These barriers are not absolute barriers to the passage of chemicals into the central nervous system; rather, they represent a site that is less permeable than most other areas of the body.

The passage of chemicals into the brain, in general, follows the same principle as for transfer across other cells in the body. The chemicals that are not bound to plasma proteins are free to enter the brain. If a chemical is ionized, then it will not enter the brain; however, nonionized chemicals will enter the brain readily at a rate proportional to its lipid water partition coefficient as discussed previously.

The route of exit of chemicals from the cerebrospinal fluid differs from the route of entrance because the chemicals leave the cerebrospinal fluid by bulk fluid flow through the villi of the arachnoids. In addition, certain chemicals may be removed from the cerebrospinal fluid by specialized active transport processes similar to those that exist for organic ions in the tubules.

Placental Barrier: The exhaustive knowledge of principles of transfer of chemicals across the placenta is important because many xenobiotics can cross the placenta and exert their toxic effects on the fetus. They may induce fetal deaths and even congenital anomalies. The passage of chemicals across the placental membranes occurs primarily by simple diffusion; carrier-mediated transport is generally restricted to endogenous substrates. Again, the same factors, especially the lipid water partition coefficient, are important determinants in the placental transfer. However, the concentration of chemicals in the various tissues of the fetus will be determined by the ability of the individual tissue to concentrate the chemicals, which may be dependent on the plasma—protein concentration and binding affinity for various chemicals.

Blood—Testes Barrier: Like the other barriers, the blood—testes barrier is a specific consequence of intercellular tight junctions interposed either directly or indirectly between the blood and another distinctive fluid compartment. It occurs between Sertoli cells in the seminiferous epithelium. The tight junction, which is part of the elaborate Sertoli cell junctional complex, consists of an extraordinary number of lines of membrane fusion in parallel array. This barrier has an important protective role in safeguarding the germ line from noxious influences originating from within and from outside. The barriers also help in shielding meiotic cells from environmental mutagens and in the prevention of autoimmune orchitis.

7.4.2 TRANSFER ACROSS OTHER MEMBRANES

The general mechanisms apply to the passage of xenobiotics through other body membranes, such as those concerned with the ocular fluid, mammary glands, and salivary glands. The mechanisms of transport of substances across these membranes are still incompletely understood, and only some general principles may be important determinants for these fluids.

7.4.3 FACTORS AFFECTING DISTRIBUTION AND TISSUE RETENTION

As discussed previously, several factors such as blood flow, volume of distribution, enzyme induction, chemical interaction, age and sex differences, and genetic factors play a great role in tissue distribution and tissue retention of xenobiotics.

In this section, emphasis is given only to binding with proteins and storage in various body tissues.

Binding to Plasma Proteins: The binding of foreign compounds, and particularly of drugs to plasma proteins, is important because the bound compound is temporarily localized, can seldom cross biological membranes or diffuse into tissues, and has pharmacological effects or toxic actions that are reduced or abolished. Of the plasma proteins that bind foreign compounds, albumin has the capacity to bind many compounds; however, other plasma proteins, such as globulins, are also involved. The binding of foreign compounds may be affected by several factors such as species variation, changes in pH, and hormonal influences.

The binding of drugs or chemicals to plasma proteins are sometimes very important because a chemical strongly bound to plasma protein will have a long duration of action. For example, suramin, an effective agent in the therapy of trypanosomiasis, is strongly bound to plasma protein. A single dose of the drug confers protection for 3 months or more.

The binding of xenobiotics to plasma proteins is also of special importance to toxicologists because severe toxic reactions can result if the agent is displaced from the plasma protein. In vitro studies showed that warfarin (rat killer) was partly displaced from human albumin by acidic drugs, such as phenylbutazone and sulphaphenazole, but not by a basic drug such as atropine. Such observations have clinical implications because patients receiving a coumarin anticoagulant, like warfarin, may lead to hemorrhage if given a drug, like phenylbutazone, that displaces it from plasma proteins. Unfavorable chemical interactions are frequently due to such displacement phenomena.

Storage in Body Fat: Extremely lipid-soluble foreign compounds tend to localize in adipose tissue by partitioning between intracellular lipid and body water. For example, organochlorinated pesticides such as DDT that, because of their worldwide usage, may attain an almost constant level in the body because of equilibrium between rates of absorption, bio-transformation, and excretion. Thus, a compound that has a high lipid/water partition coefficient may be stored in the body fat to a large extent and may not affect obese persons as much as lean ones.

Storage in the Brain Tissues: Certain compounds have high affinity for the brain tissue. For example, central nervous system drugs (such as the barbiturates and thiopentone) and psychotropic drugs (such as chlordiazepoxide and chlorpromazine) have been found to enter the brain rapidly after IV administration in animals.

Storage in Erythrocytes: Some pharmacological agents, such as p-nitro-aniline, become localized in the erythrocyte by binding with hemoglobin. Similarly, another toxic agent, triethyl tin, has been reported to be bound rapidly to rat hemoglobin. Experiments with radioactive arsenic have shown that more than 90% was present in blood, probably bound to hemoglobin. Localization within the erythrocyte has been observed with other inorganic ions, such as lead, cadmium, and others.

Other Tissues as a Storage Depot: The components of some tissues have a particular affinity for certain foreign compounds. The antibiotic tetracycline is taken up in bone and it presumably binds calcium. Approximately 90% of the lead in the body is found in the skeleton. Another chemical, cadmium, has been found in the kidney and liver. IV-administered charcoal is taken up in the spleen. Carbon monoxide has a very high affinity for hemoglobin, and paraquat (herbicide) accumulates in the lung. As a result, the biological half-life of such compounds can be very long.

Other transcellular fluids, such as aqueous humor, endolymph, and joint fluids, do not generally accumulate chemicals and constitute only minor storage depots in the body. The luminal fluid of the thyroid serves as the major storage depot for iodine in the body and can concentrate drugs such as perchlorate and some other ions.

7.4.4 BINDING TO BIOLOGICAL MACROMOLECULES AND TOXIC EFFECTS

The binding of certain xenobiotics to important cellular constituents may have serious consequences for animals because reversible binding may prevent or replace participation of true substrate. Certain chemically reactive foreign compounds thus may readily bind irreversibly to macromolecules such DNA, RNA, or proteins, particularly enzymes. For example, several carcinogens are thought to be associated with DNA, which is the genetic material of the cell, thereby affecting proper transcription of the genetic code and associated mechanisms of growth control. Detailed discussion of this mechanism is outside the scope of this chapter.

The interaction of foreign compounds such as mercurial and organophosphorus compounds with enzymes has been used to modify or destroy enzyme activity, thereby affecting the biotransformation of chemicals.

7.4.5 REDISTRIBUTION

After the initial distribution of chemicals within the body, it may later redistribute to areas of lower blood flow and tissues when more binding sites become available. For example, immediately after absorption, inorganic lead is localized in the erythrocytes, liver, and kidney. The lead is later redistributed to the bone and substitutes for calcium in the crystal lattice. A month later, 90% of the lead left in the body is localized in the bones.

7.5 EXCRETION

Excretion may be defined as a process by which toxicants and/or their metabolites are irreversibly transferred from the body to the external environment. Thus, excretion is one of the primary mechanisms of protecting the body from the toxic effects of toxicants through the elimination of these compounds from the body. Compounds that are rapidly eliminated are less likely to accumulate in tissues and damage critical cells. Although the terms elimination and excretion are sometimes used synonymously, the former term encompasses all the processes that decrease the amount of parent compound in the body, including biotransformation. Excretion by principal organs is called renal excretion; excretion by organs other than the kidneys is known as extrarenal or nonrenal excretion.

7.5.1 RENAL EXCRETION

The kidneys are the most important route of excretion of foreign compounds and their metabolites from the body. Renal excretion occurs by three different mechanisms: glomerular filtration, active tubular secretion of ionized substances, and passive tubular reabsorption of unionized substances.

Glomerular filtration produces an ultra filtrate of the body plasma that contains foreign compounds and their metabolites in approximately the same concentrations as those occurring in the blood. Once the compound has filtered at the glomeruli, it may remain within the tubular lumen and be excreted, or it may be passively reabsorbed across the tubular cells of the nephron into the blood stream. Those molecules that are reabsorbed do not appear in the urine to any extent. However, lipid-insoluble ionized molecules, such as conjugates of foreign compounds, are poorly reabsorbed and are thus more readily excreted than their precursors via the kidneys.

The compounds can also be excreted from the plasma by passive diffusion through the tubule into the urine. Like other biological membranes, the tubular epithelium, particularly in the distal tubule, behaves as a lipoprotein barrier, allowing the transfer of lipid-soluble, nonionized molecules. Lipid-soluble compounds present in the glomerular filtrate in the nonionized form are therefore reabsorbed into the blood stream, whereas compounds of low lipid solubility are only partially reabsorbed. Moreover, compounds that are more highly ionized in the urine than in the blood plasma tend to diffuse across the tubular epithelium from the blood into the glomerular filtrate. Thus, when the tubular urine is more alkaline than the plasma, weak acids are readily transferred into the urine; conversely, weak bases are transferred when the tubular urine is more acidic. The rate of renal excretion of weak organic electrolytes is therefore largely dependent on the pH of the urine. The rate of excretion of amphetamine, for example, was 20-times greater in human subjects with urine pH of 5 than in others with urine pH of 8.

Foreign compounds can also be excreted into the urine by active tubular secretion. There are two secretory processes: one for organic anions (acids) and the other for organic cations (bases). The compounds excreted by active transport are highly ionized and may be transferred into the tubular urine against high concentration gradients. It is unlikely that the active transport mechanisms can distinguish between strong and weak organic electrolytes, and the lipid-insoluble ionic forms of both are probably excreted by these mechanisms. The compounds actively secreted include anions, such as penicillin-G, p-aminohippuric acid, probenecid, and chlorothiazide, and cations, such as tetra-ethyl-ammonium, tolazoline, hexamethonium, and *N*-methyl-nicotinamide.

Substances secreted by the same active transport mechanism compete with each other for the mechanism, and the excretion rate of one compound can be reduced by administration of another. This phenomenon has been useful in pharmacological manipulations to inhibit excretion of drugs and thus to maintain the therapeutic blood levels of the other. One example is the competitive effect of probenecid and carinamide on the excretion of penicillin.

In newborn infants, especially premature infants, many functions of the kidney are incompletely developed. The chemicals are not eliminated as rapidly and thus they are more toxic in the newborn than in the adult. For example, the elimination half-time for insulin is approximately three-times longer in an adult than in an infant, suggesting partial impermeability of the glomerular membrane or, more likely, less renal blood flow relative to the body water volume.

7.5.2 BILIARY EXCRETION

The blood from the GI tract passes through the liver before it reaches the general systemic circulation. The liver can remove the compounds from the blood and prevent their distribution to other parts of the body. Because the liver is the site where the metabolism of most of the compounds occurs, the compound and the metabolites may be excreted directly into the bile without re-entering the blood stream to be excreted by the renal system. A chemical may be excreted by liver cells into the bile and thus passes into small intestine. If the properties of the chemicals or their metabolites are favorable for the intestinal reabsorption, then a cycle may result (enterohepatic cycle) in which biliary secretion and intestinal reabsorption continue until renal excretion finally eliminates the compounds from the body.

The biliary route of excretion plays a major role in the elimination of anions, cations, and nonionized molecules containing both polar and lipophilic groups. During these processes, the chemicals enter the bile primarily through active secretion. Simple diffusion is another possible route of entry, but this would not appear to be of major significance because the compound is lipid-soluble and can pass from the parenchymal cells into the bile; it would probably be reabsorbed by the intestine.

The prototype of the organic anions transport system is the bromosulfalein (BSP). This has long been used as a test of liver function. The removal of BSP is decreased after liver injury and returns to normal as liver function is restored.

There is a distinct mechanism for the biliary excretion of organic cations. Ethobromide, a quaternary derivative of procaine amide, is a good example. The secretion of this drug is competitively decreased by other quaternary ammonium compounds (mepiperphenidol, benzomethamine, oxyphenonium, *N*′-methyl-nicotinamide), and these drugs are secreted into the bile.

The liver also has a transport system for the excretion of nonionized molecules containing both polar and lipophilic groups. In addition to these three transport systems for organic compounds, the liver probably has another transport system for the excretion of metals. For example, lead is excreted into the bile against the large bile/plasma concentration ratio and an apparent biliary transport maximum exists. A similar mechanism for other metals remains to be determined.

The biliary excretion of foreign compounds varies with species and is generally highest in the dog and rat. Biliary excretion is also dependent on molecular size and increases as the molecular weight of the compound increases. The increase in biliary excretion that occurs with an increase in molecular weight is paralleled by a decrease in excretion in the urine. This is well illustrated by the substituted fluorescein dyes.

The hepatic excretory system is not fully developed in the infants, which is why some compounds are more toxic in infants than in adults. More information is required to determine if increased toxicity of some compounds in infants is due to this reason.

7.5.3 GASTROINTESTINAL TRACT

Many compounds are excreted in the feces. The excretion may be because the agent/compound is not absorbed after oral ingestion, the agent/compound was excreted into the bile, or it is excreted by the GI tract. Some ionized foreign compounds in circulating blood can be excreted into the gut, provided that the concentration gradient is favorable; the connection with the value of pKa is a determinative factor. They appear to be excreted by passive diffusion. However, organic acids and very weak bases (pKa 0.3), which would be only slightly ionized at a pH of l, are not excreted in the gastric juice.

7.5.4 EXPIRED AIR

Many volatile compounds that enter the body are excreted unchanged in the expired air. For example, fluorobenzene, carbon monoxide, as well as certain alcohols and other volatile agents are excreted by this route. These are all probably eliminated by simple diffusion, and their elimination depends on blood gas solubility. Gases with low blood/gas solubility such as benzene and nitrous oxide are excreted at rapid rate, whereas the chemicals that have higher blood/gas solubility such as bromobenzene or ethanol are excreted very slowly by the expired air.

7.5.5 SWEAT

In general, very small amounts of chemicals are excreted in sweat. However, diethyl di-thiol-iso-phthalate, a drug used for leprosy and applied to human subjects, is largely excreted in the sweat.

After oral administration to human subjects, the sweat/plasma concentration ratios of various sulphonamides that were excreted in sweat were highest with compounds that were least ionized at a pH of 7.4, suggesting that the sweat gland epithelium is readily permeable to un-ionized molecules only.

7.5.6 SALIVA

Some sulfonamides are excreted in the parotid saliva of humans. Other drugs such as pentobarbitone or some acidic drugs are excreted in higher concentrations in the parotid saliva of ruminants, which is alkaline. Further studies are required to determine whether this route is responsible for the secretion of other foreign compounds from human or animal systems.

7.5.7 MILK

Certain foreign compounds and their metabolites are partly excreted in the milk of lactating mammals. The compounds are excreted in the milk by simple diffusion because the milk is more acidic (pH 6.5–6.7) than plasma; basic compounds may be present in greater concentrations but the reverse may occur for acidic compounds. Several compounds, such as DDT, thiouracil, tetracycline, and erythromycin, have been reported to be excreted in milk.

7.5.8 VAGINAL SECRETIONS

The role of excretion of chemicals though vaginal secretions is not clear. However, hippuric acid, the glycine conjugate of benzoic acid, has been reported in the estrus secretion of cows. Further information is required regarding the excretion of other foreign compounds through vaginal secretions.

7.5.9 OTHER ROUTES

Only very limited information is available regarding the other routes of elimination such as lachrymal fluid, intestinal fluid, tracheobronchial secretions, and others.

CHAPTER

Biotransformation

8

CHAPTER OUTLINE

8.1 INTRODUCTION

Biotransformation is a key body defense mechanism whereby chemical reactions transform xenobiotic compounds in the body. The term metabolism is used for chemical transformation of xenobiotics and endogenous nutrients (eg, proteins, carbohydrates, and fats) within or outside the body.

8.2 FUNCTIONS OF BIOTRANSFORMATION

Biotransformation performs the following functions:

1. It causes conversion of an active compound to a less active compound, which is called inactivation or detoxification. Examples are phenobarbitone to p-hydroxyphenobarbitone and DDT to metabolite products DDE and DDA.

Fundamentals of Toxicology. DOI: http://dx.doi.org/10.1016/B978-0-12-805426-0.00008-1

2. It causes conversion of an active compound to a more active metabolite(s), which is called bioactivation. Examples are malathion to malaoxon or parathion to paraoxon and acetonitrile to cyanide.
3. It causes conversion of an inactive compound (ie, pro-drug or precursor compound) to an active metabolite(s), which is called activation. Examples are phenacetin to paracetamol and thiocyanates to cyanide.
4. It causes conversion of an active compound to an equally active metabolite(s) (no change in the activity). Examples are dichrotophos to monochrotophos and digitoxin to digoxin.
5. It causes conversion of an active compound to active metabolite(s) with entirely pharmacological/toxicological activity (change in activity). Examples are Iproniazid (antidepressant) to isoniazid (antitubercular) and aflatoxin B1 (hepatotoxin) to aflatoxin M1 (carcinogen).

8.3 XENOBIOTIC METABOLIZING ENZYMES

The liver is the primary site for metabolism of almost all xenobiotics because it is relatively rich in a large variety of enzymes. This is called hepatic metabolism. Metabolism by other organs is of lesser importance (extrahepatic metabolism) because low levels of metabolizing enzymes are present in such tissues. The relative amount of these enzymes located in different tissues such as liver, lung, kidney, intestine, skin, testes, placenta, adrenals, and nervous tissues is presented in Table 8.1.

These enzymes can be divided into two main groups:

1. Microsomal enzymes
2. Nonmicrosomal enzymes

Microsomal Enzymes: These enzymes are present in the endoplasmic reticulum (ER) (especially smooth) of liver and other tissues. When the cell is homogenized and differentially centrifuged, the ER breaks down to small vesicles known as microsomes. All enzymes present are called microsomal enzymes.

Nonmicrosomal Enzymes: Enzymes occurring in organelles/sites other than microsomes are called nonmicrosomal enzymes. These are usually present in the cytoplasm, plasma, and mitochondria.

Table 8.1 Tissue Localization of Xenobiotic-Metabolizing Enzymes

Relative Amount	Tissue
High	Liver
Medium	Lung, kidney, intestine
Low	Skin, testes, placenta, adrenals
Very low	Nervous system tissues

8.4 PATHWAYS OF BIOTRANSFORMATION

The major transformation reactions for xenobiotics are divided into two phases known as phase I and phase II.

8.4.1 PHASE I REACTIONS (NONSYNTHETIC OR NONCONJUGATIVE PHASE)

Phase I reactions modify the compound's structure by adding a functional group. This allows the substance to interact with a reactive group, such as −OH, SH, $-NH_2$, or −COOH. Most of these reactions involve different types of microsomal enzymes, except a few that involve nonmicrosomal enzymes. Phase I reactions usually yield products with decreased activity. However, some may give rise to products with similar or even greater activity. These reactions, along with their examples, are summarized in Tables 8.2 and 8.3.

8.4.1.1 Oxidation

Oxidation is the most common reaction and may take place in a number of ways, such as hydroxylation, deamination, desulfurization, dealkylation, or sulfoxide formation (Table 8.4).

In the biotransformation of lipophilic xenobiotics, microsomal oxidation is the most prominent reaction in which microsomal enzymes associated with smooth endoplasmic reticulum of hepatocytes are involved and the enzyme cytochrome P450, a heme protein, which is a part of an enzyme system termed the mixed function oxidase (MFO) system, plays an important role. The role of hepatic microsomal P450 is very important in determining the intensity and duration of the action of drugs and detoxification of toxic chemicals. The cytochrome P450 is a family of hemoprotein oxidoreductases. The heme ion in cytochrome P450 is usually in the ferric (Fe^{3+}) state. When reduced to the ferrous (Fe^{2+}) state, it can bind ligands such as O_2 and carbon monoxide (CO). This CO derivative of the reduced form shows absorption maximum at 450 nm, from which cytochrome P450 derives its name.

This enzyme has a specific requirement for reduced nicotinamide adenine dinucleotide phosphate (NADPH) and molecular oxygen. The basic reaction catalyzed by cytochrome P450 is mono-oxygenation, in which one atom of oxygen is incorporated into a substrate, RH, and the other is reduced to water with reducing equivalents derived from NADPH, as follows:

$$RH + O_2 + NADPH + H^+ \rightarrow ROH + H_2O + NADP^+$$

The other enzyme systems of phase I biotransformation (Table 8.2) are involved in metabolism when the appropriate functional groups are available; for example, alcohol dehydrogenase is involved in the biotransformation of

Table 8.2 Types of Phase I Biotransformation Reactions With Examples

Types of Reactions	Enzyme	Example
A. Oxidation		
1. Dealkylation a. N-dealkylation b. O-dealkylation c. S-dealkylation	Microsomal	OP and carbamate insecticides; phenacetin, codeine, methyl parathion; 6-methyl mercaptopurine (respectively)
2. Desulfuration	Microsomal	Malathion
3. Hydroxylation a. Aliphatic hydroxylation b. Aromatic hydroxylation c. Heterocyclic ring hydroxylation d. N-hydroxylation	Microsomal	Butacarb; arene, acetanilide; nicotine; paracetamol (respectively)
4. Oxidation (oxide formation) a. N-oxidation b. S-oxidation	Microsomal	Nicotine; fenthion (respectively)
5. Epoxidation or epoxide formation	Microsomal	Heptachlor
6. Deamination	Microsomal	Amphetamine
7. Alcohol oxidation	Microsomal and nonmicrosomal	Ethanol
8. Aldehyde oxidation	Nonmicrosomal	Acetaldehyde
9. Miscellaneous oxidative halogenations	Microsomal and nonmicrosomal	Chloroform
B. Reduction		
1. Azo reduction 2. Nitro reduction 3. Carbonyl reduction	Microsomal; microsomal and nonmicrosomal; nonmicrosomal (respectively)	Azo compounds, prontosil; nitro, parathion; aliphatic aldehyde and ketone (respectively)
C. Hydrolysis		
1. Hydrolysis of esters 2. Hydrolysis of amides 3. Hydrolytic dehalogenation	Microsomal	Malathion (estrases); dimethoate

alcohols and aldehydes, and monomine oxidase is a flavine adenine dinucleotide (FAD)-containing enzyme that catalyzes the oxidative deamination. Epoxide hydrolases are enzymes that add water across epoxide bonds to form diols. A number of carboxyl esterases are responsible for biotransformation of certain

Table 8.3 Phase 1 Reactions and the Activity of Metabolite

Process	Xenobiotics	Metabolite
Detoxification	Pentobarbital	p-Hydroxypentobarbital
	Procaine	p-Aminobenzoate
Active xenobiotics to active metabolite	Phenylbutazone	Oxyphenbutazone
	Aspirin	Salicylic acid
	Chloroform	Phosgene
	Aniline	p-Amino phenol

Table 8.4 Some Examples of Oxidation of Xenobiotics

Xenobiotic		Metabolite
Acetanilide	$\xrightarrow{\text{hydroxylation}}$	Paracetamol
Codeine	$\xrightarrow{\text{dealkylation}}$	Morphine or norcodeine
Amphetamine	$\xrightarrow{\text{Hydroxylation}}$	p-Hydroxyamphetamine
Amphetamine	$\xrightarrow{\text{Oxidation and deamination}}$	Benzoic acid
Ethanol	$\xrightarrow{\text{Non-microsomal oxidation}}$	Acetaldehyde
Histamine	$\xrightarrow{\text{Deamination}}$	Imidazoleacetaldehyde
Adrenaline	$\xrightarrow{\text{Monoamine oxidase–}}$	3,4- dihydroxymandelic acid

compounds including organophosphates. The extent to which these metabolic reactions take place appears to vary with the species.

8.4.1.2 Reduction

Reduction is acceptance of one or more electrons(s) or their equivalent from another substrate. Detoxification of xenobiotics via reactive routes is much less important than the oxidative systems in higher animals and plants, but it is gaining importance in the environment. Biotransformation by reduction is also capable of generating polar functional groups such as hydroxyl and amino groups, which can undergo further biotransformation or conjugation. Many reductive reactions are the exact opposite of oxidative reactions:

$$\text{Alcohol dehydrogenation} \leftrightarrow \text{carbonyl reduction}$$

$$\text{N-oxidation} \leftrightarrow \text{Amine oxide reduction}$$

The N-containing functional groups that commonly undergo bioreduction are nitro oxide, azo oxide, and N-oxide. Such reactions are usually the reverse of oxidation. Reductive reactions involve anaerobic conditions, require NADPH, and are almost certainly mediated by FAD-containing enzymes. Aldehydes and ketones may be reduced to corresponding alcohol and nitro compounds may be reduced to amines (Table 8.2). A few of these examples are given as:

$$\text{Parathion} \xrightarrow{\text{Nitro reduction}} \text{Aminoparathion}$$

$$\text{Prontosil (azo dye)} \xrightarrow{\text{Azo-reduction}} \text{Sulfanilamide}$$

$$\text{Methadone} \xrightarrow{\text{Carbonyl reduction (aliphatic ketone)}} \text{Methadol}$$

8.4.1.3 Hydrolysis

Hydrolysis is the process of cleaving of a foreign compound by the addition of water. It occurs in the cytoplasm and in smooth endoplasmic reticulum. It is an important metabolic pathway for compounds with an ester linkage (—CO, O—) or an amide (—CO, HN—) bond. The cleavage of esters or amides generates nucleophilic compounds that undergo conjugation.

Hydrolytic reactions differ from oxidative and reductive reactions in three aspects:

1. The reaction does not involve change in the state of oxidation of the substrate.
2. The reaction results in a large chemical change in the substrate brought about by loss of relatively large fragment(s) of the molecule.
3. The hydrolytic enzymes that metabolize xenobiotics are the same that act on endogenous substrates, and their activity is not confined only to the liver; they are found in many other organs, including kidneys and intestine.

Hydrolytic enzymes catalyze a number of functional groups like esters, amides, and hydrazides (Table 8.2).

For example, esterases hydrolyze esters and amides to corresponding carboxylic acids, alcohols, or amines as follows:

Pethidine	to	Pethidinic acid
Procaine	to	p-Aminobenzoic acid
Acetylcholine	to	Choline + acetic acid

8.4.2 PHASE II REACTIONS OR CONJUGATION/SYNTHETIC REACTIONS

Phase II reactions (conjugation/synthetic reactions) include reactions that catalyze conjugation of xenobiotics or their phase I metabolites with endogenous substances with a water-soluble molecule. In phase II, most of the reactions involve nonmicrosomal processes (except a few that involve microsomal enzymes). Due to biotransformation, the water solubility of a compound is typically increased, and this is an important step toward the excretion of lipid-soluble toxicants. Water-soluble compounds that are small enough to pass through the renal glomerulus can usually be excreted relatively rapidly through the urine without biotransformation. Biotransformed toxicants will often have reduced toxicity compared to the parent compounds. In some cases, however, biotransformation increases toxicity. Biotransformation enzymes have broad substrate specificity. Therefore, they are able to transform a wide range of substrates.

Synthetic reactions may take place when a xenobiotic or a polar metabolite of phase I metabolism containing –OH, –COOH, $–NH_2$, or –SH group undergoes further transformation to generate nontoxic products of high polarity, which are highly water-soluble and readily excretable by combining with some hydrophilic endogenous moieties (Table 8.5). Conjugating agents are glucuronic acid, acetyl, sulfate, glycine, cysteine, methionine, and glutathione, which conjugate with different functional groups of xenobiotics, as shown in Table 8.6.

Most of the phase II biotransforming enzymes are located in the cytosol, with the exception of uridine diphosphate glucuronyl transferase (UDPGT), which is a microsomal enzyme. Phase II reactions proceed faster than the phase I reactions. Therefore, the rate of elimination of a compound whose excretion depends on

Table 8.5 Conjugation Reactions and Different Functional Groups of Xenobiotics

Conjugation Reaction	Functional Groups of Xenobiotics	Conjugate
Glucuronide	–OH, – COOH, $– NH_2$,	
Glucuronic acid		
conjugation	–SH	
Sulfate ester formation	–OH, $– NH_2$	Sulfate
Methylation	–OH, $– NH_2$, – SH	Methyl group
Acetylation	$–NH_2$, $– SO_2$, $– NH_2$	Acetyl group
Glutathione conjugation	–F, Cl, – Br	Glutathione
Amino acid conjugation	–COOH	Glycine, taurine

Table 8.6 Types of Phase II Biotransformation Reactions With Examples

Type of Reaction	Enzymes	Example
Glucuronide conjugation	Nonmicrosomal (cytosol)	Benzoic acid
Sulfate conjugation	Nonmicrosomal (cytosol)	Phenol
Methyl conjugation	Nonmicrosomal (cytosol)	Pyridine
Glutathione conjugation and mercapturic acid formation	Nonmicrosomal (mitochondria)	Naphthalene
Acetyl conjugation	Nonmicrosomal	Para-amino salicylic acid
Conjugation with amino acids	Nonmicrosomal	Amino acid glycine, glutamine
Conjugation with thiosulfate	Nonmicrosomal	Cyanide with thiosulfate

biotransformation by cytochrome P450 enzymes followed by phase II conjugation is generally determined by a first-order reaction.

Conjugation reactions may be divided into electrophilic (conjugations involving glucuronide, sulfate, acetate, glycine, glutathione, and methyl transfer) or nucleophilic conjugations involving only glutathione.

The conjugating moieties do not react directly with the xenobiotics or the metabolites of phase I reactions; rather, they do so either in an activated form (usually nucleotides) or with an activated form of the xenobiotics. The reaction between the nucleotide and the xenobiotics is catalyzed by an enzyme. The conjugation reaction requires a conjugating agent, a nucleotide containing either the conjugating agent or the xenobiotics, and a transferring enzyme. Depending on the occurrence of conjugating agents or the amount of the transferring enzyme, variations in conjugating reactions occur in different species of animals. However, phase I reactions are ubiquitous throughout mammalian species. Hence, certain synthetic reactions are either slow or absent in some species of animals; for example, glucuronide synthesis takes place at a slow rate in cats, acetylation is absent in dogs and foxes, and sulfate conjugation is low in pigs.

8.4.2.1 Glucuronide conjugation

Formation of glucuronides is quantitatively most important. It is performed by the smooth endoplasmic reticulum–bound glucuronyl transferase. Glucuronic acid is donated by uridine diphosphate glucuronic acid (UDPGA), which serves as an endogenous substrate for the enzyme glucuronyl transferase. Substrates for glucuronide formation are phenols, alcohols, carboxylic acids, amines, hydroxylamines, and mercaptans. Glucuronides are mainly excreted via bile, hydrolyzed in gut, and then may be reabsorbed and delivered again to the liver, where conjugation may occur again. Glucuronide synthesis is slow in cats due to a low level of glucuronyl transferase, but it is absent in certain breeds of fish due to deficiency of the nucleotide UDPGA.

8.4.2.2 Sulfate conjugation

Another common phase II reaction is sulfate conjugation. The enzymes involved are cytoplasmic sulfotransferases, a group of soluble enzymes located primarily in the liver, kidneys, intestines, lungs, and brain. The endogenous donor of the sulfate group 3′ phosphoadenosine 5′ phosphosulfate (PAPS) serves to transfer the sulfuryl group to an nucleophilic position (O, N, or S). This process yields ethereal sulfates of various aromatic and aliphatic hydroxyl compounds (eg, phenols, alcohols, chloramphenicol, steroids [androgens and estrogens]). The n-hydroxy compounds are substrates for conjugation with sulfate. Sulfate conjugation involves the transfer of SO_3^- (not SO_4^-) from PAPS to the xenobiotic, and conjugates are mainly excreted in urine. Sulfate conjugation capacity is limited in pigs due to deficiency of the enzyme sulfotransferase.

8.4.2.3 Methyl conjugation

Methyl conjugation is generally a minor pathway of biotransformation. The cofactor for methylation is S-adenosyl methionine (SAM). Methylation reactions are catalyzed by cytoplasmic enzyme methyl transferase. Substrates are phenols, catechols, aliphatic and aromatic amines, and sulfhydryl-containing compounds.

8.4.2.4 Glutathione conjugation

Glutathione conjugation is an important detoxification mechanism. Glutathione (GSH) is a tripeptide found in most of the tissues, especially in high concentrations in the liver, and plays an extremely important role in protecting hepatocytes, erythrocytes, and other cells against toxic injury. It is involved in enzymatic and nonenzymatic reactions. Nonenzymatically, it acts as a low-molecular-weight scavenger of reactive electrophilic xenobiotics and competes with DNA, RNA, and proteins in capturing electrophiles.

Enzymatic reactions involving glutathione are catalyzed by the enzyme glutathione-S-transferase. It catalyzes the reaction between glutathione and aliphatic of aromatic epoxides and halides. Glutathione conjugates formed in the liver are excreted intact in bile or they are converted to mercapturic acids in the kidneys, which are highly water-soluble and excreted in urine.

Glutathione-S-transferase also catalyzes reactions of organic nitrates with glutathione. Nitrates are reduced to nitrite, which interacts with amines and results in the formation of carcinogenic nitrosamines. Depletion of glutathione predisposes to hepatotoxicity and mutagenicity.

8.4.2.5 Acetyl conjugation

N-acetylation is the major route of biotransformation for xenobiotics containing an aromatic amine (R-NH_2) or a hydrazine group (R-NH-NH_2) (eg, isoniazid, sulfonamides, etc.). It is performed by cytoplasmic enzymes *N*-acetyltransferases found in the liver and other tissues. The acetyl donor is acetyl coenzyme A. Acetylation decreases water solubility as well as lipid solubility. Dogs and foxes do not acetylate the aromatic amino group because they lack the enzyme arylamine acetyl transferase due to the presence of a factor in blood that decreases the arylamine acetyl transferase.

8.4.2.6 Conjugation with amino acids or amino acid conjugation

Conjugation with amino acids is performed by mitochondrial enzymes and *N*-acetyl transferases. Substrates for such conjugation are carbolic acids. Xenobiotics containing the carboxylic acid group conjugate with the $-NH_2$ group of amino acids such as glycine, glutamine, taurine, and others. However, the xenobiotics containing an aromatic hydroxylamine group conjugate with serine and proline. Other acceptor amino acids for xenobiotic conjugation are ornithine, arginine, histidine, serine, and aspartic acid.

Bile acids are endogenous substrates for glycine and taurine conjugation. Amino conjugates are primarily eliminated in urine. Conjugation with amino acids varies with species and also with xenobiotics; for example, bile acids conjugate with glycine and taurine in most species, except cats and dogs, in which these conjugate with taurine only. Benzoic acid conjugates with glycine in most species, except in birds and reptiles, in which it conjugates with ornithine.

8.4.2.7 Conjugation with thiosulfate

Conjugation with thiosulfate is an important reaction in the detoxification of cyanide. Conjugation of cyanide ions involves transfer of sulfur atom in the presence of a mitochondrial enzyme rhodanese to form inactive thiosulfate. The thiosulfate formed is much less toxic than the cyanide (true detoxification) and it is excreted in urine.

$$CN^- + S_2O_3^{-2} \xrightarrow{\text{Rhodanese}} SCN^- + SO_3^{-2}$$

Cyanide thiosulfate Thiocyanate sulfate

Conjugation of cyanide with thiosulfate

8.5 COMPLEX NATURE OF BIOTRANSFORMATION

Phase I and phase II pathways and various reactions are often discussed separately, but in body toxicants they generally undergo several types of biotransformation reactions simultaneously with a number of enzyme systems acting consecutively or concurrently on a substrate or metabolite of that substrate. Thus, many metabolites can be formed from a single substrate simultaneously or one after the other in the body. For example, benzene biotransformation results in a number of metabolites from different metabolic pathways.

8.6 INDUCTION AND INHIBITION OF METABOLIZING ENZYMES

8.6.1 INDUCTION OF ENZYMES

Several drugs and chemicals have the ability to increase the metabolizing activity of enzymes, called enzyme induction. These chemicals known as enzyme inducers mainly interact with DNA and increase the synthesis of microsomal enzyme proteins, especially cytochrome P450 and glucuronyl transferase. As a result, there is enhanced metabolism of endogenous substances (eg, sex steroids) and xenobiotic metabolites by microsomal enzymes. Some compounds (eg, carbamazepine and rifampicin) may stimulate their own metabolism; this phenomenon is called auto-induction or self-induction.

Microsomal enzyme induction by drugs and chemicals usually requires repetitive administration of the inducing agent over a period of several days and the induction, once started, may continue for several days. Metabolizing enzyme induction has great clinical importance because it affects the plasma half-life and duration of action of xenobiotics.

8.6.2 INHIBITION OF ENZYMES

Contrary to metabolizing enzyme induction, several drugs and chemicals have the ability to decrease the metabolizing activity of certain enzymes, called enzyme inhibition. Enzyme inhibition can be either nonspecific of chromosomal enzymes or specific of some nonmicrosomal enzymes (eg, monoamine oxidase, cholinesterase, and aldehyde dehydrogenase). The inhibition of hepatic microsomal enzymes mainly occurs due to administration of hepatotoxic agents, which causes either an increase in the rate of enzyme degradation (eg, carbon tetrachloride and carbon disulfide) or a decrease in the rate of enzyme synthesis (eg, puromycin and dactinomycin). Enzyme inhibition may also produce undesirable xenobiotic interactions.

8.7 BIOACTIVATION AND TISSUE TOXICITY

Formation of harmful or highly reactive metabolites from relatively inert/nontoxic chemical compounds is called bioactivation or toxication. The bioactive metabolites often interact with the body tissues to precipitate one or more forms of toxicities, such as carcinogenesis, teratogenesis, and tissue necrosis (Table 8.7).

The bioactivation reactions are generally catalyzed by cytochrome P450-dependent mono-oxygenase systems, but some other enzymes, like those in intestinal flora, are also involved in some cases. The reactive metabolites primarily belong to three main categories: electrophiles, free radicals, and nucleophiles. The formation of electrophiles and free radicals from relatively harmless substances/xenobiotics accounts for most toxicities (Fig. 8.1).

Table 8.7 Selective Examples of Bioactive Metabolites of Xenobiotics Responsible for Toxic Effect

Compound	Active Metabolite	Toxic Effect
Carbon tetrachloride	Trichloromethyl radical	Lipid peroxidation
Chloroform	Phosgene	Hepatic necrosis
Paracetamol	Imidoquinone derivative	Hepatic necrosis
Acrylonitrile	Cyanide	Histotoxic hypoxia
Benzene	Muconic aldehyde	Bone marrow injury
Ethanol	Acetaldehyde	Hepatic fibrosis
Isopropyl alcohol	Acetone	Cardiotoxicity
Methanol	Formaldehyde	Ocular toxicity
Methylene chloride	Carbon monoxide	Hypoxia
Nitrate	Nitrite	Methemoglobin formation

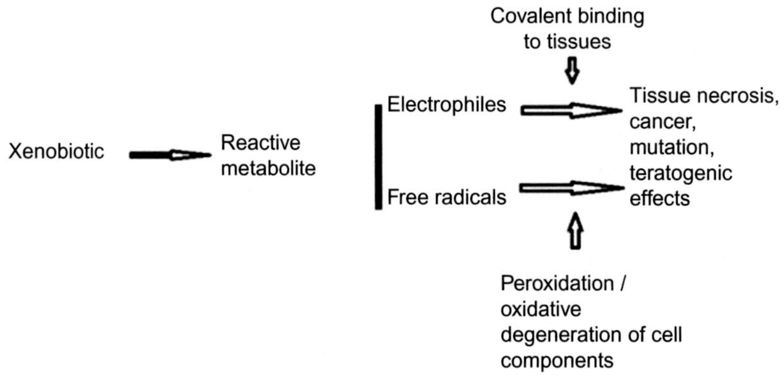

FIGURE 8.1

Bioactivation of xenobiotics through various reactive pathways.

8.7.1 ELECTROPHILES

Electrophiles are molecules that are deficient in electrons pair with a positive charge, which allows them to react by sharing electron pairs with electron-rich atoms in nucleophiles. Important electrophiles are epoxides, hydroxyamines, nitroso and azoxy derivatives, nitrenium ions, and elemental sulfur. These electrophiles form covalent binding to nucleophilic tissue components such as macromolecules (proteins, nucleic acids, and lipids) or low-molecular-weight cellular constituents to precipitate toxicity. Covalent binding to DNA is responsible for carcinogenicity and tumor formation.

8.7.2 FREE RADICALS

Free radicals are molecules that contain one or more unpaired electrons (odd number of electrons) in their outer orbit. Radicals are formed by accepting or losing an electron. They may be positively charged (cation radical), negatively charged (anion radical), or neutral (neutral radical). Free radicals are generally formed via NADPH cytochrome P450 reductase or other flavin-containing reductases. Xenobiotics that, on metabolic activation, yield free radicals are quinines, acrylamines, nitroaryls, and carbon tetrachloride. Most free radicals are organic. They produce toxicity by peroxidation of cellular components. For example, carbon tetrachloride forms trichloromethyl radicals, which cause peroxidation of polysaturated lipids and covalently bind to proteins and unsaturated lipids. An important class of free radicals is inorganic free radicals, such as hydrogen peroxide and superoxide anions (O_2^-). These oxidative moieties can cause tremendous tissue damage, leading to mutation or cancer. Their potential toxicity is far greater than that of electrophiles.

8.7.3 NUCLEOPHILES

Nucleophiles are molecules with electron-rich atoms. Formation of nucleophiles is a relatively uncommon mechanism for toxicants. Examples of toxicity induced through nucleophiles include formation of cyanides from amygdalin, acrylonitrile, and sodium nitroprusside and generation of carbon monoxide from dihalomethane. Although some nucleophiles like cyanide and carbon monoxide are reactive, many other nucleophiles are activated by conversion to electrophiles.

8.7.4 OTHER PATHWAYS

Certain compounds are biotransformed to potentially toxic metabolites by pathways other than those discussed here. These include oxidation of ethanol by nonmicrosomal dehydrogenase to acetaldehyde, a metabolite responsible for some of the manifestations of alcohol toxicity. Artificial sweetener cyclamate is converted by intestinal bacteria to cyclohexamine, which is very toxic and induces teratogenicity and carcinogenicity (urinary bladder tumor). Similarly, nitrite, a potent respiratory toxicant, is formed from nitrate by bacterial reduction in the intestine.

CHAPTER

Principles and basic concepts of toxicokinetics

9

CHAPTER OUTLINE

9.1 INTRODUCTION

Toxicokinetics refers to the study of absorption, distribution, metabolism/biotransformation, and excretion (ADME) of toxicants/xenobiotics in relation to time. The basic kinetic concepts for the absorption, distribution, metabolism, and excretion of chemicals in the body system initially came from the study of drug actions or pharmacology; therefore, this area of study is traditionally referred to as pharmacokinetics. Toxicokinetics represents the extension of kinetic principles to the study of toxicology and encompasses applications ranging from the study of adverse drug effects to investigations on how disposition kinetics of exogenous chemicals derived from either natural or environmental sources (generally referred to as xenobiotics) govern their deleterious effects on organisms, including humans.

An important parameter in toxicokinetics is the time course of blood or plasma concentration of the toxicant with time. The purpose of this chapter is to introduce the basic concepts of toxicokinetics to those who want to gain firsthand knowledge in the field of toxicokinetics. Therefore, principles of basic concepts used in toxicokinetics have been briefly discussed.

Fundamentals of Toxicology. DOI: http://dx.doi.org/10.1016/B978-0-12-805426-0.00009-3

9.2 ESSENTIALS OF TOXICOKINETICS/PHARMACOKINETICS PRINCIPLES

The knowledge of kinetic principles is essential in therapeutics because it shows the relationship between the pharmacological or toxicological effects of a drug/toxicant and the concentration of the drug/toxicant in the body. These principles are useful for determining the following factors:

1. the extent and rate to which pharmacokinetic parameters (ADME) occur in body;
2. the dose and dosing schedule of the drug and their modification according to individual needs;
3. the drug concentrations that produce therapeutic and toxic effects;
4. the drug concentration in various body fluids and tissues, and accumulation of the drug or its metabolites in the body;
5. the half-life ($T_{½}$) and duration of action of the drug;
6. the effect of the disease state on various pharmacokinetic parameters;
7. in the case of animals, the withdrawal time for meats, eggs, and dairy products when the drug is administered to food-producing animals;
8. the nature and extent of drug interactions.

9.3 PLASMA DRUG CONCENTRATION VERSUS TIME

When a drug is administered by an oral or extravascular (EV) route (intramuscular (IM), subcutaneous (SC), intraperitoneal (IP), etc.), it slowly enters the systemic circulation. Plasma drug concentration gradually increases to a maximum (peak level). As the drug is being absorbed into blood, it is distributed to body tissues and eliminated. The ascending portion of the curve to the left of the peak represents the absorption phase because in this phase, the rate of absorption is greater than the rates of distribution and elimination. The descending section of the curve to the right of the peak generally represents the elimination phase because in this phase, the rate of elimination exceeds the rate of absorption (Fig. 9.1). The rate or velocity with which absorption and elimination processes occurs is given by respective slopes of the curve and is expressed by the absorption rate constant (K_a) and elimination rate constant β (beta), respectively. A typical plasma concentration curve obtained after a single oral dose of a drug and the relationship of the drug concentration − time curve and various pharmacological/toxicological parameters are depicted in Fig. 9.1. These parameters are also applicable to toxicants.

Fig. 9.1 clearly indicates some important parameters essential for the determination of drug regimens. The parameters are briefly described here:

Minimum Effective Concentration (MEC): The minimum concentration of drug in plasma required to produce the desirable pharmacological/therapeutic response. In case of antimicrobials, the term minimum inhibitory concentration (MIC)

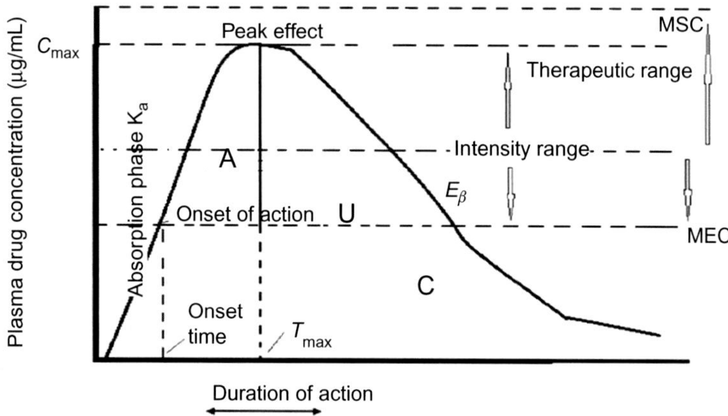

FIGURE 9.1

Plasma concentration–time profile of drug/toxicant after oral administration of a single dose of a toxicant. C_{max}, maximum/peak plasma concentration; *MEC*, minimum effective concentration; *MSC*, maximum safe concentration; T_{max}, time of peak concentration; *AUC*, area under curve; K_a, absorption rate constants (absorption phase); and E_β, elimination rate constant (elimination phase).

is used, which may be defined as the minimum concentration of antimicrobial agent in plasma required to inhibit the growth of micro-organisms.

Maximum Safe Concentration (MSC) or Minimum Toxic Concentration (MTC): The concentration of drug in plasma above which toxic effects are produced. A concentration of drug above MSC is said to be a toxic level. The drug concentration between MEC and MSC represents the therapeutic range.

Maximum Plasma Concentration/Peak Plasma Concentration (C_{max} or C_{pmax}): The point of maximum concentration of drug in plasma. The maximum plasma concentration depends on the administered dose and rates of absorption (absorption rate constant, K_a) and elimination (elimination rate constant, β). The peak represents the point of time when absorption equals the elimination rate of the drug. It is often expressed as µg/mL.

Area Under Curve (AUC): The total integrated area under the plasma drug concentration – time curve. It expresses the total amount of drug that enters the systemic circulation after administration of the drug.

Peak Effect: The maximal or peak pharmacological effect produced by the drug. It is generally observed at peak plasma concentration.

Time of Maximum Concentration/Time of Peak Concentration (t_{max}): The time required for a drug to reach peak concentration in plasma. The faster the absorption rate, the lower is the t_{max}. It is also useful in assessing efficacy of drugs used to treat acute conditions (eg, pain) that can be treated by a single dose. It is expressed in hours.

Onset of Action: The beginning of the pharmacological response produced by the drug. It occurs when the plasma drug concentration just exceeds the MEC.

Onset Time: The time required for the drug to start producing a pharmacological response. It usually corresponds to the time for the plasma concentration to reach MEC after administration of the drug.

Duration of Action: The time period during which the pharmacological response is produced by the drug. It usually corresponds to the duration when the plasma concentration of the drug remains above the MEC level.

9.4 ORDERS OF RATE PROCESSES

Before discussing various models used in toxicokinetics analysis, it is pertinent to know the various rate processes that will be encountered during ADME. For example, when a toxicant or xenobiotic is administered by an oral or EV route (IM, SC, IP, etc.), it slowly enters the systemic circulation and the plasma drug concentration gradually increases to a maximum (peak level). As the toxicant/drug is being absorbed into blood, it is distributed to body tissues and may also simultaneously be eliminated. If one assumes that the concentration of a chemical in blood or plasma is in some describable dynamic equilibrium with its concentrations in tissues, then changes in plasma toxicant concentration should reflect changes in tissue toxicant concentrations, and relatively simple kinetic models can adequately describe the behavior of that toxicant in the body system.

The following are commonly encountered rate processes in toxicokinetics:

1. Zero-order process
2. First-order process
3. Mixed-order process.

9.4.1 ZERO-ORDER PROCESS/ZERO-ORDER KINETICS

Zero-order process (zero-order kinetics or constant-rate kinetics) may be defined as a toxicokinetics process whose rate is independent of the concentration of the xenobiotic/chemical; that is, the rate of the toxicokinetics process remains constant and cannot be increased further by increasing the concentration of the xenobiotic.

9.4.2 FIRST-ORDER PROCESS/FIRST-ORDER KINETICS

First-order process (first-order kinetics or linear kinetics) may be defined as a toxicokinetics process whose rate is directly proportionate to the concentration of the xenobiotic/chemical (ie, the greater the concentration, the faster is the process).

9.4.3 MIXED-ORDER PROCESS/MIXED-ORDER KINETICS

Mixed-order process (mixed-order kinetics, nonlinear kinetics, or dose-dependent kinetics) may be defined as a toxicokinetics process whose rate is a mixture of both zero-order and first-order processes. The mixed-order process follows zero-order kinetics at a high concentration and the first-order kinetics at a lower concentration of the xenobiotic. This type of kinetics is usually observed with increased or multiple doses of some chemicals.

9.5 TOXICOKINETICS MODELS

For a toxicokinetics analysis, the choice of model used depends on the intended application and the available data. Commonly used models are classic toxicokinetics (traditional), noncompartment models/noncompartment analysis, and physiological models.

9.5.1 CLASSIC TOXICOKINETICS

Classic toxicokinetics modeling (traditional) is a mathematical description and depends on the time course of toxicant disposition in the whole organism. In this approach, the body is represented as a system of one or two compartments (sometimes more than two compartments), even though the compartments do not have exact correspondence to anatomical structures or physiologic processes. These empirical compartmental models are almost always developed to describe the kinetics of toxicants in readily accessible body fluids (mainly blood) or excreta. This approach is particularly suited for human studies, which typically do not provide organ or tissue data.

This is the simplest way of gathering information on absorption, distribution, metabolism, and elimination of a compound and to examine the time course of blood or plasma toxicant concentration over time. If one assumes that the concentration of a chemical in blood or plasma is in some describable dynamic equilibrium with its concentrations in tissues, then changes in plasma toxicant concentration should reflect changes in tissue toxicant concentrations and relatively simple kinetics models can adequately describe the behavior of that toxicant in the body system.

The advantages of these models are:

1. they do not require information on tissue physiology or anatomic structure;
2. they are useful in predicting the toxicant concentrations in blood at different doses;
3. they are useful in establishing the time course of accumulation of the toxicant, either in its parent form or as biotransformed products during continuous or episodic exposures, and in defining concentration–response (vs dose–response) relationships; and
4. they provide help/guidance in the choice of effective dose and design of dosing regimen in animal toxicity studies.

Classic toxicokinetics models typically consist of a central compartment representing blood and tissues that the toxicant can readily access and equilibration is achieved almost immediately after its introduction, along with one or more peripheral compartments that represent tissues in slow equilibration with the toxicant in blood. An infinite number of compartments exist in the body (each organ, tissue, or body fluid can form a compartment); tissues with approximately similar chemical distribution characteristics are pooled to form kinetically homogeneous hypothetical compartments. These compartments are called open models because there is no restriction to the movement of chemicals between compartments as chemicals freely move from one compartment to another. Schematic representations of one-, two-, and three-compartment models are summarized in Fig. 9.2.

9.5.1.1 One-compartment open model

The one-compartment open model is the simplest model, which considers the whole body as a single, kinetically homogeneous unit. In this model, the final distribution equilibrium between the chemical in plasma and other body fluids is attained rapidly and maintained at all times.

Intravenous Administration: In case of IV bolus administration of any chemical, the chemical distributes instantaneously in the body and the entire dose of the chemical enters the body and is distributed immediately via circulation to all tissues (Fig. 9.2). In such a situation, the xenobiotic concentration–drug time curve will be obtained as a straight line on semi-logarithmic paper showing mono-phasic exponential decline (Figs. 9.3 and 9.4). In this model, the decline in plasma concentration of the xenobiotic occurs only due to elimination of the chemical from the body; therefore, the phase is called the elimination phase. The distribution phase is normally neglected in calculations because distribution is so rapid that it cannot be shown on the graph. The extrapolated zero-time intercept of linear elimination phase gives the coefficient B, and the elimination rate constant is given by β. The value of B is an estimate of zero-time concentration (C_0 or C_p^0) of the chemical in plasma (Fig. 9.4).

In the one-compartment model, the most straightforward toxicokinetics assessment entails quantification of the blood or, more commonly, plasma concentrations of a toxicant at several time points after an IV bolus injection. Often, the data obtained fall on a straight line when they are plotted as the logarithms of plasma concentrations versus time; the kinetics of the toxicant is said to conform to a one-compartment model (Fig. 9.4).

Mathematically, this means that the decline in plasma concentration over time profile follows a simple exponential pattern, as represented by the following mathematical expressions:

For example, if

$$C = B \times e^{-\beta \times t}$$

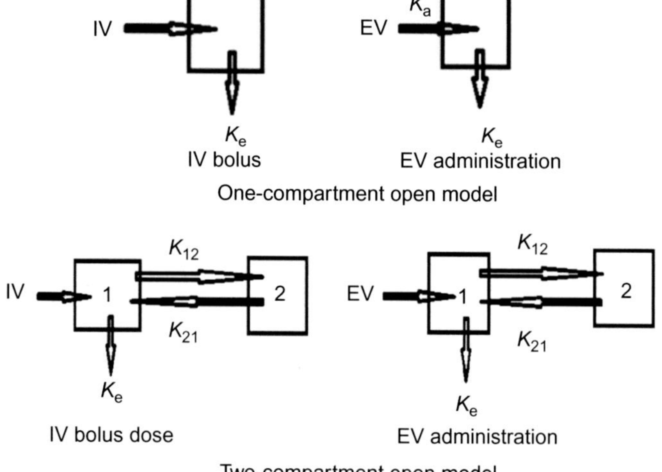

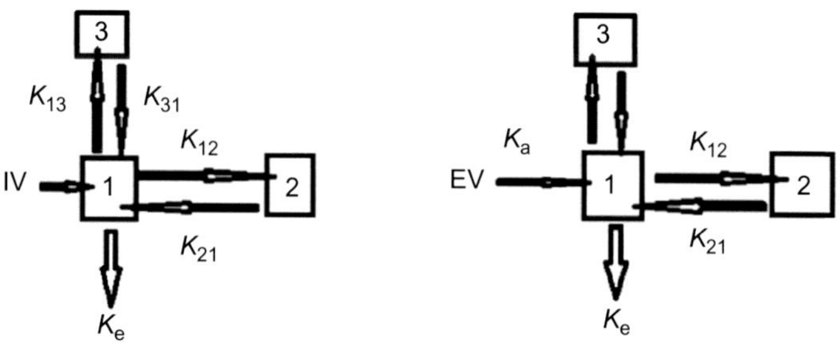

FIGURE 9.2

Schematic representation of various compartmental (one, two, and three) models: *IV*, intravenous; *EV*, extravenous route (intramuscular (*IM*), subcutaneous (*SC*), intraperitoneal (*IP*), etc.); K_a, first absorption rate constant; K_e, first-order elimination rate constant (from central compartment); K_{12}, first-order rate constant for the toxicant transfer central (1) to peripheral (2) compartments; K_{21}, first-order rate constant for the toxicant transfer peripheral (2) to central (1) compartments; K_{13}, first-order rate constant for the toxicant transfer central (1) to peripheral (3) compartments; K_{31}, first-order rate constant for the toxicant transfer peripheral (3) to central (1) compartments.

or its logarithmic transform

$$\log C = \log B - \frac{\beta \times t}{2.303}$$

where C is the plasma toxicant concentration at time t after injection, then B is the coefficient unit of plasma concentration achieved immediately after injection, and β is the exponential constant or elimination rate constant with dimensions

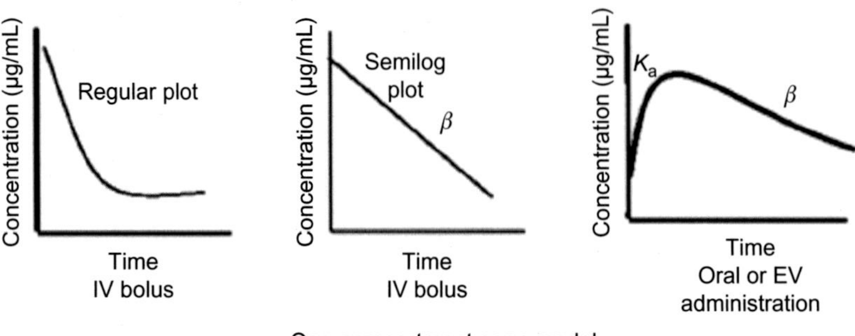

FIGURE 9.3

Graph showing one-compartment open model following intravenous (IV) bolus and oral or extravascular (EV) route of a single dose of toxicant. After IV bolus, the curve is a straight line on semi-logarithmic paper and shows monophasic decline. In contrast to IV bolus, after oral or EV administration (instead of a straight line), there are two exponents (ie, absorption and elimination phase).

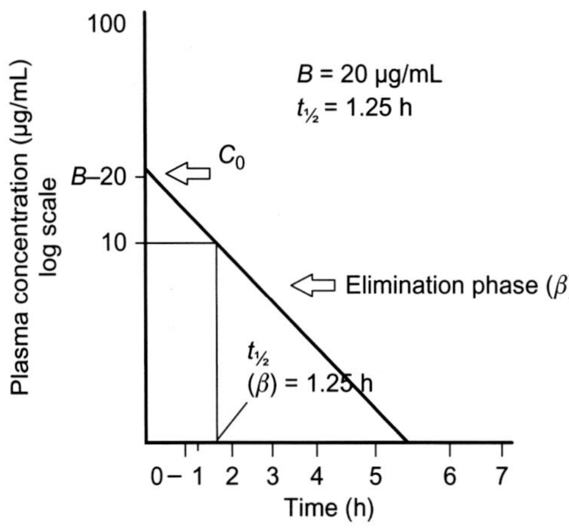

FIGURE 9.4

Semi-logarithmic graph exhibiting kinetic behavior conforming to one compartment model. Plasma concentration profile after intravenous bolus administration.

of reciprocal time (eg, min^{-1} or h^{-1}). The constant 2.303 in this equation is needed to convert the natural logarithm to the base-10 logarithm. It can be seen from the equation that the elimination rate constant can be determined from the slope of the log C versus time plot (ie, $\beta = -2.303 \times \text{slope}$).

The elimination rate constant β represents the overall elimination of the toxicant, which includes biotransformation, exhalation, and/or excretion pathways. When elimination of a toxicant from the body occurs in an exponential fashion, it signifies a first-order process; that is, the rate of elimination at any time is proportional to the amount of toxicant remaining in the body (ie, body load) at that time. This means that after an IV bolus injection, the absolute rate of elimination (eg, mg of toxicant eliminated per minute) continually changes over time. Soon after introduction of the dose, the rate of toxicant elimination will be at its highest. As elimination proceeds and the body load of the toxicant is reduced, the elimination rate will decline.

Therefore, it is evident that a constant percentage of toxicant present in the body is eliminated over a given time period regardless of dose or the starting concentration, and it is more intuitive and convenient to refer to an elimination $T_{1/2}$, which is the time it takes for the original blood or plasma concentration to decrease by 50% or to eliminate 50% of the original body load.

By substituting $C/B = 0.5$ into the equation, we obtain the following relationship between $T_{1/2}$ and β:

$$T_{1/2} = \frac{0.693}{\beta}$$

where 0.693 is the natural logarithm of 2. Simple calculations reveal that it would take approximately four half-lives for >90% of the dose to be eliminated, and approximately seven half-lives for > 99% elimination. Thus, given the elimination $T_{1/2}$ of a toxicant, the length of time it takes for near-complete washout of a toxicant after discontinuation of its exposure can easily be estimated.

Extravascular Administration: When a xenobiotic is administered by an oral or EV route (eg, IM, SC, IP etc.), absorption is a prerequisite for its action. If it is distributed according to the one-compartment open model, the rate of change of concentration of the xenobiotic is described by two exponents: an absorption component (K_a) and an elimination exponent (β) (Fig. 9.3).

9.5.1.2 Two-compartment open model

The two-compartment open model assumes that the body is composed of two compartments: the central compartment and the peripheral compartment. The central compartment (compartment 1) consists of blood and highly perfused organs like liver, kidney, lungs heart, and brain; the less perfused tissues like skin, muscles, bone, and cartilage comprise the peripheral compartment (compartment 2). The drug/toxicant, when directly administered by the IV route, goes into the central compartment. After it is absorbed, it is distributed to various organs and rapidly equilibrates. Elimination of the chemical occurs from the central compartment because the main organs involved in drug elimination (eg, liver and kidneys) are located there. The distribution of drugs to the peripheral compartment is through blood (central compartment) and occurs slowly. It is assumed that the chemical transfer from the central compartment to the peripheral compartment, and the transfer back from the peripheral compartment to the central compartment occurs by first-order process and is defined by rate constant (K). The subscript indicates the direction of the chemical movement; for example, K_{12} refers to drug movement from compartment 1 (central compartment) to compartment 2 (peripheral compartment), and the reverse is true for K_{21} (Fig. 9.2). The two-compartment open model adequately describes the disposition kinetics of most of the chemicals in humans and animals.

Intravenous Administration: After the IV bolus administration that follows the two-compartment kinetic model, the decline in plasma concentration is bi-exponential; when the plasma xenobiotic concentration–time curve is plotted on a semi-logarithmic paper, the plasma concentration declines rapidly during the first phase, followed by a slow terminal decline (Fig. 9.5). The initial steep decline in the concentration is attributed mainly to distribution of drug from the central compartment to the peripheral compartment, and the terminal slow decline is mainly due to elimination from the central compartment. The linear terminal portion of the curve is called the elimination phase. Resolving the bi-exponential curve into its components by the methods of residuals (feathering technique) yields a second linear segment called the distribution phase. The extrapolated zero-time intercepts of linear distribution phase (residual line) is denoted by α, and the elimination is denoted by β (Fig. 9.6).

After rapid IV bolus of some toxicants, the semi-logarithmic plot of plasma concentration versus time does not yield a straight line, but rather a curve that implies more than one dispositional phase (Fig. 9.5). In these instances, it takes some time for the toxicant to be taken up into certain tissues and to then reach an equilibration with the concentration in plasma; therefore, a multi-compartmental model is needed for the description of its kinetics in the body (Fig. 9.3).

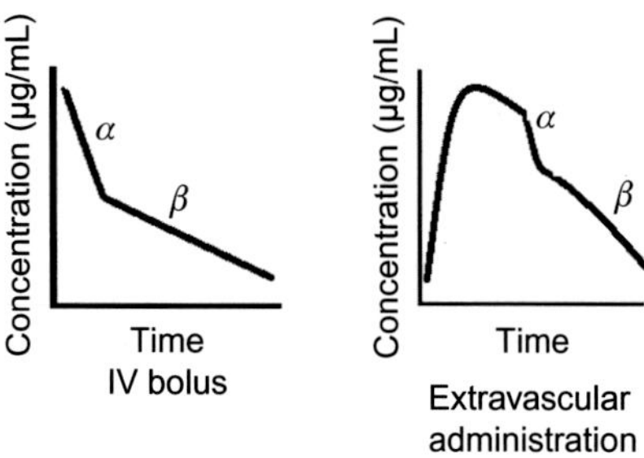

FIGURE 9.5

Graph showing two-compartment open model following intravenous bolus and extravascular administration of a single dose of toxicant (curve is bi-exponential). Linear terminal portion is elimination phase β.

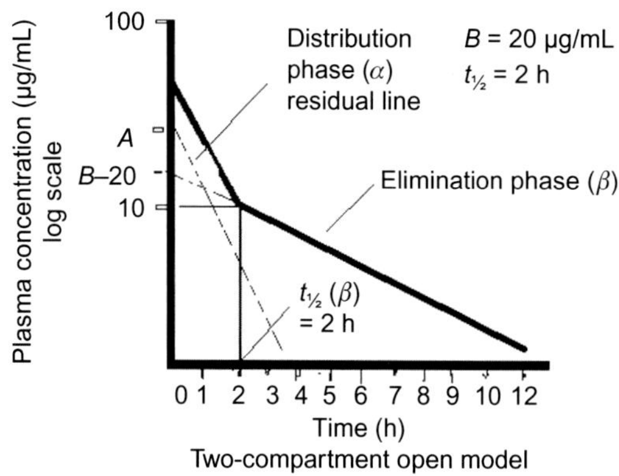

FIGURE 9.6

Semi-logarithmic graph depicting the plasma drug concentration–time profile after intravenous bolus administration of a single dose (example of two-compartment model).

For example, a two-compartment model can be represented by the following bi-exponential equation, as shown in Fig. 9.6.

$$C = A \times e^{-\alpha \times t} + B \times e^{-\beta \times t}$$

where C is the plasma toxic concentration at time t after injection. A and B are coefficients in units of toxicant concentration, and α and β are the respective exponential constants for the initial and terminal phases in units of reciprocal time. The initial (α) phase is often referred to as the distribution phase, and the terminal (β) phase is referred to as the postdistributional or elimination phase. Fig. 9.6 shows a graphical resolution of the two exponential phases from the plasma concentration–time curve.

The sum of A and B coefficients gives the initial concentration of the chemical in the plasma (C_0 or C_p^0). For the two-compartment model, α is the rate constant for distribution and β is the rate constant for elimination; they are expressed in units of reciprocal time (min^{-1}). β is used for the rate constant for elimination from the entire body. The coefficients (A and B) and rate constants (α and β) are calculated from the experimental data by least regression analysis.

For any chemical that enters the body by an oral or EV route and is distributed according to the two-compartment model, the rate of change in the concentration of a chemical in plasma is described by three exponents: K_a, an absorption exponent; α, a distribution exponent; and β, an elimination exponent (Fig. 9.5).

Different exponential equations described here serve as the basis to calculate physiologically relevant pharmacokinetic parameters that reflect the various kinetic processes.

Likewise, plasma concentration–time profile kinetics of a toxicant exhibiting three or more compartments (multi-compartments) of kinetics can be characterized by multi-exponential equations. This aspect is beyond the scope of this chapter.

9.5.1.3 Determination of other kinetic parameters

Absorption and Bioavailability: After oral or EV routes, often only a fraction of the total dose to which an animal or human is exposed gets absorbed systemically. This fraction is referred to as the bioavailability (F) and is calculated by comparing the areas under the plasma time/concentration curves for the toxic compound administered IV versus the typical route of exposure. These data are not readily available for most toxic compounds, although the relative bioavailability from different routes (eg, oral versus dermal) is often known.

As shown in Fig. 9.1, bioavailability is determined by measuring the area under the plasma drug concentration versus time curve (AUC) after oral or EV routes. This is compared with AUC measured after IV bolus administration of the same drug.

If the AUCs for both curves are equal, then bioavailability is 100% ($F = 1$). The equation for the same is given as:

$$\text{Bioavailability} = \frac{\text{AUC oral} \times \beta'}{\text{AUC IV} \times \beta} \times 100 \quad \text{or} \quad F = \frac{\text{AUC oral} \times \beta'}{\text{AUC IV} \times \beta}$$

where β and β' are elimination rate constants after IV bolus and EV routes and F is the bioavailability fraction (fraction of the administered dose that enters the systemic circulation).

Bioavailability is a useful parameter that is used to predict the drug efficacy after different routes of administration.

The influence of the route of administration of a drug/toxicant on bioavailability is generally in the following order:

IV > oral route > topical route

AUC: The area under the curve can be calculated in several ways. The most common method is by dividing the Y intercept by the slope (rate constant) of the respective component. Thus, for a one-compartment model, AUC = B/β; for a two-compartment model, AUC = $A/\alpha + B/\beta$, and so on.

Two-compartment model for IV bolus injection:

$$\text{AUC} = A/\alpha + B/\beta$$

Two-compartment model for EV routes (oral, IM, SC, IP, etc.):

$$\text{AUC} = B/\beta - A'/K_a$$

Other measures of the rate and extent of absorption, such as the absorption rate constant (K_a), maximum measured concentration in plasma (C_{max}), and time after exposure when maximum concentration is measured (T_{max}), have been discussed previously in this chapter.

Volume of Distribution (V_d): The total volume of fluid in which a toxic substance must be dissolved to account for the measured plasma concentrations is known as the apparent V_d. If a compound is distributed only in the plasma fluid, then the V_d is small and plasma concentrations are high. Conversely, if a compound is distributed to all sites in the body, or if it accumulates in a specific tissue such as fat or bone, then the V_d becomes large and plasma concentrations are low. Hence, the assumption is made that the body behaves as a single homogenous compartment with respect to the toxicant and V_d because it provides an estimate of the extent or magnitude of distribution of a toxicant/drug in the body. The value of V_d is characteristic of a chemical and usually constant over a wide range for a given species of animals. The value of V_d may be determined either by the extrapolation method or by the area method using the following equations.

$$V_d = \frac{Dose\ (D)}{C}$$

where D is the amount of drug in the body and C is the plasma drug concentration. The extrapolation method is the simplest, but it is less accurate. This is obtained by extrapolating the linear terminal phase (elimination phase, β) of the plasma drug concentration–time curve to the Y axis (Fig. 9.6). The value of B (or C_0) thus obtained is substituted in the aforementioned equation.

$$V_d = \frac{Dose\ (D)}{B} \quad or \quad \frac{Dose\ (D)}{C_0}$$

where B is the zero-time intercept of terminal elimination phase.

The AUC method provides a more satisfactory way of calculating the V_d parameter. It can be estimated as follows:

For drugs given as an IV bolus injection:

$$V_d = \frac{Dose\ (D)}{AUC \times \beta}$$

For drugs given by EV routes:

$$V_d = \frac{Dose\ (D) \times F}{AUC \times \beta}$$

where F is the fraction of dose absorbed in the system.

Clearance: Total body clearance (Cl) is the parameter that reflects the body's inherent ability to eliminate a xenobiotic through organs of elimination. The value of this parameter represents the volume of blood cleared of the toxic substance per unit of time. If the total absorbed dose is known, then Cl can be calculated using the following equation. Many times the absorbed dose is not known, and the calculated value of this parameter reflects not only Cl but also an unknown value for bioavailability (F).

Clearance can be calculated as follows:

$$Cl = \frac{Dose\ (D)}{AUC\ 0-\infty}$$

where AUC $0-\infty$ is the area under the plasma time/concentration curve extrapolated to infinity.

Because body clearance relates plasma concentration with the rate of drug elimination, it can also be calculated according to the following formula.

$$Cl = \frac{\text{Rate of elimination}}{\text{Plasma drug concentraion}}$$

Pharmacologically, body clearance is obtained as the product of V_d and overall elimination rate constant (β). If $T_{½}$, V_d, and β are known, then the Cl can be determined as follows:

$$Cl = \beta \times V_d$$

$$or = \frac{0.693,\ V_d(area)}{T_{1/2}}$$

The equation shows that the half-life changes inversely (and proportionately) with the clearance of drug, that is, as the body clearance increases, the half-life of the drug decreases.

Half-Life: A compound's half-life in plasma ($T_{½}$ or $t_{½}$) is a composite parameter that is dependent on the body's inherent ability to eliminate the compound (Cl) and the extent to which the compound is distributed through the body (V_d). $T_{½}$ may be defined as the time taken for the concentration of a compound/toxicant in plasma to decline by ½ or 50% of its initial value (or it may be defined as the time required for the body to eliminate half of the chemical). This value is determined during the elimination phase of a chemical; therefore, it is called the elimination half-life. Occasionally, the term plasma half-life is inversely related to the elimination rate constant, β (ie, the faster the elimination, the shorter the half-life), and is expressed in hours or minutes. Mathematically, it is illustrated in the following equation:

$$T_{1/2} = \frac{In2}{\beta} = \frac{0.693}{\beta}$$

where *In2* is the natural logarithm of 2 (or 0.693). Half-life of a drug/chemical can also be readily obtained from the β-slope of the plasma chemical concentration–time profile as depicted in Fig. 9.6. The elimination half-life can also be obtained from clearance (Cl) and apparent V_d according to the following formula:

$$T_{1/2} = \frac{0.693,\ V_d}{Cl}$$

Occasionally, the term half-life is used for purposes other than the elimination of drugs/chemicals. These may include absorption half-life (time during which 50% of the administered chemical is absorbed), distribution half-life (time during which 50% of the administered chemical is distributed), and biological effect half-life (time during which 50% of the pharmacological effect produced by a drug is declined). These terms are not generally used.

Relationship of Elimination Half-Life to Clearance and Volume: Elimination $T_{½}$ is probably the most easily understood pharmacokinetic concept and is an important parameter because it determines the persistence of a toxicant following discontinuation of exposure. Elimination half-life also governs the rate of accumulation of a toxicant in the body during continuous or repetitive exposure and is dependent on both volume of distribution and clearance. $T_{½}$ can be calculated from V_d and Cl:

$$T_{1/2} = \frac{0.693,\ V_d}{Cl}$$

It is well known that for a fixed V_d, $T_{½}$ decreases as Cl increases, because the chemical is being removed from this fixed volume faster as clearance increases. Conversely, as the V_d increases, $T_{½}$ increases for a fixed Cl because the volume of fluid that must be cleared of chemical increases but the efficiency of clearance does not.

9.5.1.4 Flip-flop kinetics

Flip-flop kinetics refers to when the rate of absorption of a compound is significantly slower than its rate of elimination from the body. Therefore, the compound's persistence in the body becomes dependent on absorption rather than elimination processes. This sometimes occurs when the route of exposure is dermal. Fig. 9.7 indicates a comparison of toxicants with a slow rate of absorption to those with a rapid rate of absorption, demonstrating "flip-flop" kinetics, whereby persistence of the compound is dependent on the rate of absorption rather than the rate of elimination.

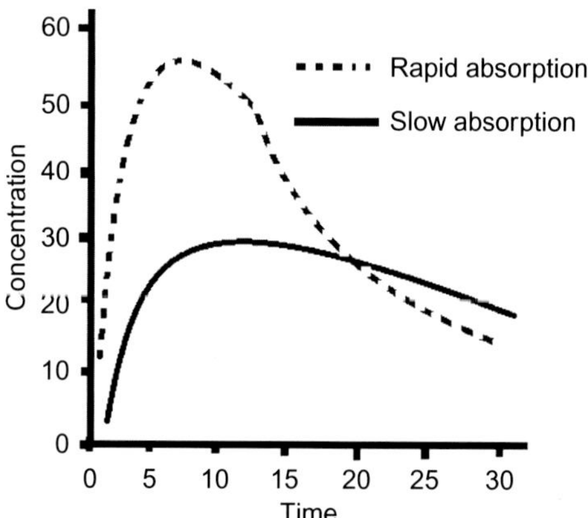

FIGURE 9.7

Concentrations of toxicants comparing a slow rate of absorption to a rapid rate of absorption, demonstrating "flip-flop" kinetics, where persistence of the compound is dependent on the rate of absorption, rather than the rate of elimination.

9.5.1.5 Saturation toxicokinetics

As already mentioned, the distribution and elimination of most toxicants occur by first-order processes. Under first-order elimination kinetics, the elimination rate constant, apparent volume of distribution, clearance, and half-life are expected not to change with increasing or decreasing dose (ie, dose-independent). However, for some toxicants, as the dose of a toxicant increases, its V_d and/or Cl may change. This is generally referred to as nonlinear or dose-dependent kinetics because biotransformation, active transport processes, and protein binding have finite capacities and can be saturated.

As the dose is escalated and the concentration of a toxicant at the site of metabolism approaches or exceeds the K_M (substrate concentration at one-half V_{max}, the maximum metabolic capacity), the increase in the rate of metabolism becomes less than proportional to the dose and eventually approaches a maximum at exceedingly high doses. The transition from first-order to saturation kinetics is important in toxicology because it can lead to prolonged persistence of a compound in the body after an acute exposure and excessive accumulation during repeated exposures. In addition to the complication of dose-dependent kinetics, there are chemicals with clearance kinetics that change over time (ie, time-dependent kinetics). A common cause of time-dependent kinetics is auto-induction of xenobiotic metabolizing enzymes; that is, the substrate is capable of inducing its own metabolism through activation of gene transcription. This phenomenon is very common with some drugs that lead to enzyme induction, thereby shortening the elimination half-life.

9.5.1.6 Steady-state concentration

Steady-state concentration (C_{ss}) is defined as the time during which the concentration remains stable or consistent when the drug is given repeatedly or continuously (IV infusion). The time to reach steady-state is a function of $T_{½}$ and is achieved when the rate of the drug entering the systemic circulation equals the rate of elimination. For most drugs, the C_{ss} is reached in approximately five half-lives. The time to reach steady-state is independent of dose size, dosing interval, and number of doses. In case of multiple dosing, when a drug is administered in a fixed dose at fixed intervals, the plasma concentration increases exponentially to a plateau or steady-state with a half time of increase that is equal to the $T_{½}$ of the drug. As indicated previously, 50% of the steady-state level is achieved in one $T_{½}$, 75% (50 + 25) is achieved in two, 87.5% is achieved in three, and more than 99% is achieved in seven half-lives. In practice, a useful estimate of time to reach a steady-state is obtained by the following equation:

$$\text{Time to 95\% steady state} = 4.3 \times t_{1/2}$$

Therefore, the shorter the half life, the more rapidly the steady-state is reached, and vice versa.

9.5.1.7 Accumulation

Chronic exposure to a chemical leads to its cumulative intake and accumulation in the body. For the chemical that follows first-order elimination kinetics, the elimination rate increases as the body burden increases. For a one-compartment model, an exponential increase in plasma concentration is expected during continuous exposure, and the time it takes for a toxicant to reach steady-state is governed by its elimination half-life.

Therefore, accumulation is the ratio of maximum plasma concentration following the dose at steady-state compared with that following the first dose (ie, $C_{ss\cdot max}/C_{1max}$). The extent to which a chemical accumulates in the body during multiple dosing is a function of exposure or dosing interval and elimination of half-life, but it is independent of dose size. If the elimination half-life is equal to dosing interval, then at steady-state level the chemical will accumulate twofold ($C_{ss\cdot max}/C_{1max} = 2$). When the dosing interval is less than $T_{½}$, the degree of accumulation will be greater and the chemical may show toxic responses.

9.5.1.8 Three-compartment open model

The toxicokinetics behavior of some chemicals that have a high affinity for a particular tissue and are under redistribution is best interpreted according to a three-compartment open model. The body is thought of as consisting of three compartments: one central and two peripheral compartments. The central compartment (compartment 1) comprises plasma and highly perfused organs, whereas peripheral compartments 2 and 3 comprise moderately (eg, skin and muscles) and poorly perfused tissues (eg, bone, teeth, ligaments, hair, and fat) respectively. If any chemical is administered by IV, then it is first distributed immediately into the highly perfused tissues (compartment 1) and then slowly into the moderately perfused tissues (compartment 2); thereafter, it is distributed very slowly to the poorly perfused tissues (compartment 3). If the plasma level—time profile is plotted on a semi-logarithmic graph, it gives a tri-exponential appearance.

Sometimes three or even four exponential terms are needed to fit a curve to the plot of log C versus time. Such compounds are viewed as displaying characteristics of three- or four-compartment open models. The principles underlying such models are the same as those applied to the two-compartment open model, but the mathematics is more complex and beyond the scope of this chapter.

9.5.2 NONCOMPARTMENT MODELS/NONCOMPARTMENT ANALYSIS

Noncompartment models and noncompartment analysis are another approach used to study the time course of drugs in the body. They do not require the assumption of a specific compartment model, and they consider the time course of drug concentration in plasma as a statistical distribution curve and derive kinetic parameters from simple algebraic equations. A detailed description of drug disposition characteristics is not required. The disadvantage of this method is that it often deals with averages and provides limited information regarding plasma concentration–time profile.

9.5.3 PHYSIOLOGICAL-BASED TOXICOKINETICS

Physiologically based toxicokinetics (PBTK) models are mathematical stimulations of physiological processes that determine the rate and extent of xenobiotics/ toxicant absorption, distribution, metabolism, and excretion. The primary difference between physiologic compartmental models and classic compartmental models lies in the basis for assigning the rate constants that describe the transport of chemicals into and out of the compartments. In classic kinetics, the rate constants are defined by the data; thus, these models are often referred to as data-based models. In PBTK models, the rate constants represent known or hypothesized biological processes, and these models are commonly referred to as physiologically based toxicokinetics models.

The advantages of PBTK models compared with classic models are:

1. these models can describe the time course of distribution of toxicants to any organ or tissue.
2. they allow estimation of the effects of changing physiologic parameters on tissue concentrations.
3. the same model can predict the toxicokinetics of chemicals across species by allometric scaling, and complex dosing regimens and saturable processes such as metabolism and binding are easily accommodated.

The disadvantages are:

1. much more information is needed to implement these models compared with classic models.
2. the mathematics can be difficult for many toxicologists to handle.
3. values for parameters are often ill-defined in various species, strains, and disease states.

Nevertheless, PBTK models are conceptually sound and are potentially useful tools for gaining rich insight into the kinetics of toxicants beyond what classic toxicokinetics models can provide. However, the PBTK models are fundamentally complex compartmental models; these generally consist of a system of tissue or organ compartments that are interconnected by the circulatory network. If necessary, each tissue or organ compartment can further be divided into extracellular and intracellular compartments to describe the movement of the toxicant at the cellular level. The exact model structure, or how the compartments are organized and linked together, depends on both the chemical and the organism being studied.

9.5.3.1 Compartments of PBTK models

The first step in the construction of a PBTK model is determining the purpose of the model and what internal tissue doses are needed to answer the specific scientific questions being asked. Once that is done, a schematic diagram is constructed that consists of each of the tissue compartments of interest, a plasma compartment, and a compartment or compartments representing the rest of the physiological system. It is often necessary to include more than one compartment to represent the remaining portions of the body to reflect the differences in high and low blood-flow tissues. Compartments usually consist of three individual well-mixed regions, or sub-compartments, that correspond to specific physiologic spaces or regions of the organ or tissue. These sub-compartments are:

1. the vascular space through which the compartment is perfused with blood.
2. the interstitial space that forms the matrix for the cells.
3. the intracellular space consisting of the cells in the tissue.

Model structures can also vary with the chemicals being studied. For example, a model for a nonvolatile, water-soluble chemical that might be administered by IV injection is shown in Fig. 9.8.

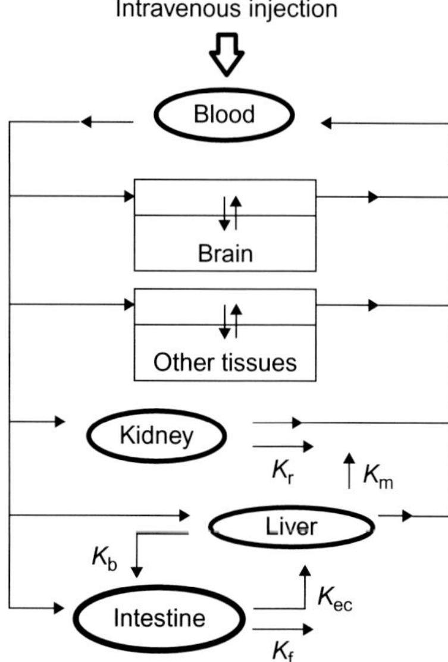

FIGURE 9.8

Schematic representation of physiologically based toxicokinetics model for a hypothetical toxicant that is soluble in water. Oval shape shows perfusion-limited compartments (kidney, liver, and intestine) and rectangular shape shows diffusion-limited compartments (brain and other tissues). The toxicant is eliminated through metabolism in the liver (K_m), biliary excretion (K_b), renal excretion (K_r) into the urine, and fecal excretion (K_f). The chemical can also undergo enterohepatic circulation (K_{ec}).

9.6 DETERMINATION OF DOSE/DOSAGE REGIMEN

Dosage regimen is defined as the manner in which a drug is administered. For some drugs like antiemetics, pre-anesthetic, anthelmintics, and others, a single dose may provide effective treatment. In such cases, there is no chance of drug accumulation and a constant therapeutic plasma concentration is not considered essential for treatment. However, for many drugs like antimicrobials, antihypertensives, and antiarrhythmics, multiple doses of drug at appropriate intervals over a period of time are required for successful therapy. In these cases, design of an optimal dosage regimen is necessary.

Irrespective of the route of administration, a dosage regimen is composed of two important variables;

1. the magnitude of each dose (dose size)
2. the frequency with which the dose is repeated (dosing interval)

Dose: Dose or dose size is a quantitative term estimating the amount of drug that must be administered to produce a particular biological response (ie, to achieve a specified target plasma drug concentration). Because the magnitude of both therapeutic and toxic responses depends on plasma drug concentration, the size of the dose should be selected so that it produces the peak plasma concentration (C_{max}) or steady-state level within the limits of therapeutic range (between minimum effective concentration and maximum safe concentration). The therapeutic plasma concentration range is obtained by careful clinical evaluation of the response in a sufficient number of appropriately selected individuals (for microbials, the range is based on the minimum inhibitory concentration for susceptible microorganisms).

The dose (D) necessary to achieve peak or maximum therapeutic concentration (C_{max}) depends on the volume of distribution (V_d) and is calculated by the following equation:

$$D = C_{max} \times V_d(\text{area})$$

When a drug is administered by a route other than the IV route, its bioavailability (F) may be less than 1.0 and must be taken into account:

$$D = C_{max} \times V_d(\text{area})/F$$

Because the dose size for drugs that do not accumulate depends on the V_d, the dose must be increased or decreased proportionately with changes in V_d to establish the required plasma drug concentration.

Dosing Interval: Dosing interval is the time interval between doses. It ensures maintenance of plasma concentration of a drug within the therapeutic range for the entire duration of therapy. Dosing interval should be selected primarily by concentration of the fluctuations in drug concentration (ratio C_{max}/C_{min}) that can be tolerated without excessive toxicity or loss of efficacy and the overall elimination rate constant (β).

The dosing interval is determined by the time (T_{max}) it takes for the maximum plasma concentration (C_{max}) to decrease to a point below which the desired response no longer occurs (MEC, C_{min}).

$$T_{max} = \frac{In\,[C_{max}/C_{min}]}{\beta}$$

where In is the natural logarithm. On the basis of the aforementioned equation, if C_{min} for a drug is equal to the half of C_{max} (ie, $C_{max}/C_{min} = 2$), then the dosing interval is equal to the half-life of the drug. Accordingly, for most drugs, a dosing interval equal to or less than the elimination half-life is:

$$T_{max} = \frac{In[C_{max}/C_{min}]}{\beta} = \frac{In2}{\beta} = t_{1/2}$$

and is recommended for therapeutic purposes. For a given fluctuation (ratio C_{max}/C_{min}), the similar ratio of β (ie, the longer the half-life, the longer will be the dosing interval. Therefore, dosing interval is related primarily to the half-life of the drug.

9.7 CONCLUSION

Knowledge of toxicokinetics data and knowledge of compartmental modeling are useful for deciding what dose or dosing regimen of a chemical are to be used in the planning of toxicology studies. For many chemicals, blood or plasma chemical concentration versus time data can be adequately described by one- or two-compartment models (traditional or classical models). In some instances, more sophisticated models with increased numbers of compartments such as physiological-based toxicokinetics models will be needed to describe blood or plasma toxicokinetics data.

The parameters of the classic compartmental models are usually estimated by statistical fitting of data to the model equations using nonlinear regression methods. A number of software packages are available for both data fitting and simulations with classic compartmental models. The data generated from toxicokinetics analysis helps in seeking an understanding of the dynamics of a toxic event (eg, what blood or plasma concentrations are achieved to produce a specific response, how accumulation of a chemical controls the onset and degree of toxicity, and the persistence of toxic effects after termination of exposure). Toxicokinetics also helps to select the dosage regimen and dosing interval of drugs/chemicals required for successful therapy and/or experimental studies.

UNIT III

CHAPTER

Toxicological testing: genesis

10

CHAPTER OUTLINE

10.1 INTRODUCTION

Today, toxicity testing of a chemical for the purposes of human health risk assessment, as might be expected, is not a routine aspect of toxicology. It is actually one of the most controversial subjects because of the requirement of animals in large quantities. Among the many areas of controversy is the use of animals for experimental purposes. Extrapolation of animal data to humans, extrapolation from high-dose to low-dose effects, and the increasing cost and complexity of testing protocols may not be beneficial. New tests are constantly being devised and are often added to testing requirements already in existence. Most testing can be subdivided into in vivo tests for acute, sub-chronic, or chronic effects and in vitro tests for genotoxicity or cell transformation, although other tests are used. Any chemical that has been developed or is being introduced into commerce is subject to toxicity testing to satisfy the regulations of one or more regulatory agencies.

Fundamentals of Toxicology. DOI: http://dx.doi.org/10.1016/B978-0-12-805426-0.00010-X

The compounds produced as waste products of industrial processes (eg, combustion products) are also subjected to testing.

10.2 LAWS AND REGULATIONS

There is a wide range of laws and regulations that shape the role of toxicology in society. One of the first laws dealing with toxicology, passed in 82 BC by the Roman Emperor Sulla, was intended to deter intentional poisonings because women were poisoning men to acquire their wealth. In 1880, food poisonings spurred Peter Collier, chief chemist of the US Department of Agriculture, to recommend passage of a national food and drug law. The United States, in the year 1938, enacted the Federal Food, Drug, and Cosmetic Act following an incident in which elixir sulfanilamide, which contains the poisonous solvent diethylene glycol, killed 107 people, many of whom were children.

Toxicology is the responsibility of national government agencies such as the US Food and Drug Administration (FDA), the US Environmental Protection Agency (EPA), and several other agencies in Japan and other countries. In 2006, Europe moved forward with Registration, Evaluation, and Authorization of Chemicals (REACH), a legislation that requires testing and evaluation of chemicals before their introduction into commerce in European Union (EU) countries. This aspect has been dealt with in detail under REACH legislation in this chapter. The purpose of the implementation of these legislations is to protect the health and well-being of the people and environment.

10.2.1 REGULATION IN THE UNITED STATES

A turning point in the regulations governing the US FDA occurred in 1962, when a new sleeping pill, thalidomide, was shown to cause birth defects. Infants in Europe and Australia whose mothers used thalidomide while pregnant were born with birth defects. Fortunately, the FDA kept this drug off the American market despite the best efforts of industry to have the drug approved. Following this incident, in 1966, regulations and guidelines for reproduction studies evaluating the safety of drugs were introduced. This statutory law significantly strengthened the FDA's control regarding approval of new drugs.

Also, in 1962, Rachel Carson published her landmark book *Silent Spring*, which dramatically documented the impact of chemicals on the environment and raised concerns about the effect of pesticides on human health. In a delayed political response, the EPA was created in 1970 to administer a variety of laws to protect human health and the environment. The EPA is responsible for monitoring and regulating pesticides, industrial chemicals, hazardous waste, drinking water, air pollutants, and other environmental hazards.

To provide basic knowledge to beginners, general guidelines for the manufacture and use of drugs and cosmetics and regulatory statutes involved in regulation internationally are discussed.

The pharmaceutical industry is one of the most regulated industries in the United States, Europe, and Japan. A multitude of regulations, guidelines, and restrictions apply to every phase of pharmaceutical business, research, development, manufacturing, and marketing. The US FDA guidelines were updated in 1974. These guidelines were again revised in 1980. In the 1990s, a few toxicology guidelines relating to pharmaceutical products were published.

Toxicological testing, regulated by statute, is performed by many groups: industrial, governmental, academic, and others. Regulation, however, is performed by a narrow range of governmental agencies, each charged with the formulation of regulations under separate laws and with their administration. The guidelines for the manufacture and use of drugs and regulatory statutes involved in the regulation of toxic chemicals in the United States are summarized in Tables 10.1 and 10.2, respectively. The industrialized countries also have laws and agencies for the regulation of toxic chemicals.

10.2.2 GUIDELINES FOR DRUGS

The objective of all toxicity testing is the elimination of potential risks to humans; most of the testing is performed on experimental animals. This is necessary because our current knowledge of quantitative structure activity relationships (QSAR) does not permit accurate extrapolation to new compounds. Human data are difficult to obtain experimentally for ethical reasons but are necessary for deleterious effects such as irritation, nausea, allergies, odor evaluation, and other higher nervous system functions. Some insight may be obtained in certain cases from occupational exposure data. Such data, however, often tend to be inconclusive; they are irregular and not clearly defined regarding the composition of the toxicant or the exposure levels because multiple exposures are common.

Table 10.1 Chronology of US Guidelines for Use and Manufacture of Drugs and Chemicals

1966	FDA guidelines for reproduction studies for safety evaluation of drugs
1968	FDA general guidelines for animal toxicity studies
1974	Pharmaceutical manufacturers association toxicity testing guidelines
1976	National Cancer Institute Bioassay Protocol
1978	EPA pesticide guidelines
1978	Good Laboratory Practices
1979	TSCA draft health effects test guidelines
2005	Patent regime law

Table 10.2 Major Regulatory Agencies for Control and Use of Toxic Chemicals in the United States

FDA, foods, drugs, and cosmetics: Food and Drugs Act, 1906
Food, Drugs, and Cosmetics Act (FDC), 1938
Pesticides: Fungicides, Insecticides & Rodenticides Act (FIFRA), 1947
Water pollutants: Federal Water Pollution Control Act, 1948
CEQ, environmental impacts: National Environmental Policy Act (NEPA), 1969
OSHA, workplace: Occupational Safety and Health (OSH) Act, 1970
EPA, air pollutants: Clean Air Act, 1970
Ocean dumping: Marine Protection, Research, and Sanctuaries Act (MPRSA) or Ocean Dumping Act, 1972
CPSC, dangerous consumer products: Consumer Product Safety Act (CPSA), 1972
Drinking water: Safe Drinking Water Act, 1974
DOT, transport of hazardous materials: Hazardous Materials Transportation Act (HMTA), 1975
Toxic chemicals: Toxic Substances Control Act (TSCA), 1976
Hazardous wastes: Resource Conservation and Recovery Act (RCRA), 1976
Abandoned hazardous wastes: Superfund (CERCLA), 1980
Food Quality Protection Act (FQPA), 1996
FDA: Food Safety Modernization Act, 1997

EPA, *Environmental Protection Agency;* CEQ, *Council for Environmental Quality (now Office of Environmental Policy);* OSHA, *Occupational Safety and Health Administration;* FDA, *Food and Drug Administration;* CPSC, *Consumer Product Safety Commission;* DOT, *Department of Transportation.*

Clearly, any experiments involving humans must be performed under carefully defined conditions after other tests are completed.

For a variety of reasons, extrapolation of information from experimental animals to humans presents complex problems, including differences in metabolic pathways, dermal penetration, mode of action, and others. However, experimental animals present numerous advantages in testing procedures. These advantages include the following:

1. the possibility of clearly defined genetic constitution and their amenity to controlled exposure
2. controlled duration of exposure
3. the possibility of detailed examination of all tissues following necropsy

Although all tests are not required for all potentially therapeutic drugs/chemicals, any of the tests shown in Table 10.3 may be required by the regulations imposed under a particular law. The particular set of tests required depends on the predicted or actual use of the chemical, the predicted or actual route of exposure, and the chemical and physical properties of the chemical. The details of these tests are discussed in subsequent chapters.

Table 10.3 Summary of Toxicity Tests Required by Regulatory Authorities

I. *Chemical and physical properties*

For the chemical in question, probable contaminants from synthesis as well as intermediates and waste products from the synthetic process

II. *Exposure and environmental fate*
   - A. Degradation studies—hydrolysis, photodegradation, etc.
   - B. Degradation in soil, water, under various conditions
   - C. Mobility and dissipation in soil, water, and air
   - D. Accumulation in plants, aquatic animals, wild terrestrial animals, food plants, animals, etc.

III. *In vivo tests*
   - A. Acute
     1. LD_{50} and LC_{50}—oral, dermal or inhaled
     2. Eye irritation
     3. Dermal irritation
     4. Dermal sensitization
   - B. Sub-chronic
     1. 30- to 90-day feeding
     2. 30- to 90-day dermal or inhalation exposure
   - C. Chronic/reproduction
     1. Chronic feeding (including oncogenicity tests)
     2. Teratogenicity
     3. Reproduction (multigeneration)
   - D. Special tests
     1. Neurotoxicity
     2. Potentiation
     3. Metabolism
     4. Pharmacodynamics
     5. Behavior

IV. *In vitro tests*
   - A. Mutagenicity—prokaryote (Ames test)
   - B. Mutagenicity—eukaryote (*Drosophila*, mouse, etc.)
   - C. Chromosome aberration (*Drosophila*, sister chromatid exchange, etc.)

10.2.3 TOXIC SUBSTANCES CONTROL ACT OF THE UNITED STATES

The need to control chemical contamination was recognized in 1976, when the US Congress passed the Toxic Substances Control Act (TSCA) to "prevent unreasonable risks of injury to health or the environment associated with the manufacture, processing, and distribution of the product for commercial use, or for disposal of chemical substances." The act provides the EPA with the authority to require reporting, record-keeping and testing requirements, and restrictions relating to chemical substances and/or mixtures.

Certain substances are generally excluded from the TSCA, including, among others, food, drugs, cosmetics, and pesticides. The TSCA addresses the production, importation, use, and disposal of specific chemicals, including polychlorinated biphenyls (PCBs), asbestos, radon, and lead-based paint.

The Office of Pollution Prevention and Toxics (OPPT) manages programs under the Toxic Substances Control Act and the Pollution Prevention Act. Under these laws, the EPA evaluates new and existing chemicals and their risks, and it finds ways to prevent or reduce pollution before it gets into the environment.

10.2.4 REACH REGULATION OF EUROPEAN COUNTRIES

The new EU regulatory framework for Chemicals, REACH, was enacted on June 1, 2007. The aim of REACH is to enhance the protection of human health and the environment. This will be achieved by passing more responsibility for the management of chemicals to the industry.

REACH establishes European-wide uniform legal standards. It replaces the former evaluation of existing substances and the notification of new chemical substances. It has implications for producers, importers, formulators, distributors, and users of chemicals, as well as those producing and/or importing articles. Manufacturers and importers of a substance in quantities less than 1 ton (1000 kg) per year are not subjected to registration.

One of the main reasons for developing and adopting the REACH regulation was that a large number of substances have been manufactured and placed on the market in Europe for many years, sometimes in very high amounts, and yet there has been limited information on the hazards that they might pose to human health and the environment. It was considered that there is a need to fill these information gaps to help to ensure that the industry is able to assess hazards and risks and to identify and implement the necessary risk management measures to protect human health and the environment.

Data sharing is a core principle of REACH, and one of its aims is to require that testing in vertebrate animals is not repeated. Registrants use the data sharing mechanism to avoid unnecessary animal testing. The legislation provides several mechanisms to ensure the sharing of data; companies may need to inquire if data have already been submitted on their substance, share information from animal studies, and, with some exceptions, submit joint registration dossiers with other registrants for the same substance. Thus, one of the objectives of the REACH regulation is to promote non-animal test methods.

The new EU chemicals legislation applies to all industry sectors dealing with chemicals and along the entire supply chain. It makes companies responsible for the safety of chemicals they place on the market. The classification, labeling, and packaging (CLP) regulation ensures that the hazards presented by chemicals are clearly communicated to workers and consumers in the EU through classification and labeling of chemicals.

The new estimates for the number of substances falling under REACH range from 68,000 to 101,000 chemicals (substantially exceeding the previous estimates of 29,000 substances). The latter estimates were, however, based on data before 1994, and both expansion of the EU and growth of the chemical industry since have contributed to higher numbers today.

Several groups of substances are either outside the scope or exempted from certain aspects of REACH, such as the following: pharmaceutical products for human or veterinary use; food or feed stuff additives; animal nutrition; and substances like glucose, water, several natural substances, unintended reaction products, non-isolated intermediates, and polymers,

In brief, the principle of "one substance one registration" set by REACH requires that cooperation between potential registrants must be established and data must be shared and submitted jointly. This is a core principle within REACH intended to prevent duplicated testing in vertebrate animals.

10.3 INTERNATIONAL HARMONIZATION

To decrease the cost of testing and have harmonization, the proceedings of an International Conference on Harmonization (ICH), Guideline on Detection of Toxicity to Reproduction for Medicinal Products, is the only publication with any major impact on the industry. With the introduction of ICH, it has become mandatory that all the regulatory studies, both in vivo and in vitro, if performed as per the guidelines of the Organization for European Cooperation and Development (OECD), are acceptable by the US FDA and Japan.

Good Laboratory Practice (GLP) regulations came into existence in 1978 in the United States and in 1981 in OECD countries. Adherence to these principles permits international acceptability of safety testing data from different countries. With the product patent regime enforced in 2005, the drug industry, chemical industry, pesticide industry, and food industry have oriented themselves to find new trade opportunities.

The World Trade Organization (WTO) strongly emphasizes good practices through the chapter on technical barriers. This means that companies not following good practices in testing, safety studies, manufacturing, and others will lose their market share.

10.4 ROLE OF ANIMAL TESTING

The role of various regulation agencies is to ensure a high level of protection of human health and the environment from hazardous effects of chemicals. The regulations represent the balance established in the legislative process between the need for generating new information on hazardous properties using animal tests and the aim of avoiding unnecessary animal testing. It therefore establishes the principle that testing on vertebrate animals shall be a last resort.

Companies producing or importing chemical substances have to ensure that they can be used safely. This is achieved by using and, when necessary, generating information on the intrinsic properties of substances to assess their hazards for classification and risk assessment and to develop appropriate risk management measures to protect human health and the environment.

A key motivation for developing these regulations is to fill information gaps for the large number of substances already in use in the world, because for many such substances there was inadequate information on their hazardous properties and the risks their use may pose. Without a comprehensive set of information on the essential hazardous properties of higher-volume chemical substances, registrants cannot undertake a chemical safety assessment that will recommend appropriate risk management measures to avoid or limit exposure. In particular, information on properties such as organ toxicity after long-term exposure, the potential to induce cancer, toxicity to the developing fetus, toxicity to reproductive functions, or long-term aquatic toxicity are often not available for such substances.

10.5 STANDARD INFORMATION REQUIREMENTS

Each registrant has to provide all relevant and available information on the intrinsic properties of the substance in their registration dossier.

When data for a basic (core) set of information addressing a number of intrinsic properties of a substance as specified in a regulation is not available, registrants are responsible for generating these data and providing them in their registration dossier. Depending on the property concerned, the standard information requirements may specify information that can be obtained from standard tests. Depending on the test specified, bacteria, cultured cells, or animals are normally used.

The core information is intended to show, for example, whether a single exposure, or one lasting a few hours or days, has the potential to cause serious harm to human health or the environment. Information from other tests, for example, for bacterial cells, may be able to provide an indication regarding the potential of a substance to cause cancer.

Sometimes there are additional information requirements. At these levels, more detailed and extensive information is required and can be obtained using higher-tier studies. If data gaps have been identified and cannot be filled, other registrants will have to conduct higher-tier studies to fulfill the requirements of the registrant country. However, before such testing can begin, testing proposals must be submitted and prior approval from the respective authority must be received.

10.6 RECENT TRENDS

10.6.1 AVOID UNNECESSARY TESTING

To reduce the use of animals, several different mechanisms have been evolved by each country. For example, the United States, European countries, Japan, and other countries avoid unnecessary animal tests; in particular, data sharing, the use of alternative test methods, and other approaches are used to predict the properties of substances. However, the filling of data gaps means that some new animal testing will be necessary.

10.6.2 ALTERNATE APPROACHES

Over the past few years, a number of in vitro test methods that are suitable for test purposes have been adopted and incorporated in the test methods regulation. However, there are currently no in vitro tests, ex vivo tests, or test batteries that can act as a like-for-like replacement of higher-tier toxicology studies, such as those investigating carcinogenicity, ex vivo mutagenicity, or reproductive toxicity. However, they may be useful as part of a weight of evidence (WoE) approach or as a basis for classification under CLP; thus, depending on the case, they can render testing on animals unnecessary.

Animal tests can be avoided if the hazardous properties of a substance can be predicted using computer models, sometimes referred to as in silico methods such as using the quantitative structure activity relationship (QSAR) or the structure activity relationship (SAR) approach. At present, such in silico predictions cannot be used alone to predict a number of the toxicological properties (long-term toxicity, carcinogenicity, mutagenicity, and reproductive toxicity), although they may be useful as part of a WoE approach or as a basis for classification under CLP.

Properties of substances can be predicted using information from tests on analogs by the "read-across" approach, or for a group of substances using the "category" approach. The registrant is responsible for making the scientific arguments that these predicted properties are adequate for REACH in terms of providing comparable information of the animal studies on the registered substance. Read-across and categories are the most promising approaches to predict the long-term toxicological and carcinogenic, mutagenic, and reprotoxic (CMR) properties of substances for REACH and CLP. However, it should be noted that sufficient information must be available to support these predictions.

Furthermore, newly developed alternative in vitro test methods undergo validation to assess their relevance and reliability. The European Centre for the Validation of Alternative Methods (ECVAM) validates alternative methods that replace, reduce, and refine the use of animals in scientific procedures. Regulatory acceptance of validated alternative methods will be facilitated and streamlined by the new mechanism of "preliminary analysis of regulatory relevance" (PARERE).

These consultation networks of the European Commission involve EU Member State contact points and relevant agencies and committees, such as the European Chemical Agency (ECHA).

10.6.3 CHEMINFORMATICS

Cheminformatics (also known as *chemoinformatics*, chemioinformatics, and chemical informatics) is the use of computer and informational techniques applied to a range of problems in the field of chemistry. These in silico techniques are used in, for example, pharmaceutical companies during the process of drug discovery. A major focus for the future of computational toxicology will be integration and analysis of large data sets. There are several databases, each with differing content, architecture, and searchability, that make the task of integration extremely difficult.

In fact, this is a relatively new field of information technology that focuses on the collection, storage, analysis, and manipulation of chemical data. The chemical data of interest typically include information on small molecule formulas, structures, properties, spectra, and activities (biological or industrial). Cheminformatics originally emerged as a vehicle to help the drug discovery and development process; however, cheminformatics now plays an increasingly important role in many areas of biology, chemistry, and biochemistry. The intent of this unit is to give readers some introduction into the field of cheminformatics and to show how cheminformatics not only shares many similarities with the field of bioinformatics but also enhances much of what is currently done in bioinformatics. For example, bioinformatics resources (ie, databases and software) are of growing importance to understanding or predicting drug metabolism, especially with respect to the absorption, distribution, metabolism, excretion, (ADME), and toxicity (T) of both existing drugs and potential drug leads. Detailed descriptions and critical assessments of a number of potentially useful bioinformatics/cheminformatics databases and predictive ADMET software tools are provided. Additionally, several pharmaceutically important applications of both the databases and software are highlighted. Given the rapid growth in this area and the rapid changes that are taking place, special emphasis is placed on freely available or web-accessible resources.

10.6.4 NANOMATERIALS

A new field of research has emerged: nanotoxicology. Nanomaterials are structures with characteristic dimensions between 1 and 100 nm that exhibit a variety of unique and tunable chemical and physical properties that have engineered nanoparticles central components in an array of emerging technologies. Nanomaterials can have unique physiochemical properties that result from the combination of their small size, chemical composition, surface structure, solubility, shape, and aggregation. For example, nanoscale titanium dioxide found in sunscreen is invisible when rubbed on your nose, unlike standard titanium, which is white. This occurs because the small particle size changes the interaction with visible light. Another important characteristic of nano-sized particles is the vastly increased surface area, which is important because it increases the interaction with light or other chemicals. These particles can also be coated with other chemicals to reduce clumping of the material or add special properties. For example, additional chemicals may be added to sunscreen to increase absorption of ultraviolet light. Nanomaterials come in a variety of substances, such as metals (eg, silver, nickel, iron), oxides (eg, titanium and zinc), carbon-based materials (eg, nanotubes, fullerenes), quantum dots, and macromolecules, all with their unique properties and uses. Nanotubes have many uses; they can be used in filtration systems, for encasing medicines for drug delivery, or for constructing ultra-strong and ultra-light material such as that used for tennis rackets or golf clubs.

Nanotechnology has opened the door to new therapies with enhanced absorption and distribution, but these properties also raise the prospect of increased harm from toxic reactions. Human exposure to nanoparticles can occur during their development, production, use, and disposal. Nanomaterials show useful properties such as electronic reactivity and tissue permeability that are not provided by micromaterials. Thus, nanomaterials are expected to be innovative materials for the development of medicine and cosmetics.

Nanomaterials have a much higher ratio of surface area to weight than conventional materials, and this property can affect mechanisms of action, biodistribution, and pharmacokinetics. Because of their tiny size, nanomaterials have special properties that make them ideal for a range of commercial and medical uses. However, the pharmacokinetics, long-term fate, and potential toxicity of functional nanomaterials should be well examined before any novel nanomaterials can be translated into the clinic.

Studies that would be characterized as "classic" pharmacokinetics for drugs or chemicals have not been conducted for most of the manufactured nanomaterials.

According to available literature, the continuing evaluation of the health implications of exposure to nanomaterials is essential before the commercial benefits of these materials can be fully realized.

10.7 GOOD LABORATORY PRACTICES

GLP is a quality system concerned with the organizational processes and conditions under which nonclinical health and environmental safety studies are planned, performed, monitored, recorded, archived, and reported. The principles of GLP need to be applied to the nonclinical safety testing of test items such as pharmaceuticals, pesticides, cosmetics, drugs, feed additives, industrial chemicals, and others. The test items can also be of natural or biological origin and, in some circumstances, may be living organisms.

10.7.1 BACKGROUND

During the 1970s, the US FDA found that several scientific reports on animal studies were unreliable. The investigations of the US FDA in several toxicology laboratories in the United States demonstrated a certain lack of organization and poor management. This prompted the federal agencies of other countries to introduce regulations regarding the conduct of safety toxicology studies. As has been stated previously, the principles of GLP regulations were introduced in 1978 in the United States and in OECD countries in 1981. Adherence to these principles ensures international acceptability of safety testing data from different countries. The metamorphosis has begun; many contract research organizations (CROs) are being set up and discovery research has started taking roots in several countries. Many foreign companies have started outsourcing research and testing work to companies located in India and other countries or to their own companies with joint ventures in those countries.

10.7.2 PRINCIPLES OF GOOD LABORATORY PRACTICES

The principles of GLP promote the development of quality test data for mutual acceptance among countries. Adaptation of these principles will help to overcome trade differences by signing the Memoranda of Understanding between different (chemical) trading nations. The worldwide recognition of GLP principles required the OCED member countries sign an agreement of Mutual Acceptance of Data (MAD). This has dispensed with repeat testing that is beneficial to human and animal welfare and, at the same time, reduces the costs for industry and governments.

The implementation of GLP is facilitated by a specific set of requirements with regard to:

- Organization and personnel in the test facility
- Quality assurance program
- Adequate size, construction, and location
- Standard apparatus, materials, and reagents
- Adaptation of appropriate acceptable approved testing procedures
- Standard operating procedures (SOPs)
- Standard safety testing programs
- Creation of archives

OECD has published a series of documents on the principles of GLP and compliance monitoring (number 1 to 14). These documents can be downloaded from the OECD website (http://www/oecd.org/ehs).

CHAPTER

Toxicological testing: in vitro models

11

CHAPTER OUTLINE

11.1 INTRODUCTION

As has been stated previously, toxicological testing laboratories now have to comply with strict official controls and inspections regarding animal use at any time and that can be reinforced by relevant legislation. The toxicological testing using in vivo systems has already been discussed in the previous chapter. The main objective of this chapter is to outline the major aspects of in vitro models used in toxicity testing and to give a brief overview of endpoint determination. The principal focus is to highlight some of the current in vitro models available in toxicity testing.

11.2 ANIMAL WELFARE LEGISLATION

Animal welfare legislation is currently applicable in most countries to help prevent misuse of animals in toxicological testing. Implementation of these laws help improve animal welfare and prevention of cruelty to animals, including animal housing (eg, breeding, handling and feeding). It also has a great role in the

Fundamentals of Toxicology. DOI: http://dx.doi.org/10.1016/B978-0-12-805426-0.00011-1

regulatory toxicity testing guidelines, by applying humane endpoints and decreasing the number of animals required.

Handling laboratory animals and administering toxicological compounds are stressful procedures. There has been an attempt to apply the highest ethical standards not only by introducing an excellent environment and social and complex housing but also by reducing and improving techniques used on laboratory animals. Implanted biosensors are now available that permit the continuous telemetric monitoring of physiological and biochemical parameters in experimental animals. These techniques have been proven useful in toxicological studies not only to minimize the artifacts due to animal handling and restraint but also to improve animal welfare. In addition, noninvasive and currently expensive methods such as magnetic resonance imaging (MRI) and nuclear magnetic resonance spectroscopy are available for the visualization of pathological findings and the determination of the distribution of a test chemical in laboratory animals, respectively, which further contribute to improved animal welfare.

11.3 IN VITRO MODELS

There are several advantages of the use of in vitro cellular models due to the following reasons:

1. Relatively inexpensive
2. Easy to maintain and manipulate compared to animal models
3. Allow the study of direct cellular effects of toxins on specific cell or tissue types in a controlled environment

However, the main disadvantage of in vitro systems over animal models is the lack of systemic effects such as an appropriate balance and supply of growth factors and a system of xenobiotic metabolism and elimination of toxins. There are a number of types of cell culture available for in vitro testing that offer various degrees of complexity and relatedness to the in vivo situation. These tests, in order of increasing complexity and genetic similarity to the tissue of origin, are summarized in Table 11.1. These include permanent cell lines (primary cultures and organotypic or whole organ cultures), which are described herein.

11.3.1 PERMANENT CELL LINES

Permanent cell lines are mitotic and can be finite, established, or clonal in nature. They have the advantage of being relatively easy and inexpensive to maintain compared to animals, and they are amenable to cryopreservation under liquid nitrogen. However, if maintained through high numbers of divisions, then there

Table 11.1 Organization of a Tiered System for In Vitro Toxicity Testing (Tests in Order of Increasing Complexity and Genetic Similarity to the Tissue of Origin)

Culture Type	Suitability
Mitotic cell lines	Studies of basal toxicity (eg, membrane damage, viability, etc.) and cell proliferation
Differentiating cell lines	Screening and mechanistic studies of developmental toxicity, target cell-specific toxicity
Primary cell cultures	Developmental or target cell-specific toxicity; genetically more similar to target system but generally heterogeneous and short-lived
Organotypic/whole organ cultures	Tissue slices or cultures organs that can maintain cell interactions and tissue function

is an increasing likelihood of genetic drift that might affect phenotypic properties of relevance to toxicity testing.

11.3.2 PRIMARY CULTURES

Finite cell lines are normally derived from primary cultures and can survive for 40–50 divisions before finally dying (eg, fibroblasts). Established cell lines are effectively immortal, having been transformed with a virus, a mutagen, or spontaneously. These are generally tumor-like in nature; some widely used examples include mouse 3T3 fibroblasts, HeLa cells, and Chinese hamster ovary (CHO) cells. However, several cell lines can be induced to differentiate, making them potentially useful models of specific stages of development, for example, the use of nerve growth factor or retinoic acid to induce a neuronal phenotype in cultures of rat PC12 pheochromocytoma and human SH-SY5Y neuroblastoma cells, respectively.

Clonal cell lines are derived from the mitotic division of a single cell seeded in a sterile microtiter plate by limiting dilution, as used in the cloning of hybridoma cell lines. Thus, cell lines can be cloned to exhibit a specific trait (eg, high levels of specific receptors, drug resistance, etc.). Although a homogeneous response to toxin treatment might then be expected from such a cell line, there is the risk of losing other features of a more heterogeneous population.

A more recent development has been the use of stem cell lines as models for developmental toxicity testing. These cell lines are normally maintained in growth media containing mitogens, and they can be induced to differentiate into different cell types (eg, cardiomyocytes, pancreatic and neural cells) by removal of mitogens and/or the addition of specific trophic factors. Embryonic stem cells (ESCs) have the potential to differentiate into any cell type, whereas progenitor cells are already committed to follow a specific developmental pattern.

Table 11.2 Examples of Cell Culture Systems Used to Model Specific Types of Toxicity

Type of Toxicity	Cell Culture System(s)
Dermal toxicity	Keratinocyte and fibroblast cell lines; excised rat skin and human models
Hepatic toxicity	Human hepatoma HepG2 cell line and subclones expressing CYP1A1, cell lines engineered to express single human or animal P450, primary hepatocyte cultures, longer-term collagen sandwich cultures, liver slices and isolated perfused liver
Neurotoxicity	Differentiating neural cell lines (eg, human SH-SY5Y and rat PC12 neuroblastoma); primary cultures, whole rat brain reaggregates, and organotypic brain slice cultures
Developmental toxicity	Whole rat embryo cultures, rat limb bud reaggregate cultures, and mouse embryonic stem cell lines
Immunotoxicity	Antibody production and activation/proliferation of lymphocytes
Genotoxicity	Mammalian cell gene mutation and chromosome aberration tests

11.3.3 ORGANOTYPIC OR WHOLE ORGAN CULTURES

Another way to address this issue may be to develop organotypic cultures, a postmitotic system containing predifferentiated cells prior to the addition of toxin. In this case, tissue slices (typically 200 μm thickness) are cut from fresh tissue on a microtome and then subsequently rinsed and cultured in growth medium with agitation, as discussed. Such slices maintain the complexity of cell–cell interactions and extracellular matrix composition of the original tissue; in some cases, they can survive up to several weeks. Nevertheless, even this kind of cellular system lacks the systemic interaction with the immune and circulatory systems that would occur in vivo. Therefore, this is not a complete substitute for in vivo testing. However, using cell cultures as part of a tiered system of increasing complexity from in vitro to in vivo measurements would improve throughput, decrease costs, and allow drastic reduction in the use of live animals when screening compounds for potential toxic effects. Some examples of cell culture systems (in vitro toxicity) currently in use to model specific types of toxicity are indicated in Table 11.2.

11.4 IN VITRO EMBRYOTOXICITY TESTING

As has been discussed in the previous chapter, the regulatory guidelines such as EPA, ICH, and OECD define the specific endpoints to detect adverse effects of drugs or chemicals on reproduction and fertility. These guidelines specify only the organs and tissues to be evaluated grossly, weighed, and microscopically examined; they do not specify sample size and do not indicate parts of appropriate tissues to be examined. These studies rely primarily on fertility parameters to assess the reproductive performance rather than histopathology.

Although general toxicity studies have no such recommendations, it has been shown that reproductive toxicity measures including histopathology from the repeat dose toxicity studies are the most sensitive endpoints in predicting reproductive toxicity. At the same time, assessing the reproductive health of a population and its different professional groups requires the application of rapid test systems that allow potential pathogens to be searched for by multidirectional testing of environmental objects and biosubstrates (blood and its components, tissue fluids, amniotic fluids, etc.) and that predict the potential hazards they pose to the reproductive function of humans, particularly their embryonic development. The aforementioned facts point to the necessity of developing test systems designed to assess the effect of exposure not only on specific chemical substances but also on a combination of unfavorable factors of human embryogenesis.

11.4.1 PRINCIPLES OF IN VITRO EMBRYOTOXICITY TESTING

The in vitro test system represents a flexible system (battery) of different tests in the framework of a single or a few compatible test models. This system makes it possible to gain additional information and should not be considered as an alternative to the standard toxicity test for pregnant animals described previously.

The basic aim of testing is to give a prognosis of the hazard of a test substance for human embryogenesis. Dealing with one or another test system, we should realize its potential and tend to include it in the most informative tests; however, we should not expect more than it is able to provide. We should keep in mind the following:

- there are no universal animal testing systems
- single tests, including specialized, are unable to reflect the entire diversity of embryo responses to exposure
- the system of testing should include approaches for testing as much as possible developmental processes and allow general conclusions regarding the embryo development
- the test system should allow one not only to assess the embryotoxic activity of a test substance but also to reveal its *embryotoxic properties*, where activity is only one of these properties
- the system should allow testing water-soluble and poorly water-soluble substances, as well as gaseous substances
- the possibility of using the metabolic activation/inactivation system should be available

- the possibility of using the intrinsic metabolic resource of the test model is desirable
- genetic modifications of the test model are desirable
- the system should be able to accept human pharmacokinetics/toxicokinetics data and allow the use of human fluids and tissues (blood, amniotic fluids, abortive material, etc.).
- in vitro methods allow the embryotoxic activity of a substance to be tested directly on an embryo, irrespective of how the structure and activity of the substance have been modified in the mother's organism

This last point is quite important because the pharmacokinetics of a substance in a body is not infrequently individual (genetically determined) and reflects the specific features of a species, animal strain, and concrete specimen.

11.4.2 USE OF IN VITRO MODELS/ALTERNATIVE TEST METHODS

A number of alternative test methods have been developed to reduce the number of whole animals used in studies and/or to obtain more rapid information concerning the potential of a compound to be a reproductive/developmental toxicant. Validation of many of the methods has been problematic because they do not address the contribution of maternal factors or multiorgan contributions to outcomes. Some of these alternative methods include the use of cell or embryo culture. For example, the micromass culture involves the use of limb bud cells from rat embryos grown in micromass culture for 5 days. The processes of differentiation and cell proliferation are assessed. In the Chernoff/Kavlock assay, pregnant rodents are exposed during organogenesis and allowed to deliver. Postnatal growth, viability, and gross morphology of litters are recorded (detailed skeletal evaluations are not performed). Other alternative tests involve the use of nontraditional test species such as *Xenopus* embryos (FETAX) and *Hydra*. *Xenopus* embryos, which are exposed for 96 h and then evaluated for morphological defects, viability, and growth. The cells of *Hydra* aggregate to form artificial embryos. The dose response in these "embryos" is compared to that of the adult *Hydra*. The chick embryotoxicity screening test (CHEST) is another alternative method used for screening chemicals. The most attractive test models use mammals such as mouse and rat embryos (Table 11.2).

11.4.3 RAT/MICE EMBRYOS AS A MODEL

Using rat/mice embryos as a model is a rapid method to estimate the embryotoxic properties of chemicals. Use of preimplantation embryos provide both cytological and embryological test models because they contains few cell structures or self-determined systems and integrated (whole) organisms. Based on the model, it is possible to estimate both cytotoxic and embryotoxic effects after pathogenic influence has occurred. Most information on the pathogenic effects of various factors can be gained by studying embryos developing in vitro during the initial organogenesis stages, which are the most sensitive to damaging agents.

During this period, one can observe organ anlage and differentiation directly in the culture (fusion of the paired heart rudiments and initiation of heart beating, anlage of fore and hind limbs, head brain segments, auditory and ophthalmic placodes, somitogenesis, etc.).

The use of postimplantation rat/mice embryos allows assessment of not only embryotoxic effects but also potential genotoxic effects of pathogenic factors by using the most sensitive genotoxicity tests, such as the sister chromatide exchange (SCE) frequency assay. Simultaneous assessment of these effects in the framework of a single model makes it possible to inter-relate the embryotoxic and mutagenic impacts. Naturally, the SCE frequency assay does not exhaust genotoxicity testing approaches; in addition, the micronuclear test can be used.

11.4.4 USE OF CULTURED EMBRYOS

This technique involves direct introduction of a test agent into the culture medium. After incubation, induced effects and toxic and ineffective levels of the test sample are estimated. Work with embryo cultures has certain features that seem to be decisive. Embryo in vitro culturing (ie, in the absence of the mother's organism) makes it possible to assess a direct hazard that the test agent poses to the developing fetus, irrespective of possible (genetic or functional) fluctuations of the mother's organism. Direct exposure of in vitro cultured embryos allows one:

- to perform morphofunctional assessment of embryo development
- to determine the threshold and effective concentrations
- to determine the time–concentration effect function
- to compare obtained data with human pharmacokinetics data
- to give a prognosis for human embryogenesis

The morphofunctional assessment of embryo development in culture is performed by measuring the principal development parameters related to growth processes (craniocaudal size, total protein content), embryo body differentiation (somitogenesis, development of brain and heart compartments, limb rudiments, vision and hearing organs hyoid arches, mandibular and maxillary processes, etc.), morphofunctional processes (neurulation, embryo turning, allantoic growth and establishment of chorio-allantoic connection, formation of blood islets, vasculogenesis, hematopoiesis, initiation of yolk circulation, etc.). In practice, a semi-quantitative (grade) system is not infrequently used to characterize the degree of development of one or another rudiment or the completeness of morphogenetic processes.

The evaluation of preimplantation embryos is analyzed in terms of the numbers of live, dead, and abnormal (dysmorphogenic) ones that have reached certain stages of development.

Among the dead are deformed, fragmented nuclei and nuclei with dull cytoplasm. Anomalies have been detected in the continuing development of embryos in culture. After culturing, mature embryos are evaluated for cell mass, proliferative activity, and cell death, as expressed by the number of pycnotic nuclei.

The result of cultivation allows determination of the effective embryotoxic concentration and threshold concentration (the minimum effective and noneffective) for various (if there is a need) effects (embryolethality, teratogenic effect, growth restriction, impact on the proliferative activity of cells, effect on a particular morphogenetic process).

11.4.5 ENDPOINT DETERMINATION FOR IN VITRO TESTING SYSTEMS

A good in vitro testing system should be sensitive but at the same time yield minimum false-positive and false-negative results. It should have at least the following endpoint measurements:

1. Should show dose–response relationships for a given toxin
2. Should reflect and should be predictive of the in vivo pattern of toxicity for a given group of agents
3. Should be objective and reproducible
4. Should have internal controls

It will be useful if the testing system involves rapid assays of toxicity and allows simultaneous testing of multiple compounds and/or doses. The testing system should also be relatively inexpensive and should involve technology and skills that are easily transferable to other laboratory personnel.

To achieve an ideal testing system, a battery of endpoint measurements may be included to minimize the occurrence of false-negative and false-positive results.

11.5 CONCLUSION

A major issue facing toxicological science today is how to convert experimental data from in vivo and in vitro models into knowledge about molecular mechanisms of toxicity and safe levels of exposure to the agents tested. A number of animal models that have been used for many years for screening purposes have been gradually reduced. Scientists have played an important role in the development of legislation and guidelines relating to the use and replacement of laboratory animals in toxicity assessment. The generally accepted approach to screen compounds for toxicity is to use a multitiered system, starting with simple monocultures of specific cell types, followed by co-cultures that simulate metabolic effects and/or cell–cell interactions in the whole organism, before performing final testing on animals. Further, development of improved in vitro systems will eventually minimize the use of animals for toxicity studies.

CHAPTER

Toxicological testing: In vivo systems

12

CHAPTER OUTLINE

Fundamentals of Toxicology. DOI: http://dx.doi.org/10.1016/B978-0-12-805426-0.00012-3

12.1 INTRODUCTION

The importance of toxicological testing is critical for new pharmaceuticals and other new chemical entities such as agrochemicals and industrial chemicals required for use in our daily lives. In some cases, basic research can produce data that eventually lead to the ban of certain chemicals because they were proven to be unsafe. This has led to increased demand for safety screening to ensure successful drug development and safe chemicals before they become available for general use. Part of this screening process includes the internationally recognized in vivo or in vitro toxicological tests. Toxicological testing laboratories now have to comply with strict official controls and inspections on animal use at any time, and they can be reinforced by relevant legislation. The toxicological testing using in vivo test systems are summarized in this chapter.

12.2 ADMINISTRATION OF TOXICANTS

Regardless of the chemicals tested for acute or chronic toxicity, all in vivo testing requires reproducible results. As has been discussed previously, the nature and degree of the toxic effect can be affected by several variables, including the route of administration. The differences in variation in toxicity due to the route of administration could be at the portals of entry or due to effects on toxicokinetic/pharmacokinetic processes. For example, intravenous (IV) may give rise to a concentration high enough to saturate some rate-limiting process, whereas oral/per os (PO), intramuscular (IM), or subcutaneous (SC) routes may distribute the dose over a longer time and avoid such saturation (for details, the reader is referred to a chapter dealing with toxicokinetics). To eliminate the effects of handling and other stresses, as well as the effects of the solvents or other carriers, it is usually better to compare treated animals with both solvent-treated and untreated or possibly sham-treated controls.

12.2.1 ROUTES OF ADMINISTRATION

- *Oral*: Oral administration is often referred to as administration PO. Compounds can be administered mixed in the diet, dissolved in drinking water, by gastric gavage, by controlled-release capsules, or by gelatin capsules. In the first two cases, either a measured amount can be provided or access can be ad libitum (available 24 h per day). In gastric gavage, the test material is administered through a stomach tube or gavage needle; if a solvent is necessary for preparation of dosing solutions or suspensions, then the vehicle is also administered to control animals.
- *Dermal*: Dermal administration is required for estimation of toxicity of chemicals that may be absorbed through the skin, as well as for estimation of

skin irritation and photosensitization. Compounds are applied, either directly or in a suitable solvent, to the skin of experimental animals after hair has been removed by clipping. Often, dry materials are mixed with water to make a thick paste that can be applied in a manner that ensures adequate contact with the skin. Frequently, the animals must be restrained to prevent licking and, hence, oral uptake of the material. Solvent and restraint controls should be considered when stress is involved. Skin irritancy tests may be conducted on either animals or humans, with volunteer test panels used for human tests.

- *Inhalation*: The respiratory system is an important portal of entry. The alternative method, direct instillation into the lung through the trachea, presents problems of reproducibility as well as stress; therefore, it is generally unsatisfactory. Inhalation toxicity studies are conducted in inhalation chambers. For rat studies, a particle size of 4 μ is usually used. Animals are normally exposed for a fixed number of hours each day and a fixed number of days each week. Exposure may be via the nose only, whereby the nose of the animal is inserted into the chamber through an airtight ring, or the whole body, whereby animals are placed inside the chamber.
- *Injection*: Methods of injection include IV, IM, intraperitoneal (IP), and SC. Infusion of test materials over an extended period is also possible. Again, both solvent controls and untreated controls are necessary for proper interpretation of the results.

12.2.2 CHEMICAL AND PHYSICAL PROPERTIES

The information obtained regarding chemical and physical properties can be used in many ways, such as:

- Identification of expected hazards or poisoning episodes and determination of stability in light, heat, freezing, and oxidizing or reducing agents may enable preliminary estimates of persistence in the environment as well as indicate the most likely breakdown products that may also require testing for toxicity.
- Establishment of such properties as the lipid solubility or octanol/water partition coefficient may enable preliminary estimates of rate of uptake and persistence in living organisms.
- Vapor pressure may indicate whether the respiratory system is a probable route of entry.
- Knowledge of the chemical and physical properties must be acquired to develop analytical methods for the measurement of the compound and its degradation products.
- If the chemical is to be used for commercial purposes, then similar information is needed on intermediates in the synthesis or by-products of the process because both are possible contaminants in the final product.

12.2.3 EXPOSURE AND ENVIRONMENTAL FATE

Data on exposure and environmental fate will provide information that may be useful in the prediction if the chemical is toxic. These tests are primarily useful for chemicals released into the environment such as pesticides, and they include the rate of breakdown, the rate of leaching, and the rate of movement toward groundwater. The results of these tests are then used by a variety of extrapolation techniques to estimate hazard to humans.

12.3 IN VIVO TESTS

12.3.1 ACUTE AND SUBCHRONIC TOXICITY TESTS

Acute toxicity test methods measure the adverse effects that occur within a short time after administration of a single dose of a test substance. This testing is performed principally in rodents and is usually done early in the development of a new chemical or product to provide information on its potential toxicity. This information is used to protect individuals who are working with the new material and to develop safe handling procedures for transport and disposal. The information gained also serves as the basis for hazard classification and labeling of chemicals in commerce. Acute toxicity data can help to identify the mode of toxic action of a substance and may provide information on doses associated with target organ toxicity and lethality that can be used in setting dose levels for studies of repeated doses. This information may also be extrapolated for use in the diagnosis and treatment of toxic reactions in humans. The results from acute toxicity tests can provide information for comparison of toxicity and dose–response among members of chemical classes and can help in the selection of candidate materials for further work. They are further used to standardize certain biological products such as vaccines. The results of acute toxicity tests have a wide variety of regulatory applications. These include determination of the need for child-proof packaging, determination of re-entry intervals after pesticide application, establishment of the requirements and basis for training workers in chemical use, determination of requirements for protective equipment and clothing, and decision making about general registration of pesticides or their restriction for use by certified applicators. Acute oral toxicity may be used in risk assessments of chemicals for humans and nontarget environmental organisms. The various national and international regulatory authorities have used different hazard classification systems in the past. In light of the importance of hazard classification, Organization for European Cooperation and Development (OECD) recently harmonized criteria for hazard classification for global use. For example, the five harmonized categories for acute oral toxicity (in mg/kg body weight) are 0–5, 5–50, 50–300, 300–2000, and 2000–5000.

12.3.2 ACUTE ORAL TOXICITY TESTING

Acute oral toxicity testing is focused on the dose that kills half of the animals (ie, the median lethal dose or LD_{50}), the timing of lethality following acute chemical exposure, and observing the onset, nature, severity, and reversibility of toxicity. The LD_{50} concept was developed by Trevan in 1927. Original testing methods were designed to characterize the dose–response curve by using several animals (usually at least five per sex) at each of several test doses. Data from a minimum of three doses is required. The LD_{50} values are presented as estimated doses (mg/kg) with confidence limits. The simplest method for the determination of the LD_{50} is a graphic one and is based on the assumption that the effect is a quantal one (all or none), that the percentage responding in an experimental group is dose-related, and that the cumulative effect follows a normal distribution. As a result of much recent controversy, the LD_{50} test has been the subject of considerable regulatory attention, and as a result changes in requirements have been promulgated. These changes are intended to obtain more information while at the same time using fewer animals. Recently, attention has been focused on developing alternatives to the classical LD_{50} test to reduce the number of animals used or to refine procedures to make exposures less stressful to animals. OECD adopted several alternative methods for determining acute oral toxicity. A discussion on the recent guidelines issued by OECD is beyond the scope of this chapter.

12.3.3 EYE IRRITATION

The eye irritation test used includes all variations of the Draize test, and the preferred experimental animal is the albino rabbit. The test consists of placing the material to be tested directly into the conjunctival sac of one eye, with the other eye serving as the control. The lids are held together for a few seconds, and the material is left in the eye for at least 24 h. After that time it may be rinsed out; in any case, the eye is examined and graded after 1, 2, and 3 days. Grading is subjective and based on the appearance of the following: the cornea, particularly regarding opacity; the iris, regarding both appearance and reaction to light; the conjunctiva, regarding redness and effects on blood vessels; and the eyelids, regarding swelling. Fluorescein dye may be used to assist visual examination because the dye is more readily absorbed by damaged tissues, which then fluoresce when the eye is illuminated. Each end point in the evaluation is scored on a numerical scale, and chemicals are compared on this basis. In addition to the "no-rinse" test, some protocols also investigate the effect of rinsing the eye 1 minute after exposure to determine if this reduces the potential for irritation. In addition, eyes may be graded for up to 21 days after administration of an irritating test material to evaluate recovery. The eye irritation test is probably the most criticized by advocates of animal rights and animal welfare, primarily because it is inhumane. Attempts to solve the dilemma have taken two forms: to find substitute in vitro tests and to modify the Draize test so that it becomes not only more humane but also more predictive for humans.

12.3.4 DERMAL IRRITATION AND SENSITIZATION

The tests for dermal irritation caused by topical application of chemicals fall into three general categories:

1. primary irritation
2. cutaneous sensitization
3. phototoxicity and photosensitization

Because many foreign chemicals come into direct contact with the skin, including cosmetics, detergents, bleaches, and many others, these tests are considered essential to the proper regulation of such products. Less commonly, dermal effects may be caused by systemic toxicants.

Primary Irritation: In the typical primary irritation test, the backs of albino rabbits are clipped free of hair and an area of approximately 5 cm^2 on each rabbit is used in the test. This area is then treated with either 0.5 mL or 0.5 g of the compound to be tested and then covered with a gauze pad. The entire trunk of the rabbit is wrapped to prevent ingestion. After 4 to 24 h, the tape and gauze are removed and the treated areas are evaluated for erythematous lesions (redness of the skin produced by congestion of the capillaries) and edematous lesions (accumulation of excess fluid in SC tissue), each of which is expressed on a numerical scale. After an additional 24 to 48 h, the treated areas are again evaluated.

Cutaneous Skin Sensitization: Cutaneous skin sensitization tests are designed to test the ability of chemicals to affect the immune system in such a way that a subsequent contact causes a more severe reaction than the first contact. Skin sensitization tests generally follow protocols that are modifications of the Buchler (dermal inductions) method or the Magnesson and Kligman (intradermal inductions) method. The test animal commonly used in skin sensitization tests is the guinea pig; animals are treated with the test compound in a suitable vehicle, with the vehicle alone, or with a positive control such as 2,4-dinitrochlorobenzene (a relatively strong sensitizer) or cinnamaldehyde (a relatively weak sensitizer) in the same vehicle. During the induction phase, the animals are treated for each of 3 days evenly spaced during a 2-week period. This is followed by a 2-week rest period followed by the challenge phase of the test. This consists of a 24-h topical treatment performed as described for primary skin irritation tests. The lesions are scored on the basis of severity and the number of animals responding (incidence). If there is a greater skin reaction in the animals given induction doses compared to those given the test material for the first time, then intradermal injections together with Freund's adjuvant (a chemical mixture that enhances the antigenic response) and the challenge by dermal application, or tests in which both induction and challenge doses are topical but the former is accompanied by intradermal injections of Freund's adjuvant, are used. It is important for compounds that cause primary skin irritation to be tested for skin sensitization at concentrations low enough that the two effects are not confused.

Phototoxicity and Photosensitization: Phototoxicity tests are designed to evaluate the combined dermal effects of light (primarily UV light) and the chemical in question. Tests have been developed for both phototoxicity and photoallergy. In both cases, the light energy is believed to cause a transient excitation of the toxicant molecule, which, on returning to the lower energy state, generates a reactive, free-radical intermediate. In phototoxicity, these organic radicals act directly on the cells to cause lesions, whereas in photoallergy they bind to body proteins. These modified proteins then stimulate the immune system to produce antibodies, because the modifications cause them to be recognized as foreign or "nonself" proteins. These tests are basically modifications of the tests for primary irritation and sensitization, except that following application of the test chemical, the treated area is irradiated with UV light. The differences between the animals treated and irradiated and those treated and not irradiated is a measure of the phototoxic effect.

12.3.5 SAFETY PHARMACOLOGY STUDIES

Safety pharmacology studies are conducted to investigate the potential undesirable pharmacodynamic effects of a test article on physiological functions in relationship to exposure. These tests are typically conducted as part of the development of new drugs. The objectives of safety pharmacology studies are threefold:

1. to identify undesirable effects of a test article that may have relevance to its use in humans
2. to evaluate a test article for possible effects observed in toxicology or clinical studies
3. to investigate the mechanism underlying any undesirable effects of the test article

Safety pharmacology consists of a core battery of studies with follow-up studies as indicated by preliminary findings. The core studies are designed to target vital organ systems, particularly the central nervous system (CNS), cardiovascular system (CVS), and pulmonary system. These studies are typically conducted using small numbers of rats and dogs. In the study for pulmonary function, respiratory rate, minute volume, and tidal volume are measured. In the cardiovascular telemetry study, end points include heart rate, blood pressure, and electrocardiogram evaluation. In telemetry studies, a radio transmitter is implanted in all animals to permit continuous monitoring for 24 h pretest and 24 h after dosing. A cardiopulmonary study can also be conducted in which respiratory rate, minute volume, tidal volume, blood pressure, heart rate, electrocardiogram, and body temperature are monitored in restrained animals for typically 2 h after dosing. For a detailed protocol for the safety evaluation of pharmaceutical products, the reader is referred to the subsequent chapter.

12.3.6 SUBCHRONIC TESTS

Subchronic tests are conducted orally in the rat or dog for 28 or 90 days. Such tests provide information on essentially all types of chronic toxicity other than carcinogenicity and are usually believed to be essential for establishing the dose regimens for prolonged chronic studies. They are frequently used as the basis for the determination of the no observed effect level (NOEL). This value is often defined as the highest dose level at which no deleterious or abnormal effect can be measured, and it is often used in risk assessment calculations. Subchronic tests are also useful for providing information on target organs and on the potential of the test chemical to accumulate in the organism. Subchronic studies are usually conducted using three or occasionally four dose levels. The highest should produce obvious toxicity but not high mortality, and the lowest should provide no toxicity (NOEL), whereas the intermediate dose should give effects clearly intermediate between these two extremes. Although the doses can be extrapolated from the acute test, such extrapolation is difficult, particularly in the case of compounds that accumulate in the body; frequently, a 14-day range-finding study is performed. The route of administration should ideally be the expected route of exposure in humans. Subchronic studies are usually conducted with 10 to 20 males and 10 to 20 females of a rodent species at each dose level and 4 to 8 of each sex of a larger species, such as the dog, at each dose level (studies should be conducted on two species, ideally a rodent and a nonrodent). The information required from subchronic tests varies somewhat from one regulatory agency to another. However, the requirements are basically similar to each other. Some clinical tests or blood chemistry analyses may indicate a particular target organ; if necessary, the same can be examined in greater detail.

The tissues listed in Table 12.1 plus any lesions, masses, or abnormal tissues are embedded, sectioned, and strained for light microscopy. Paraffin embedding and staining with hemotoxylin and eosin are the preferred routine methods, but special stains may be used for particular tissues or for a more specific examination of certain lesions. Electron microscopy may also be used for more specific examination of lesions or cellular changes after their initial localization by more routine methods.

12.3.7 REPEATED-DOSE DERMAL TESTS

The 21-day to 28-day dermal tests are important when the expected route of human exposure is by contact with the skin, as is the case with many industrial chemicals or pesticides. Compounds to be tested are usually applied daily to clipped areas on the back of the animal, either undiluted or in a suitable vehicle. In the latter case, if a vehicle is used, it is also applied to the controls. Corn oil, methanol, or carboxymethyl cellulose are preferred to dimethyl sulfoxide (DMSO) or acetone. The criteria for environment, dose selection, and species selection are the same as used for 90-day feeding tests, except that fewer organs may be examined.

12.3.8 28-DAY TO 90-DAY INHALATION TESTS

Inhalation studies are indicated whenever the route of exposure is expected to be through the lungs. Animals are commonly exposed for 6 to 8 h each day, 5 days

Table 12.1 List of Tissues and Organs to be Examined Histologically in Chronic and Subchronic Toxicity Tests

Adrenals	Larynx	Salivary Gland
Bone and bone marrow	Liver	Sciatic nerve
Brain	Lungs and bronchi	Seminal vesicles
Cartilage	Lymph nodes	Skin
Cecum	Mammary glands	Spinal cord
Colon	Mandibular lymph node	Spleen
Duodenum	Mesenteric lymph node	Stomach
Esophagus	Nasal cavity	Testes
Eyes	Ovaries	Thigh muscle
Gall bladder	Parathyroids	Thymus
Ileum	Pituitary	Urinary bladder
Jejunum	Prostate	Uterus
Kidneys	Rectum	

each week, in chambers specially designed for the purpose. Environmental and biologic parameters are the same as those for other subchronic tests. Particular attention must be given to effects on the tissues of the nasal cavity and the lungs. Particles 4 μ in size are considered to be inhalable; larger particles will be cleared from the respiratory tract by ciliary action and subsequently swallowed (oral exposure) or expelled by sneezing or expectoration.

12.3.9 CHRONIC TESTS

Chronic tests are those conducted over a significant part of the life span of the test animal. The duration of a chronic study is generally 1 year or more. Typically, rats and dogs are the preferred species; for carcinogenicity studies, rats and mice are used.

12.3.10 CHRONIC TOXICITY AND CARCINOGENICITY

Descriptions of tests for both chronic toxicity and carcinogenicity are included here because the design is similar.

Chronic toxicity tests are designed to discover any of numerous toxic effects and to define safety margins to be used in the regulation of chemicals. As with subchronic tests, two species are usually used, one of which is either a rat or a mouse strain, in which case the tests are performed for 2 years or 1.5 to 2.0 years, respectively. Data are gathered after 1 year to determine chronic effects and after 1.5 years (mouse) or 2 years (rat) to determine carcinogenic potential. The nonrodent species, such as the dog, a nonhuman primate, or, rarely, a small carnivore such as the ferret, is used.

Chronic toxicity tests may involve administration in the food, in the drinking water, by capsule, or by inhalation; the first route (in food) is the most common. Gavage is rarely used. The dose used is the maximum tolerated dose (MTD); usually, two lower doses, perhaps 0.25 MTD and 0.125 MTD, are the lowest doses with a predicted no effect level. The MTD has been defined as the highest dose that causes no more than a 10% weight decrement, as compared to the appropriate control groups, and does not produce mortality, clinical signs of toxicity, or pathologic lesions. This dose is determined by extrapolation from subchronic studies. The end points used in these studies are those described for the subchronic study: appearance, ophthalmology, food consumption, body weight, clinical signs, behavioral signs, hematology, blood chemistry, urinalysis, organ weights, and pathology. Some animals may be killed at fixed intervals during the test (eg, 6, 12, or 18 months) for histologic examination. Particular attention is given to any organs or tests that showed compound-related changes in the subchronic tests.

Carcinogenicity tests have many requirements in common (physical facilities, diets, etc.) with both chronic and subchronic toxicity tests as previously described. In this study, the purity of the test chemical is of great concern. A typical test involves 50 or more rats or mice of each gender in each treatment group. Some animals undergo necropsy at intermediate stages of the test (eg, at 12 months), as are all animals found dead or moribund. All surviving animals undergo necropsy at the end of the test. Tissues to be examined are listed in Table 12.1, with particular attention given to abnormal masses and lesions.

12.4 DEVELOPMENT AND REPRODUCTIVE TOXICITY

It is well known that the reproductive system is very complex. Under unfavorable environmental conditions, the tasks of revealing, assessing, and, if possible, predicting the hazards of chemical substances in multicomponent systems with complex exposures on human embryogenesis and the genetic apparatus have assumed extreme importance.

Both the male and female reproductive physiology is under the control of hormones. In males, hypothalamus located in the brain stimulates the anterior pituitary (via the gonadotrophic hormone-releasing hormone) to release gonadotrophic hormones (luteinizing hormone (LH) and follicle-stimulating hormone (FSH)). In addition to LH and FSH, prolactin is released by the anterior pituitary. The target of LH and FSH in the male is the testis. Although LH stimulates steroidogenesis, FSH has its primary effects on the sertoli cells. The role of prolactin (which is inhibited by dopamine) is to modulate the effects of LH in the testicular tissue. Critical points within the hypothalamic-pituitary-gonadal axis may be susceptible to alterations by xenobiotics, leading to altered reproductive function and pathology.

Two major components of the testes are the seminiferous tubules (site of spermatogenesis) and the interstitial compartment. The interstitial compartment contains

Leydig cells, which produce testosterone under the influence of LH. Androgens control spermatogenesis, growth and activity of accessory sex glands, masculinization, male behavior, and various metabolic functions. Secretion of androgen by the developing fetal testes is essential for differentiation of the gonads, which includes regression of Müllerian ducts and the development of Wolffian ducts.

As described previously for the male, the female hormonal signaling is composed of four primary levels: CNS, hypothalamus, anterior pituitary, and gonads. The gonadotropin-releasing hormones of the hypothalamus stimulate the anterior pituitary to release LH and FSH. Subsequently, LH and FSH stimulate the release of estrogen and progesterone from the ovaries. Estrogen is secreted in the growing follicle and has effects on the uterus. The oocytes are formed before birth and then develop into the primary oocytes after meiosis. At the time of puberty, the release of gonadotropin stimulates the oocytes to develop into graffian follicles. Estrus is the period when the female mammal is most receptive to the male (coincides with high levels of circulating estrogen). Rodents are considered to be polyestrous and have a succession of estrus cycles. Cats are seasonally (spring, early fall) polyestrus, and dogs are monoestrus. Humans and higher primates cycle at monthly intervals. Although most mammals ovulate spontaneously, some mammals (cats and minks) undergo provoked or induced ovulation (ie, stimulated by mating). The changes in circulating hormones and the stage of follicle development during an adverse toxicant insult results in a variety of toxicological manifestations.

In general, toxicants may mimic endogenous compounds (ie, hormones), thus acting as agonists or antagonists. They may be directly cytotoxic or activated to toxic compounds. Some toxicants may have indirect effects by inhibiting key enzymes involved in steroid synthesis and can adversely affect the normal functions of the cells/organs of the reproductive system. These agents may induce a variety of outcomes, including prevention of ovulation and impairment of ovum transport, fertilization, or implantation. Endocrine disruptors may mimic endogenous hormones as well as directly destroy cellular components, leading to cell death. The class of toxicants affecting germ cells can alter the structure of genetic material (chromosomal aberrations, alterations in meiosis, DNA synthesis, and replication). Mature oocytes have a DNA repair capacity different from that of mature sperm, but this capacity decreases during the period of meiotic maturation. Therefore, the adverse effects of xenobiotics can lead to a variety of developmental and reproductive abnormalities. This chapter describes in vivo protocols for testing toxicants for their safe use. The subsequent chapter deals with alternative methods (in vitro test methods) for screening toxicants and environmental chemicals.

12.4.1 TESTING PROTOCOLS

After the thalidomide disaster in 1966, formal testing guidelines were established by the US FDA *Guidelines for Reproduction Studies for Safety Evaluation of Drugs for Human Use*. Since 1994, new streamlined testing protocols have been developed with international acceptance. This newer approach, ICH, relies on the investigator to determine the model to access reproductive/developmental toxicity. However, many scientists currently conduct and publish the US FDA version of testing (ie, segment studies). Therefore, the US FDA approach has been discussed.

The aim of developmental and reproductive testing is to examine the potential for a compound to interfere with the ability of an organism to reproduce. This includes testing to assess reproductive risk in mature adults as well as in developing individuals at various stages of life, from conception to sexual maturity. Traditionally animal studies have been conducted in three segments:

Segment (I): During a premating period, the adults are treated and continuation is optional for the female through implantation or lactation
Segment (II): Treatment of pregnant animals during the major period of organogenesis
Segment (III): Treatment of pregnant/lactating animals from the completion of organogenesis through lactation (perinatal and postnatal study)

In adults, these include development of mature egg and sperm, fertilization, implantation, delivery of offspring (parturition), and lactation. In the developing organism, these include early embryonic development, major organ formation, fetal development and growth, and postnatal growth including behavioral assessments and attainment of full reproductive function. These evaluations are usually best performed in several separate studies.

12.4.2 SINGLE- AND MULTIPLE-GENERATION TESTS

Fertility and general reproductive performance can be evaluated in single- and multiple-generation tests. These tests are usually conducted using rats. Fertility is defined as the ability to produce a pregnancy, whereas the ability to produce live offspring is known as fecundity. An abbreviated protocol for a single-generation test is shown in Fig. 12.1. In typical tests, 25 males per dose group are treated for 70 days prior to mating and 25 females per dose group are treated for 14 days before mating. The number of animals is chosen to yield at least 20 pregnant females per dose group including controls. The treatment durations are selected to coincide with critical times during which spermatogenesis and ovulation occur. In the rat, it takes approximately 70 days for spermatogonial cells to become mature sperm capable of fertilization. In the female rat, the estrus cycle length is 4 to 5 days and a 14-day dosing period is considered sufficient time to detect potential effects on hormonal or other systems that may affect ovulation. In some study designs, both males and females are treated for 70 days before mating.

Treatment of the females is continued through pregnancy (21 days) and until the pups are weaned. Pups are usually 21 days of age. The test compound is administered at three dose levels in the feed, in drinking water, or by gavage. The high dose is chosen to cause some, but not excessive, maternal toxicity (eg, an

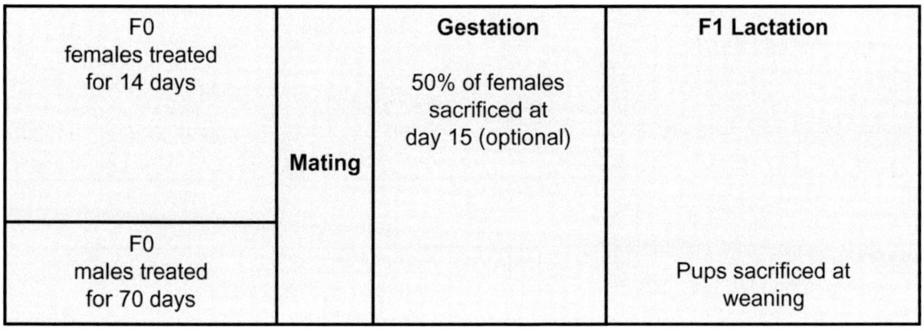

F0 females treated for 14 days	Mating	**Gestation** 50% of females sacrificed at day 15 (optional)	**F1 Lactation**
F0 males treated for 70 days			Pups sacrificed at weaning

FIGURE 12.1

Abbreviated protocol for a one-generation reproductive toxicity test.

approximate 10% decrease in body weight gain or effects on target organs). Low doses are generally expected to be no-effect levels.

After the premating period the rats are placed in cohabitation, with one male and one female caged together. Mating is confirmed by the appearance of spermatozoa in a daily vaginal smear. Day 1 of gestation is the day insemination is confirmed. The females bear and nurse their pups. After birth, the pups are counted, weighed, and examined for external abnormalities. The litters are frequently culled to a constant number (usually 8–10) after 4 days. At weaning, the pups are killed and undergo autopsy for gross and internal abnormalities. In a multigeneration study, approximately 25 per sex per group are saved to produce the next generation. Brother–sister pairings are avoided. Treatment is continuous throughout the test, which can be performed for two or, sometimes, three generations. An abbreviated protocol for a multiple generation test can be seen in Fig. 12.2.

The end points observed in these types of tests are as follows:

1. Fertility index, which is the number of pregnancies relative to the number of matings
2. The number of live births relative to the number of total births
3. Preimplantation loss, or number of corpora lutea in the ovaries relative to the number of implantation sites
4. Postimplantation loss, or the number of resorption sites in the uterus relative to the number of implantation sites
5. Duration of gestation
6. Effects on the male or female reproductive system
7. Litter size and condition, gross morphology of pups at birth, gender, and anogenital distance
8. Survival of pups
9. Weight gain and performance of adults and pups
10. Time of occurrence of developmental landmarks, such as eye opening, tooth eruption, vaginal opening in females, and preputial separation in males
11. Morphological abnormalities in weanlings

F0 Females treated for 70 days	Mating # 1	Gestation	F1A Lactation Pups sacrificed at weaning
F0 Males treated for 70 days	Mating # 2	Gestation	F1B Lactation Pups sacrificed at weaning; enough left for next generation

⇩

F1B Females continued on test	Mating # 1	Gestation	F2A Lactation Pups sacrificed at weaning
F1B Males continued on test	Mating # 2	Gestation	F2B Lactation Pups sacrificed at weaning; enough left for next generation

⇩

F2B Females continued on test	Mating # 1	Gestation	F3A Lactation Pups sacrificed at weaning
F2B Males continued on test	Mating # 2	Gestation	F3B Lactation Pups sacrificed at weaning; complete histology

FIGURE 12.2

Abbreviated protocol for a multigeneration reproductive toxicity test.

Results from single- and multiple-generation tests provide important information for assessment of test materials that may perturb a variety of systems including the endocrine system. A number of weanlings may be left to develop for further studies of behavioral and/or physiological defects (eg, developmental neurotoxicity testing).

12.4.3 TERATOLOGY

Teratology is the study of abnormal fetal development. For an agent to be labeled a teratogen, it must significantly increase the occurrence of adverse structural or functional abnormalities in offspring after its administration to the female during pregnancy or directly to the developing organism. In teratology testing, exposure to the test chemical may be from implantation to parturition, although it has also been restricted to the period of major organogenesis, the most sensitive period for inducing structural malformations. Observations may be extended throughout life, but usually they are made immediately prior to birth after a cesarean delivery. The end points observed are mainly morphologic (structural changes and malformations), although embryo–fetal mortality is also used as an end point. Fig. 12.3 shows an outline of a typical teratology study.

Teratology studies are performed in two species, a rodent species (usually the rat), and in another species, such as the rabbit (rarely in the dog or primate). Enough

Teratology		
Untreated females	Mating	Gestation
Untreated males		Pregnant females treated on days 6–15. Pups and dams sacrificed on day 20

Perinatal/postnatal			
Untreated females	Mating	Gestation	Lactation
Untreated males		Pregnant females treated on days 15–21	Females treated until weaning; pups and dams sacrificed at weaning

FIGURE 12.3

Abbreviated protocol for a teratology test and for a perinatal/postnatal toxicity test in rats.

females should be used so that, given normal fertility for the strain, there are 20 pregnant females in each dosage group. Traditionally, the timing of compound administration has been such that the dam is exposed during the period of major organogenesis, which comprises days 6 through 15 of gestation in the rat or mouse and days 6 through 18 for the rabbit. Newer study designs call for dosing until cesarean delivery. Day 1 is the day that spermatozoa appear in the vagina in the case of rats, or the day of mating in the rabbit. The test chemical is typically administered directly into the stomach by gavage, which is a requirement of the US Environmental Protection Agency (EPA) and some other regulatory agencies. This method of dosing allows a precise calculation of the amount of test material received by the animal. Studies typically have three dose levels and a control group that receives the vehicle used for test material delivery. The high dose level is chosen to be one at which some maternal toxicity is known to occur, but never one that would cause more than 10% mortality. The low dose should be one at which no maternal toxicity is apparent, and the intermediate dose(s) should be chosen as a predicted low effect level. The test is terminated by performing a cesarean delivery on the day before normal delivery is expected. The uterus is examined for implantation and resorption sites, and for live and dead fetuses, and the ovaries are examined for corpora lutea. In rodent studies, half of the fetuses are examined for soft tissue malformations and the remaining are examined for skeletal malformations. In nonrodents, all fetuses are examined for both soft tissue and skeletal malformations. The various end points that may be examined include:

1. maternal toxicity
2. embryo–fetal toxicity
3. external malformations
4. soft tissue and skeletal malformations

Careful evaluations of maternal toxicity and evaluation of parameters such as body weight, food consumption, clinical signs, and necropsy data such as organ weights are performed. Because exposure starts after implantation, conception and implantation rates should be the same in controls and at all treatment levels. Embryo–fetal toxicity is determined from the number of dead fetuses and resorption sites relative to the number of implantation sites. In addition to the possibility of lethal malformations, such toxicity can be due to maternal toxicity, stress, or direct toxicity to the embryo or fetus that is not related to developmental malformations. Fetal weight and fetal size may also be a measure of toxicity, but they should not be confused with the variations seen as a result of differences in the number of pups per litter. Smaller litters tend to have larger pups, and larger litters have smaller pups. Anomalies may be regarded as variations (that may not adversely affect the fetus, may not have a fetal outcome, or may be regarded as malformations) or as adverse effects on the fetus. For some findings there is disagreement regarding which class it belongs, such as the number of ribs in the rabbit that inherently have a large amount of variability. Common external anomalies are listed in Table 12.2 and are determined by examination of fetuses at cesarean delivery. Visceral anomalies are determined by examination of fetuses after fixation using either the dissection method of Staples or the hand-sectioning method of Wilson. Common visceral findings are listed in Table 12.3. Fetal skeletons are examined after first fixing the fetus and then staining the bone with Alizarin red.

Numerous skeletal variations occur in controls and may not have an adverse effect on the fetus (Table 12.4). Their frequency of occurrence may, however, be dose-related and should be evaluated. Almost all chemically induced malformations have been observed in control animals, and most malformations are known to be produced by more than one cause. Thus, it is obvious that great care is necessary in the interpretation of teratology studies. For an agent to be classified as a development toxicant or teratogen, it must produce adverse effects on the conceptus at exposure levels that do not induce toxicity in the mother. Signs of maternal toxicity include reduction in weight gain, changes in eating patterns, hypoactivity or hyperactivity, neurotoxic signs, and organ weight changes. Adverse effects on development under these conditions may be secondary to stress on the maternal system. Findings in the fetus at dose levels that produce maternal toxicity cannot be easily separated from the maternal toxicity. Compounds can be deliberately administered at maternally toxic dose levels to determine the threshold for adverse effects on the offspring. In such cases, conclusions can be qualified to indicate that adverse effects on the offspring were found at maternally toxic dose levels and may not be indicative of selective or unique developmental toxicity.

12.4.4 PERINATAL AND POSTNATAL EFFECTS

These tests are usually performed on rats, and 20 pregnant females per dosage group are treated during the final third of gestation and through lactation to

Table 12.2 External Malformations Commonly Seen in Teratogenicity Tests

Brain, cranium, and spinal cord	Encephalocele: protrusion of the brain through an opening of the skull; cerebrum is well-formed and covered by transparent connective tissue
	Exencephaly: lack of skull with disorganized outward growth of the brain
	Microcephaly: small head on normal size body
	Hydrocephaly: marked enlargement of the ventricles of the cerebrum
	Craniorachischisis: exposed brain and spinal cord
	Spina bifida: nonfusion of spinal processes; usually, the ectoderm covering is missing and the spinal cord is evident
Nose	Enlarged naris: enlarged nasal cavities
	Single naris: a single naris, usually median
Eye	Microphthalmia: small eye
	Anophthalmia: *lack* of eye
	Open eye: no apparent eyelid, eye is open
Ear	Anotia: absence of the external ear; Microtia: small ear
Jaw	Micrognathia: small lower jaw
	Agnathia: absence of lower jaw
	Aglossia: absence of tongue
	Astomia: lack of mouth opening
	Bifid tongue: forked tongue
	Cleft lip: either unilateral or bilateral cleft of upper lip
Palate	Cleft palate: a cleft or separation of the median portion of the palate
Limbs	Clubfoot: foot that has grown in a twisted manner, resulting in an abnormal shape or position; it is possible to have a malposition of the whole limb
	Micromelia: abnormal shortness of the limb
	Hemimelia: absence of any of the long bones, resulting in a shortened limb
	Phomelia: absence of all of the long bones of a limb; the limb is attached directly to the body

weaning (day 15 of pregnancy through day 21 postpartum). The duration of gestation, parturition problems, and the number and size of pups in the naturally delivered litter are observed. Behavioral testing of the pups has been suggested.

12.5 SPECIAL TESTS

In certain cases, some tests may be useful in current testing protocols. The following tests may be useful.

Table 12.3 Some Common Visceral Anomalies Seen in Teratogenicity Tests

Intestines	Umbilical hernia: protrusion of the intestines into the umbilical cord
	Ectopic intestines: extrusion of the intestines outside the body wall
Heart	Dextrocardia: rotation of the heart axis to the right
	Enlarged heart: either the atrium or the ventricle may be enlarged
Lung	Enlarged lung: all lobes are usually enlarged
	Small lung: all lobes are usually small; lung may appear immature
Uterus/ testes	Undescended testes: testes are located anterior to the bladder instead of lateral; may be bilateral or unilateral
	Agenesis of testes: one or both testes may be missing
	Agenesis of uterus: one or both horns of the uterus may be missing
Kidney	Hydronephrosis: fluid-filled kidney, often grossly enlarged; may be accompanied by a hydroureter (enlarged, fluid-filled ureter)
	Fused: kidneys fused, appearing as one misshapen kidney with two ureters
	Agenesis: one or both kidneys missing
	Misshapen: small, enlarged (usually internally), or odd-shaped kidneys

Table 12.4 Skeletal Abnormalities Commonly Seen in Teratogenicity Tests

Digits	Polydactyly: presence of extra digits; in mouse, six or more instead of five
	Syndactyly: fusion of two or more digits
	Oligodactyly: absence of one or more digits
	Brachydactyly: smallness of one or more digits
Ribs	Wavy: ribs may be any aberrant shape
	Extra: may have extra ribs on either side
	Fused: may be fused anywhere along the length of the rib
	Branched: single base and branched
Tail	Short: short tail, usually lack of vertebrae
	Missing: absence of tail
	Corkscrew: corkscrew-shape tail

12.5.1 NEUROTOXICITY

1. Behavioral and pharmacological tests
2. Acute and subchronic neurotoxicity tests
3. Developmental neurotoxicity tests
4. Delayed neuropathy (OPIDN)

The delayed neurotoxic potential of certain organophosphates, such as tri-o-cresyl phosphate (TOCP) or other OP compounds, is usually tested in the mature hen because the clinical signs are similar to those in humans, and such symptoms cannot be readily elicited in the common laboratory rodents.

12.5.2 POTENTIATION AND SYNERGISM

Potentiation and synergism represent interactions between toxicants that are potential sources of hazard because neither humans nor other species are usually exposed to one chemical at a time. Such tests can be conducted by comparing the LD_{50} or any other appropriate toxic end point. In the case of synergism, in which one of the compounds is relatively nontoxic when given alone, the toxicity of the toxic compound can be measured when administered alone or after a relatively large dose of the nontoxic compound.

12.5.3 TOXICOKINETICS AND METABOLISM

Knowledge of toxicokinetics and metabolism can provide valuable insights. Toxicokinetics studies are designed to measure the amount and rate of the absorption, distribution, metabolism, and excretion of a xenobiotic.

12.5.4 COVALENT BINDING

Toxicity has been associated with covalent binding in a number of ways. Organ-specific toxicants administered in vivo bind covalently to macromolecules, usually at a higher level in the target tissues than in nontarget tissues. Therefore, such tests could be useful for predicting the toxic potential of the chemical.

12.5.5 IMMUNOTOXICITY

Immunotoxicology comprises two distinct types of toxic effects. The first one is the involvement of the immune system in mediating the toxic effect of a chemical, for example, in tests for cutaneous sensitization. The second is the toxic effects of chemicals on the immune system, for example, impairment of the ability to resist infection.

Tests for immunotoxicity are not required by all regulatory agencies, except for biological active agents (see chapters: Preclinical Toxicological Investigations of Pharmaceutical Products and Preclinical Safety Evaluation of Biotechnology-Derived Products). It is an area of great interest, both in the fundamental mechanisms of immune function and in the design of tests to measure impairment of immune function.

12.6 IN VITRO AND OTHER SHORT-TERM TESTS

Toxicity tests are conducted largely in vitro with isolated cell systems. Some are short-term tests performed in vivo, and some are combinations of in vivo and in vitro systems. Their relevance in toxicity testing is discussed in the following chapter.

12.7 ECOLOGICAL EFFECTS

Tests for ecological effects include those designed to address the potential of chemicals to affect ecosystems and the population dynamics in the environment. The tests are conducted to estimate effects on field populations of vertebrates, invertebrates, and plants. The use of environmental risk assessment tests is beyond the scope of this book.

Laboratory tests There are two types of laboratory tests: toxicity determinations for wildlife and aquatic organisms and the use of model ecosystems to measure bioaccumulation and transport of toxicants and their degradation products. Among the tests included in the first category are the avian oral LD_{50}, the avian dietary LC_{50}, wild mammal toxicity, and avian reproduction.

Simulated field tests Simulated field tests consist of feeding treated prey to predators and studying the toxic effects on the predator, enabling some predictions concerning effects to nontarget organisms.

Field tests In field test situations, the effects of test chemicals are studied on the agro-ecosystem.

12.8 RISK ANALYSIS

The preceding tests for various kinds of toxicity can be used to measure adverse effects of many different chemical compounds in different species, organ, tissues, cells, or even populations, and under many different conditions.

Risk analysis involves political and legal aspects and, in toto, represents society's evaluation of the amount of risk that can be tolerated in any particular case. This aspect of risk assessment is dealt with in greater depth in Chapter 6, Hazard and Risk Assessment.

CHAPTER

Genotoxicity

13

CHAPTER OUTLINE

13.1 INTRODUCTION

Genetic toxicology is the study of the effects of chemical and physical agents on genetic material. It includes the study of deoxyribonucleic acid (DNA) damage in living cells that leads to cancer, and it also examines changes in DNA that can be inherited from one generation to the next. Thus, genetic toxicology can be defined as a branch of the field of toxicology that assesses the effects of chemical and physical agents on the hereditary material (DNA) and on the genetic processes of living cells. As such, it is important at the outset to distinguish between genotoxicity and mutagenicity. Genotoxicity covers a broader spectrum of endpoints than mutagenicity. For example, unscheduled DNA synthesis, sister chromatid exchanges, and DNA strand breaks are measures of genotoxicity, not mutagenicity, because they, themselves, are not transmissible from cell to cell or generation to generation. Mutagenicity, however, refers to the production of transmissible genetic alterations.

Fundamentals of Toxicology. DOI: http://dx.doi.org/10.1016/B978-0-12-805426-0.00013-5

13.2 HISTORICAL BACKGROUND

The origins of genetic toxicology testing started in 1900 after the rediscovery of Mandel's classic paper on the basis of inheritance. In 1901, for the first time, the term "mutation" was used to signify changes in hereditary material. The origin of genetic toxicology as an independent branch of science started in 1927, when American geneticist Hermann J. Muller (1890–1967) demonstrated that X-rays increased the rate of gene mutations and chromosome changes in fruit flies and suggested that mutations can cause cancer. The relevance of genetic toxicology is clearly evident from inheritable diseases such as phenylketonuria (an inability to metabolize phenylalanine), cystic fibrosis (lung disease), sickle cell anemia, and Tay-Sachs disease. Recent advances in molecular biology and genomic sciences have led to a greater understanding of the genetic cause of disease and paved the way to treatments. However, following World War II, it became evident that many chemical products beneficial to industrialized society might adversely affect human health and the environment. In 1971, Malling demonstrated that a mammalian liver homogenate could be added to the in vitro system to mimic in vivo metabolism. The use of these tests to predict carcinogenicity gained momentum in the mid 1970s, when McCann, Ames, and his associates published results suggesting that most carcinogens were mutagens in *Salmonella*. Recent molecular biology advances have led to an expanded awareness of the importance of genotype in susceptibility to cancer, and they promise to yield more reasoned and informed assessments of risk to present and future generations. During this period, it began as a basic research field with demonstrations that ionizing radiations and chemicals could induce mutations and chromosome alterations in plant, insect, and mammalian cells, which prompted many regulatory agencies to realize that pharmaceutical products and other chemicals must be tested before they are administered to humans or used in industry.

It was also realized that long-term animal testing resources are insufficient for evaluating the universe of chemicals to which humans and the environment may be exposed. Thus, genetic toxicology tests that assess specific mechanisms observed in the whole animal (including human) are used as initial tests for regulatory submissions because these tests have been shown to be useful in predicting the outcome of long-term animal tests.

13.3 GERM CELL MUTATION

These mutations are mainly inherited from previous generations and are expressed when an individual inherits the mutant gene from both parents. New mutations make a larger contribution to the incidence of dominant diseases than to that of recessive diseases because only a single dominant mutation is required for expression. Because genetic mechanisms are well understood, it is possible to evaluate compounds for potential genotoxic effects that are associated with mechanistically with heritable mutation (transmissible germ cell mutation). The potential consequences of somatic and germinal mutations are summarized in Fig. 13.1.

Heritable germ cell mutations and cancer are the major concerns when there is exposure to any genotoxic agent, and they provide the rationale for conducting assays to detect potential genotoxicity activity. In addition to being potential germ cell mutagens or carcinogens, there is evidence that the mutagenic events may play an important role in the cause and/or progression of human diseases other than cancer. It is now known that if a compound is genotoxic, then there is a reasonable probability that it will be a carcinogen. Types of genetic damage and methods for their detection are provided in Fig. 13.2.

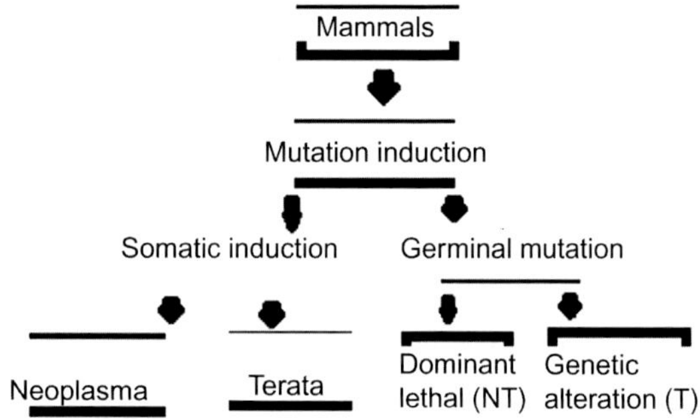

FIGURE 13.1

Potential consequences of somatic and germinal mutation. *NT*, nontransmissible; *T*, transmissible.

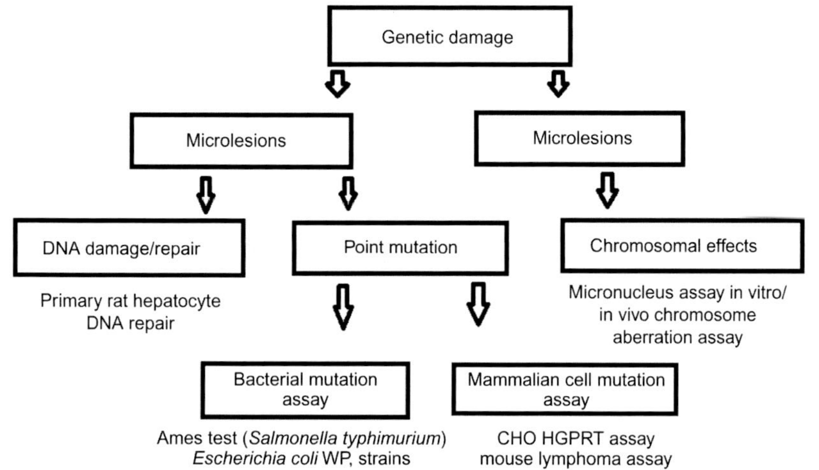

FIGURE 13.2

Types of genetic damage and methods for their detection.

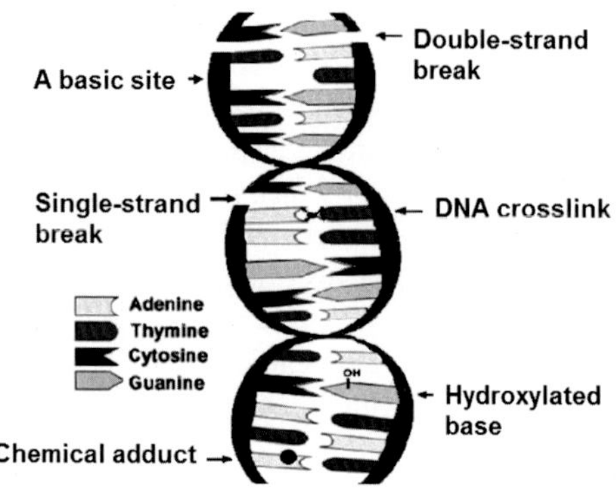

FIGURE 13.3

Schematic diagram showing common forms of DNA damage.

Genetic damage can be broadly classified as either microlesions or macrolesions (Fig. 13.3). Microlesions (not visible microscopically) are detected by measuring a cell's response to DNA damage (ie, DNA repair) or by measuring a subsequent change in the phenotype of the cell (ie, point mutation assay). Macrolesions are detected in cytogenetic assays as microscopically visible alterations in chromosomal structure/number (ie, in vitro/in vivo cytogenetics or chromosome aberration assays) or as micronuclei remaining in erythrocytes following expulsion of the nucleus (micronucleus assay).

13.4 DNA MUTATIONS

To understand cancer, it is necessary to know the cellular changes that turn a normal cell into a malignant cell that repeatedly and uncontrollably divides. This transformation occurs when there is genetic damage or an alteration in the structure of a cell's DNA, the coding machinery of life. The DNA is a double helix made of the compounds adenine (A), guanine (G), thymine (T), and cytosine (C). These chemicals are bound in long stretches as AT and CG pairs and wrapped in sugar molecules that hold them together (Fig. 13.3). Long stretches of these AT and CG combinations form genes that, when "read," produce the proteins that drive our cells. Ideally, the DNA sequence would not change except in the recombining that occurs during reproduction. However, DNA damage occurs regularly as part of the cell process and from interaction with both normal cellular chemicals and with toxic chemicals. A very robust repair mechanism rapidly and very accurately repairs the DNA damage, but if for some reason the DNA is repaired incorrectly, then a mutation occurs. The mutation is a subtle or not so subtle change in the A, G, C, or T that comprise the DNA. Many of the mutations have no effect, some have minor effects, and a small number have life-threatening effects. If a mutation occurs in the wrong place, then a cell can start to divide uncontrollably, becoming a malignant cell and causing cancer. If a mutation occurs in our germ line cells, then the mutation can be passed to our offspring. The common forms of DNA damage are summarized in Fig. 13.3.

13.5 MUTAGENS ARE CARCINOGENS

Chemicals that induce mutations in the DNA are called mutagens; when these changes lead to cancer, the chemical is called a carcinogen. Not all mutagens are carcinogens, and not all carcinogens are mutagens. In 1946, it was shown that nitrogen mustards (derived from mustard gas first used by the military in 1917 during WWI) could induce mutations in the fruit fly and reduce tumor growth in mice. Genetic toxicology developed ways to test chemical and physical agents for their mutagenic potential. In the 1970s, Bruce Ames and others developed a cellular-based test for genetic mutations. This test became known as the Ames assay. Sophisticated variations of these tests are now required by many government regulatory agencies to test chemicals for mutagenicity. Often, it is a metabolite (breakdown product) of the compound that causes cancer, not the original compound. Ideally, a foreign chemical is made less toxic when metabolized, but sometimes a chemical can be made more toxic. This more toxic chemical can then interact with cellular DNA or proteins and produce malignant cells. This process is called bioactivation. It is also possible for a chemical to encourage bioactivation or to accelerate the development of a cancer. Efforts to understand the underlying biology of cancer are ongoing. The genomic sciences are helping to explain why some people are more susceptible to cancer than others.

13.6 IMPACT ON HUMAN HEALTH

The alterations in mutations and chromosomes are important for their roles in genetic disorders, including birth defects and cancer. Therefore, mutations in both germ cells and somatic cells need to be considered when an overall risk resulting from mutations is concerned. More than 5000 diseases in humans are now known that are due to defective genes. These inherited disorders cause 20% of all infant mortalities, half of all miscarriages, and 80% of all cases of mental retardation. Until now, more than 100 different cancer genes have been identified. Therefore, mutations in both germ cells and somatic cells need to be considered when an overall risk resulting from mutations is concerned.

13.7 DNA DAMAGE AND MECHANISM

The types of DNA damage produced by radiation and chemicals are many and varied, including single-strand and double-strand breaks in the DNA backbone, crosslinks between DNA bases or between DNA bases and proteins, and chemical addition to the DNA bases. For example, ionizing radiations such as X-rays, gamma rays, and alpha particles produce DNA single-strand and double-strand breaks and a broad range of base damages. Chemicals can produce DNA alterations either directly (DNA-reactive) as adducts or indirectly by intercalation of a chemical between the base pairs (eg, 9-aminoacridine). Endogenous agents are responsible for several hundred DNA damages per cell per day (eg, 8-oxoguanine and thymine glycol). The cellular processes that can lead to DNA damage are oxygen consumption that results in the formation of reactive oxygen species (eg, superoxide $\dot{O}_2$, hydroxyl free radicals •OH, and hydrogen peroxide) and deamination of cytosines and 5-methylcytosines, leading to uracils and thymines, respectively. The spectrum of DNA damage induced by physical and chemical agents is summarized in Fig. 13.4.

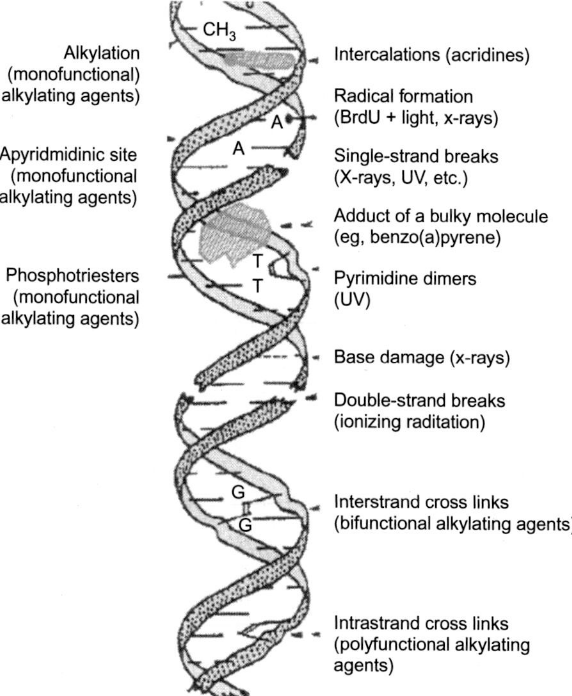

FIGURE 13.4

Schematic representation of DNA damage caused by different toxicants. Single-strand, double-strand, interstrand, intrastrand, and other kinds of damage are shown.

13.8 REGULATORY REQUIREMENTS/GUIDELINES

Until recently, the selection of specific protocols for regulatory submissions varied differently in different geographical regions. Extensive international efforts have been directed toward defining protocols for the genetic toxicology tests that have been used for chemical registration. An agreement has been reached indicating that the results obtained with a Organization for European Cooperation and Development (OECD)-defined protocol in one country will be accepted internationally. Thus, testing for the registration of chemicals and pharmaceuticals or other products will be conducted according to the OECD/SIDS (Screening Information Data Set) guidelines. Subsequently, harmonization of regulatory requirements has been considered necessary to facilitate more efficient and economical testing strategies for companies that market their products worldwide. To address this need, harmonized testing guidelines for testing of chemicals/pharmaceuticals by the US Environmental Protection Agency (EPA), for chemicals tested under the Toxic Substances Control Act (TSCA), and for pharmaceuticals have now been published by the OECD by the International Council for Harmonization (ICH). The harmonized testing approaches for regulatory submissions consist of tests for gene and chromosomal mutations.

Genotoxicity tests conducted in vitro and in vivo are designed to test any genetic damage caused directly or indirectly. Any damage to DNA in the form of gene mutation, large-scale chromosomal damage, and recombinant and numerical chromosome changes is considered essential for heritable effects and in the multistep process of malignancy. Compounds that cause such changes have the potential to cause cancer in humans.

At present, there are more than 200 assays for mutagens available, and useful information has been obtained from many of them. However, there are regulatory authorities for registration of pharmaceuticals and other chemicals, and a standard three-test genotoxicity battery has been recommended. The types of tests include: (1) in vitro bacterial reverse mutation test; (2) nonbacterial in vitro test (mammalian cell mutation or chromosomal aberration); and (3) in vivo test chromosomal aberration or micronucleus test. These harmonized testing guidelines for regulatory submissions are summarized in Table 13.1. However, a few assays for detection of genotoxicty used more commonly are provided.

13.9 ASSAYS FOR DETECTION OF GENETIC ALTERATIONS

The purpose of using in vitro and in vivo short-term testing is to provide an early warning of carcinogenic potential without the delay involved in conducting lifetime chronic feeding studies in experimental animals. Despite the numerous tests that have been devised, regulatory agencies have not yet determined that it is necessary to substitute any of them, or any combination of them, for chronic feeding studies. Genetic toxicology assays serve two inter-related but distinct purposes in

Table 13.1 Harmonized Testing Guidelines for Regulatory Submissions

	Type of Test		OECD/SIDS	TSCA	ICH
1	In vitro test				
		Bacterial reverse mutation test	Yes	Yes	Yes
2	Nonbacterial in vitro test				
		Mammalian cell mutation	Yes	Yes	Yes[a]
	OR				
		Chromosomal aberration	Yes		Yes
3	In vivo test (chromosomal effects)				
		Chromosomal aberration	Yes	Yes	Yes
	OR				
		Micronucleus	Yes	Yes	Yes

OECD, *Organization for European Cooperation and Development;* SIDS, *Screening Information Data Set;* TSCA, *Toxic Substances Control Act;* ICH, *International Council for Harmonization.*
[a]*Only the L5178Y mouse lymphoma gene and chromosomal mutation assay are recommended in the ICH guidelines.*

the toxicologic evaluation of chemicals: (1) identifying mutagens for purposes of hazard identification and (2) characterizing dose–response relationships and mutagenic mechanisms, both of which contribute to an understanding of genetic and carcinogenic risks.

13.9.1 PROKARYOTE MUTAGENICITY

Ames Test: The Ames test, developed by Bruce Ames and his coworkers at the University of California, Berkeley, depends on the ability of mutagenic chemicals to bring about reverse mutations in *Salmonella typhimurium* strains that have defects in the histidine biosynthesis pathway. These strains will not grow in the absence of histidine, but they can be caused to mutate back to the wild type, which can synthesize histidine and, hence, grow in its absence. In brief, the test is performed by mixing a suspension of bacterial cells with molten top agar.

In brief, this test contains cofactors, S-9 fraction, and the material to be tested. The mixture is poured onto Petri plates containing hardened minimal agar. The number of bacteria that revert and acquire the wild-type ability to grow in the absence of histidine can be estimated by counting the colonies that develop on incubation. To perform a valid test, a number of concentrations are tested and positive controls with known mutagens are included along with negative controls that lack only the test compound. The entire test is replicated often enough to satisfy appropriate statistical tests for significance. Parallel tests without the S-9 fraction may help distinguish between chemicals with intrinsic mutagenic potential and those that require metabolic activation. In this test, a small proportion of false-positive and false-negative results occurs. For example, certain base analogs and inorganics such as manganese are not carcinogens, but they are mutagens in the Ames test, whereas diethylstilbestrol (DES) is a carcinogen but not a bacterial mutagen.

Related tests include tests based on reverse mutations, as in the Ames test, as well as tests based on forward mutations. Examples include:

1. *Reverse mutations in Escherichia coli*: This test is similar to the Ames test and depends on reversion of tryptophane mutants, which cannot synthesize this amino acid, to the wild type. The S-9 fraction from the liver of induced rats can also be used as an activating system in this test. Other *E. coli* reverse mutation tests utilize nicotinic acid and arginine mutants.
2. *Forward mutations in S. typhimurium*: One such assay, dependent on the appearance of a mutation conferring resistance to 8-azaguanine in a histidine revertant strain, has been developed and is said to be as sensitive as the reverse mutation tests.
3. *Forward mutations in E. coli*: These mutations depend on mutation of galactose nonfermenting *E. coli* to galactose fermenting *E. coli* or the change from 5-methyltryptophane to 5-methyltryptophane resistance.
4. *DNA repair*: Polymerase-deficient, and thus DNA repair–deficient, *E. coli* has provided the basis for a test that depends on the fact that the growth of a deficient strain is inhibited more by a DNA-damaging agent than is that of a repair competent strain. The recombinant assay using *Bacillus subtilis* is conducted in much the same way because recombinant deficient strains are more sensitive to DNA-damaging agents.

13.9.2 EUKARYOTE MUTAGENICITY

Mammalian Cell Mutation: Primary cells, which generally resemble those of the tissue of origin, are difficult to culture and have poor cloning ability. Because of these difficulties, certain established cell lines are usually used. These cells, such as Chinese hamster ovary cells and mouse lymphoma cells, clone readily and do not become senescent with passage through many cell generations. Unfortunately, they have little metabolic activity toward xenobiotics and therefore do not readily activate toxicants. Moreover, they usually show chromosome changes, such as aneuploidy (ie, more or fewer than the usual diploid number of chromosomes). The characteristics usually involved in these assays are resistance to 8-azaguanine or 6-thioguanine (the hypoxanthine guanine phosphoribosyl transferase or HGPRT locus), resistance to bromodeoxyuridine or triflurothymidine (the thymidine kinase or TK locus), or resistance to ouabain (the OU or Na/K-ATPase locus). A typical test system is the analysis of the TK locus in mouse lymphoma cells for mutations that confer resistance to bromodeoxyuracil. The tests are conducted with and without the S-9 fraction from induced rat liver because the lymphoma cells have little activating ability. Both positive and negative controls are included, and the parameter measured is the number of cells formed that are capable of forming colonies in the presence of bromodeoxyuridine.

Drosophila Sex-Linked Recessive Lethal Test: The advantages of *Drosophila* (fruit fly) tests are that they involve an intact eukaryotic organism with all of its interrelated organ systems and activation mechanisms; however, at the same time, they are fast, relatively easy to perform, and do not involve mammals as test animals. The most obvious disadvantages are that the hormonal and immune systems of insects are significantly different from those of mammals and that the nature, specificity, and inducibility of the cytochrome P450s are not as well understood in insects because they are in mammals. In a typical test, males that are 2 days postpuparium and that were raised from eggs laid within a short time period (usually 24 h) are treated with the test compound in water to which sucrose has been added to increase palatability. Males from a strain carrying a gene for yellow body on the X chromosome are used. Preliminary tests determine that the number of offspring of the survivors of the treatment doses (usually 0.25 LD_{50} and 0.5 LD_{50}) are adequate for future crosses. Appropriate controls, including a solvent control (with emulsifier if one was necessary to prepare the test solution) and a positive control, such as ethyl methane sulfonate, are routinely included with each test. Individual crosses of each surviving treated male with a series of three females are made on a 0- to 2-day, 3- to 5-day, and 6- to 8-day schedule. The progeny of each female is reared separately, and the males and females of the F1 generation are mated in brother–sister matings. If there are no males with yellow bodies in a particular set of progeny, it should be assumed that a lethal mutation was present on the treated X chromosomes. A comparison of the F2 progeny derived from females inseminated by males at different times after treatment allows a distinction to be made between effects on spermatozoa, spermatids, and spermatocytes. In the Basc (Muller-5) test, the strain used for the females in the F1 cross is a multiple-marked strain that carries a dominant gene for bar eyes and a recessive genes for apricot eyes and a reduction of bristles on the thorax (scute gene) (Basc is an acronym for bar, apricot, and scute).

Related Tests: Many other tests related to the two types of eukaryote mutation tests with some variations are also used. Two distinct classes are worthy of mention. The first uses yeasts as the test organisms, and the second is the spot test for mutations in mice. One group of yeast tests includes tests for gene mutations and strains that can be used to detect forward mutations in genes that code for enzymes in the purine biosynthetic pathway; other strains can be used to detect reversions. Yeasts can also be used to test for recombinant events such as reciprocal mitotic recombination (mitotic crossing-over) and nonreciprocal mitotic recombination. *Saccharomyces cerevisiae* is the preferred organism in almost all of these tests.

13.9.3 DNA DAMAGE AND REPAIR

Many of these tests, such as those for gene mutation, chromosome damage, and oncogenicity, are developed as a consequence of damage to or chemical modification of DNA. Most of these tests, however, also involve metabolic events that occur both prior to and subsequent to the modification of DNA. Some tests, however, use events at the DNA level as end points. One of these, the unscheduled synthesis of DNA in mammalian cells, is described in some detail; the others are summarized briefly.

Unscheduled DNA Synthesis in Mammalian Cells: The principle of this test is that it measures the repair that follows DNA damage and is thus a reflection of the damage itself. It depends on the autoradiographic measurement of the incorporation of tritiated thymidine into the nuclei of cells previously treated with the test chemical. The preferred cells are usually primary hepatocytes in cultures derived from adult male rats whose cells are dispersed and allowed to attach themselves to glass coverslips.

The cells are fixed and dried, and the coverslip with the cells attached is coated with photographic emulsion. After a suitable exposure period (usually several weeks), the emulsion is developed and the cells are stained with hemotoxylin and eosin. The number of grains in the nuclear region is corrected by subtracting non-nuclear grains, and the net grain count in the nuclear area is compared between treated and untreated cells.

This test has several advantages in that primary liver cells have considerable activation capacity and the test measures an event at the DNA level. It does not, however, distinguish between error-free repair and error-prone repair; the latter itself is a mutagenic process. Thus, it cannot distinguish between events that might lead to toxic sequelae and those that do not. A modification of this test measures in vivo unscheduled DNA synthesis. In this modification, animals are first treated in vivo, and primary hepatocytes are then prepared and treated as already described.

Related Tests: For assessing DNA damage, the DNA strand length is estimated by using alkaline elution or sucrose density gradient centrifugation. This has been performed with a number of cell lines and with freshly prepared hepatocytes, in the latter case following either in vivo or in vitro treatment. It may be regarded as promising but not yet fully validated. The polymerase-deficient *E. coli* tests as well as recombinant tests using yeasts are also related to DNA repair.

13.9.4 CHROMOSOME ABERRATIONS

Tests for chromosome aberrations involve the estimation of effects on extended regions of whole chromosomes rather than on single or small numbers of genes. Primarily, they concern chromosome breaks and the exchange of material between chromosomes.

Sister Chromatid Exchange (SCE): SCE occurs between the sister chromatids that together comprise a chromosome. It occurs at the same locus in each chromatid and is thus a symmetrical exchange of chromosome material. In this regard, it is not strictly an aberration because the products do not differ in morphology from normal chromosome. SCE, however, is susceptible to chemical induction and appears to be correlated with the genotoxic potential of chemicals as well as with their oncogenic potential. The exchange is visualized by permitting the treated cells to pass through two DNA replication cycles in the presence of 5-bromo-2-deoxyuridine, which is incorporated in the replicated DNA. The cells are then stained with a fluorescent dye and irradiated with UV light, which permits differentiation between chromatids that contain bromodeoxyuridine and those that do not. The test can be performed on cultured cells or on cells from animals treated in vivo. In the former case, the test chemical is usually evaluated in the presence and absence of the S-9 activation system from rat liver. Typically, cells from a Chinese hamster ovary cell line are incubated in a liquid medium and exposed to several concentrations of the test chemical, either with or without the S-9 fraction, for approximately 2 h. Positive controls, such as ethyl methane sulfonate (a direct-acting compound) or dimethylnitrosamine (one that requires activation), as well as negative controls are also included. Test concentrations are based on cell toxicity levels determined by prior experiments and are selected in such a way that even at the highest dose excess growth does not occur. At the end of the treatment period the cells are washed, bromodeoxyuridine is added, and the cells are incubated for 24 h or more. The cells are then fixed, stained with a fluorescent dye, and irradiated with UV light. Second division cells are scored under the microscope for SCEs. The test can also be performed on cells treated in vivo, and analyses have been performed using SCEs in lymphocytes from cancer patients treated with chemotherapeutic drugs, smokers, and workers exposed occupationally. In several cases, an increased incidence of SCEs has been noted. This is a sensitive test for compounds that alkylate DNA, with few false-positive results. It may be useful for detecting promoters such as phorbol esters.

Micronucleus Test: The micronucleus test is an in vivo test usually performed in mice. The animals are treated in vivo, and the erythrocyte stem cells from the bone marrow are stained and examined for micronuclei. Micronuclei represent chromosome fragments or chromosomes left behind at anaphase. It is basically a test for compounds that cause chromosome breaks (clastogenic agents) and compounds that interfere with normal mitotic cell division, including compounds that affect spindle fiber function. Male and female mice from an outbred strain are handled by the best animal husbandry techniques, as described for acute, subchronic, and chronic tests, and are either with the solvent, 0.5 LD_{50}, or 0.1 LD_{50} of the test chemical. Animals are killed at several time intervals up to 2 days; the bone marrow is extracted, placed on microscope slides, dried, and stained. The presence of micronuclei is scored visually under the microscope.

Dominant Lethal Test in Rodents: The dominant lethal test, which is performed using rats, mice, or hamsters, is an in vivo test to determine the germ cell risk from a suspected mutagen. The test consists of treating males with the test compound for several days, followed by mating to different females each week for enough weeks to cover the period required for a complete spermatogenic cycle. Animals are maintained under optimal conditions of animal husbandry and are dosed, usually by a gavage, with several doses of less than 0.1 LD_{50}. The females are killed after 2 weeks of gestation and dissected; corpora lutea and living and dead implantations are counted. The end points used to determine the occurrence of dominant lethal mutations in the treated males are the fertility index (ratio of pregnant females to mated females), preimplantation losses (the number of implantations relative to the number of corpora lutea), the number of females with dead implantations relative to the total number of pregnant females, and the number of dead implantations relative to the total number of implantations. Mutations in sperm that are dominant and lethal do not result in viable offspring.

Related Tests: Many cells exposed to test chemicals can be scored for chromosome aberrations by staining procedures followed by visual examination with the aid of a microscope. These include Chinese hamster ovary cells in culture treated in a protocol very similar to that used in the test for SCEs, bone marrow cells from animals treated in vivo, or lymphocytes from animals treated in vivo. The types of aberrations evaluated include chromatid gaps, breaks, and deletions; chromosome gaps, breaks, and deletions; chromosome fragments; translocations; and ploidy. Heritable translocations can be detected by direct examination of cells from male or female offspring in various stages of development or by crossing the treated animals to untreated animals and evaluating fertility, with males with reduced fertility being examined for translocations, and so on. Progeny from this or other tests, such as those for dominant lethals, can be permitted to survive and then examined for translocations and other abnormalities.

13.9.5 MAMMALIAN CELL TRANSFORMATION

Most cell transformation assays utilize fibroblast cultures derived from embryonic tissue. The original studies showed that cells from C3H mouse fibroblast cultures developed morphologic changes and changes in growth patterns when treated with carcinogens. Later similar studies were performed with Syrian hamster embryo cells. The direct relationship of these changes to carcinogenesis was demonstrated by transplantation of the cells into a host animal and the subsequent development of tumors. The recent development of practical assay procedures involves two cell lines from mouse embryos, Balb/3T3 and C3H/10T1/2, in which transformation is easily recognized and scored. In a typical assay situation, cells, such as Balb/3T3 mouse fibroblasts, will multiply in culture until a monolayer is formed. At this point they cease dividing unless transformed. Chemicals that are transforming agents will, however, cause growth to occur in thicker layers above the monolayer. These clumps of transformed cells are known as foci. Despite many recommended controls, the assay is only semiquantitative. The doses are selected from the results of a preliminary experiment and range from a high dose that reduces colony formation (but not by $>50\%$) to a low dose that has no measurable effect on colony formation. After exposure to the test chemical for 1 to 3 days, the cells are washed and incubation is continued for up to 4 weeks. At that time, the monolayers are fixed, stained, and scored for transformed foci. Transformation assays have several distinct advantages. Because transplanted foci give rise to tumors in congenic hosts (those from the same inbred strain from which the cells were derived) and untransformed cells do not, cell transformation is believed to be illustrative of the overall expression of carcinogenesis in mammalian tissues. The two cell types used most (Balb/3T3 and C3H/10T1/2) respond to promoters in the manner predicted by the multistage model for carcinogenesis in vivo and may eventually be useful in the development of assays for promotion. Unfortunately, a large number of false-negative results are obtained because these cell lines do not show much activation capacity; it has not proved practical to combine them with the S-9 activation system. Furthermore, the cells are aneuploidy and may be preneoplastic in the untreated state. Syrian hamster cells, which do have considerable activation capacity, have proved difficult to use in test procedures and are difficult to score.

13.10 CONCLUSION

The development of a broad range of short-term assays for genotoxicity serves to identify many mutagens and their relationship with cancer-causing agents (carcinogens).

In the 1980s, genetic toxicology gained a better understanding of the mutagenic mechanisms underlying carcinogenicity and heritable effects. This science of genetic toxicology has begun to take advantage of the knowledge that cancer is a genetic disease with multiple steps, many of which require a mutation. However, it has been observed that the negative results in this battery usually provide a sufficient level of the absence of genotoxic potential, but the compounds giving positive results in the standard battery assay may have to be revaluated more thoroughly. If a compound tests negative in the proposed battery but shows any evidence of tumor response, then it needs more extensive testing. It should be remembered that the completion of a genotoxicty battery is required before the initiation of phase II trials. The type of genotoxicity studies routinely conducted for small molecules are not applicable to biotechnology-derived pharmaceuticals.

CHAPTER

Preclinical toxicological investigations of pharmaceutical products

14

CHAPTER OUTLINE

14.1 INTRODUCTION

The requirement of the toxicity testing of new molecule entities (NME)/chemicals will depend on a variety of considerations, and generally valid procedures cannot be proposed. As a first step, it may be useful to make an approximate estimation of toxicity based on the chemical structure and the physical and chemical properties of the substance and based on known correlations of these variables with biological activity. These considerations may be of value for decisions regarding safety measures to be taken during initial laboratory work. Extrapolation and interpolation in homologous series may also be of value for decisions regarding safety measures to be taken during initial work, but for some series of chemicals this is not applicable.

A preliminary evaluation of toxicity should start when chemicals are synthesized in the laboratory stage of development of an industrial process. The full evaluation of the chemicals involved regarding occupational and general population exposure and the assessment of possible air, water, and food contamination should be initiated later, when it has been decided to proceed with full-scale production of the chemical. Toxicity data obtained during the developmental stage of a technological process could provide information concerning the health hazards of not only raw materials and products but also various other substances used or

Fundamentals of Toxicology. DOI: http://dx.doi.org/10.1016/B978-0-12-805426-0.00014-7

produced as intermediates in the technological process, and of gaseous and other wastes. Toxicological evaluation may also help in the selection of an alternative technological process that is less hazardous to health. The phasing of toxicological studies may be useful in coordination testing at national and international levels.

Environmental and health standards will need to be defined preferentially for those chemicals that show a significant degree of toxicity and represent health hazards and that are likely to be used widely in industry, agriculture, or in consumer products.

Changes and development in industrial processes, the development of new chemicals, and changes in the use of existing chemicals may lead to new or increased hazards. This calls for a continuous re-evaluation of priorities and regulation of chemicals. The list of agencies and statutes involved in regulation of toxic chemicals in the United States has been described in previous chapters.

14.2 SAFETY EVALUATION OF PHARMACEUTICAL PRODUCTS

It is well known that for the development of an NME into a safe and efficacious pharmaceutical product, one has to spend approximately $1 billion and up to 15 years to launch the product on the market. The safety assessment of products is highly specialized, and that is grossly misunderstood by most of the lay public as well as by many medically oriented professionals. A therapeutic agent can be classified as:

1. a small molecule that is chemical in nature and has a molecular weight of less than 10,000 Da
2. a biologic agent (larger than 10,000 Da; eg, peptides, proteins, or nucleic acid (NA) derived from recombinant technology or vaccine, oligonucleotides, monoclonal antibodies, etc.)
3. a medical device either by itself or as a drug delivery combination

The initial and most important aspect of a product safety evaluation program is the series of steps depending on the objectives of any testing and research programs. It is a fact that every successful drug has to pass through both discovery and development phases that involve continuous assessment of its safety early in in vitro models involving predictive systems, metabolism, and exploratory animal studies, followed by in vitro and in vivo regulatory studies and, finally, clinical trials in humans. In general, all discovery assessments, including in silico prediction, pharmacokinetics, and metabolism, and exploratory animal studies are performed without adhering to regulations as specified by Organization for European Cooperation and Development (OECD) or the US Food and Drug Administration (FDA); principles of Good Laboratory Practice (GLP), however, follow standard protocols or references. However, it is mandatory for all regulatory studies (both

Table 14.1 An Overview of the Drug Development Process in the United States

Drug Development Process (United States)	
Discovery research	Drug candidate identification and optimization
Preclinical testing	Initial animal toxicology, safety pharmacology, PK/ADME to support IND
IND submission	
Phase I clinical trials	20–80 healthy subjects Escalating single and repeat-dose studies Safety assessment, PK/ADME, and dosage determination
Phase II clinical trials	100–300 patients with targeted disease or condition Evaluate efficacy and identify adverse reactions, optimize dosage
Phase III clinical trials	1000–3000 patients with targeted disease or condition Evaluate efficacy, monitor adverse events, and optimize dosage in an expanded, geographically dispersed, and diverse patient population
NDA submission and approval	
Phase IV postmarketing	Monitoring and reporting adverse reactions and additional studies if required

PK, *pharmacokinetics;* NDA, *new drug application;* IND, *investigational new drug application;* ADME, *absorption, distribution, metabolism/biotransformation, and excretion.*

in vivo and in vitro) to be performed as per GLP principles from the OECD or US FDA. The general guidelines and the test procedures used in the evaluations of various chemicals have been discussed in proceeding chapters. This chapter describes an overview of drug development for the safety evaluation of NME, whereas subsequent chapters discuss the test protocols required for biologic active molecules and medical devices. Table 14.1 summarizes the drug development process in the United States. Any potential for possible mutagenicity and carcinogenicity occurs early in development. The test battery typically includes two in vitro assays (bacterial reverse mutation assay or Ames test and chromosomal aberration assay or mouse tk-lymphoma test) and one in vivo mouse micronucleus induction assay. Detailed test procedures have been described in the previous chapter. The types of in vitro studies undertaken during different phases of drug development are summarized in Table 14.2.

14.2.1 DISCOVERY PHASE

The discovery phase includes various stages such as target identification, target validation, and early preclinical studies (drug candidate identification and optimization). Chemists and biologists use many tools during the discovery phase of drug research to invent the efficacious and less toxic candidates to fulfill the

Table 14.2 Types of Toxicological and Other Studies Undertaken During Different Phases of Drug Development

Development Phase	Study Type
Discovery	
	• hERG/other cardiac ion channel assays • In vitro bacterial mutagenicity screening assay • In vitro chromosome aberration screening assay • In vitro cellular toxicity
For IND and prior to phase I clinical studies	
	• Single-dose acute studies in rodents and nonrodents • 7-day dose range–finding studies in rodents and nonrodents • 2-week/4-week repeat-dose studies in rodents and nonrodents • Bacterial mutagenicity • In vitro chromosome aberrations • In vivo micronucleus • Gastrointestinal can be addressed in repeated dose studies • hERG IC_{50} • Central nervous system, respiratory, and cardiovascular safety pharmacology • Intravenous/perivascular irritation, rat or rabbit (if appropriate)
Prior to phase II clinical studies	
	• Range-finding for developmental and reproductive studies • Female fertility, rat • Embryo–fetal development, rabbit and rat • 1- or 3-month repeat-dose studies in rodents and nonrodents • ADME studies • Occupational studies (skin, eye irritation, and contact sensitization)
Prior to phase III clinical studies	
	• 6-month rodent and 6- or 9-month nonrodent repeat-dose studies • Male fertility, rat • Prenatal/perinatal toxicity, rat
For NDA	
	• Metabolite studies as appropriate • Excipient/impurity qualification studies as appropriate • 3-month mouse dose range–finding study to support carcinogenicity study (for chronic indications[a]) • Rat and mouse carcinogenicity (for chronic indications[a]) • Juvenile rat studies to support pediatric indication (if applicable) • Additional studies to address special issues (eg, immunotoxicology)

NDA, *new drug application;* IND, *investigational new drug application;* ADME, *absorption, distribution, metabolism/biotransformation, and excretion.*
[a]*Chronic indication is commonly defined as continuous treatment for 6 months or more.*

needs for therapy for a particular disease. Therefore, selection of a single compound for development requires implementation of a system for early-stage elimination of undesirable compounds while identifying compounds that have the potential to be developed as a drug. Once one or two lead compounds have been identified, it is prudent to evaluate the compound(s) using some expensive tests that have been proven to identify problems with safety and drug delivery in later development. Most large pharmaceutical companies conduct their research by using a combination of the methods to select compounds or agents that will ultimately be found effective and that are reasonably nontoxic in humans.

14.2.2 PRECLINICAL TOXICOLOGY TESTING

During the preclinical test phase, initial animal toxicology tests such as single-dose acute studies, 7-day dose range–finding studies, 2-week/4-week repeat-dose studies (using both rodent and nonrodent species), in vitro bacterial mutagenicity and chromosome aberrations, in vivo micronucleus, and hERG LC_{50} are undertaken. In addition, studies related to central nervous system, respiratory and cardiovascular safety, pharmacology (including renal and gastrointestinal), and intravenous/perivascular irritation, use the rat or rabbit (if appropriate) as part of the preclinical toxicology testing. To support the investigational studies, other studies such as absorption, distribution, metabolism, and excretion studies are used to determine pharmacologic safety.

14.2.3 PRECLINICAL DEVELOPMENT PHASE

Once a new molecule that satisfies predetermined activity criteria has been discovered and synthesized in the laboratory, a long and arduous development period begins. This period consumes approximately two-thirds of the time and cost of bringing a new drug to the market. During this period, the NME must be characterized chemically, pharmacologically, toxicologically, and clinically, and bioavailability must be determined. During clinical phase II, the following toxicological studies become part of the test protocol:

1. Range-finding for developmental and reproductive studies
2. Female fertility (rat)
3. Embryo–fetal development (rabbit and rat)
4. 1- or 3-month repeat-dose studies (in rodents and nonrodents)
5. absorption, distribution, metabolism/biotransformation, and excretion (ADME) studies
6. Occupational studies (skin, eye irritation, and contact sensitization)

Prior to phase III clinical studies:

1. 6-month rodent and 6- or 9-month nonrodent repeat-dose studies
2. Male fertility (rat)
3. Parental/perinatal toxicity (rat)

In addition, studies regarding the following tests are mandatory for all new drug applications:

1. Metabolite studies as appropriate.
2. Excipient/impurity qualification studies as appropriate
3. 3-month mouse dose range—finding study to support carcinogenicity study (for chronic indications)
4. Rat and mouse carcinogenicity (for chronic indications)
5. Juvenile rat studies to support pediatric indication (if applicable)
6. Additional studies to address special issues (eg, immunotoxicology)

14.2.4 STUDIES OF ENVIRONMENTAL SAFETY

A recent addition to the requirements imposed on the registration of a new drug is the determination of its effects on the environment. Tests must be designed to see the effects of the drug on soil, water, and animal or vegetable life. The drug must not adversely concentrate along food chains and must not accumulate in the environment.

When the comprehensive trial program and all of the various experimental studies have been conducted, and when the sponsor is satisfied about the safety and efficacy of the drug, an application is filed with the Drug Control Authority for product licensing and marketing authorization. If approved by the Drug Control Authority, then the drug is marketed for general use.

14.2.5 POSTMARKETING SURVEILLANCE

Postmarketing surveillance, sometimes called phase IV of clinical trials, is the study performed by participating clinicians and that involves patients. The study involves determination of certain unusual types of adverse reactions and toxic effects of long-term use of the drugs. The study also determines the drug utilization pattern and additional therapeutic effects. This study continues until the drug is used.

14.2.6 ESTIMATION OF THE DOSE

Extensive nonclinical data collected from a large number of acute and repeat-dose toxicity studies help to determine the initial safe and maximum recommended starting dose (MRSD) and dose range for the phase I human trials using healthy subjects (80–100) and identify any parameters for clinical monitoring for potential adverse effects. All the relevant preclinical data, including pharmacologically active dose and the full toxicological profile, and the pharmacokinetics/toxicokinetics (PK/TK) and ADME data of the therapeutic agent are considered when determining MRSD in the algorithmic process. In the calculation of MRSD, no observed adverse effect level (NOAEL) is the major element tested in animal species. For conversion of NOAEL to a human equivalent dose (HED), a species-specific conversion factor is used. The conversion should be based on the normalization of the doses to body surface area. The extrapolation of the animal dose to the human dose is performed by using the following formula:

$$\text{HED} = \text{animal dose in mg/kg} \times (\text{animal weight in kg/human weight in kg})$$

To calculate MRSD, a safety factor (usually 10) is applied to HED to increase the assurance that the first dose in humans will not cause any adverse effects. However, it can be increased when there is reason for increased concern and it can be lowered when concern is reduced because of available safe data.

14.3 CONCLUSION

It is recognized that significant advances in the harmonization of the timing of non-clinical safety studies for the conduct of human clinical trials for pharmaceuticals have already been achieved. Continued efforts are ongoing to maintain harmonization for pharmaceutical development globally. However, some differences still remain in a few areas. Regulators and industry will continue to consider these differences and work toward further improving the drug development process. In the past few years, a number of computation toxicology models have been developed (eg, in silico modeling) as alternatives to in vitro and in vivo models and in an effort to reduce animal testing; however, computational testing is not approved by regulators for pharmaceutical development at this time. Recently, the US FDA has developed an Informatics and Computational Safety Analysis program for future archiving of safety data; however, at this time, it is still a work in progress.

CHAPTER

Preclinical safety evaluation of biotechnology-derived products 15

CHAPTER OUTLINE

15.1 INTRODUCTION

Biotechnology in its broad sense is the technology involving the use of living organisms (cells, microbes, plants, and animals) to produce useful products. The application of biotechnology knowledge, and, in particular, gene technology is especially important in the pharmaceutical area because it should be instrumental in the manufacture of vaccines, development of more efficient diagnostic aids and therapeutic agents, and, ultimately, in gene therapy. The tools of biotechnology include monocloning antibodies and recombinant DNA (rDNA), peptide engineering, generation and use of various antibodies, and mammalian cell culture and transgenic animal techniques.

15.2 BACKGROUND

Several guidelines and guidance documents have been published by the various regulatory agencies relating to the assessment of biotechnology derived–products. As previously stated, specific guidelines for studies such as safety evaluation, pharmacology, and toxicology already exist for traditional pharmaceuticals.

Fundamentals of Toxicology. DOI: http://dx.doi.org/10.1016/B978-0-12-805426-0.00015-9

In contrast, guiding principles have been developed for novel biopharmaceuticals as sufficient data have accumulated for specific product classes. In addition, there is less concern regarding potential differences in metabolizing and resultant active metabolites because most biopharmaceuticals are protein-derived; as such, proteins are metabolized by proteolytic degradation, oxidation, and other methods. For biotechnology-derived products, novel routes of delivery have been more often proposed when site-directed delivery and site-specific expression may be the ultimate future goal.

15.3 REGULATORY CONSIDERATIONS

The safety evaluation of biotechnology products also challenges the ingenuity of the toxicologist. As has been mentioned, these products are usually large peptide or protein molecules that have to be administered parenterally. Furthermore, many of the products are species-specific and engineered for human use, and neutralizing antibodies are often a problem in sub-chronic animal studies. The regulatory standards for biotechnology-derived pharmaceuticals have been generally comparable among three International Conference on Harmonization (ICH) regions: the European Union, Japan, and the United States. All three regions have adopted a flexible "case-by-case" science-based approach to preclinical safety evaluation, which is needed to support clinical development and marketing authorization.

15.4 GENERAL PRINCIPLES

The nature and scope of safety evaluation studies conducted with biopharmaceuticals should reflect the basic principles of toxicology. Therefore, concerns for the general design of preclinical studies include:

1. Establishment of rationale
2. Identification of clinical indication
3. Selection of the model species (species, physiological state)
4. Selection of the dose (route, multiple, regimen)
5. Determination of exposure
6. Selection of the end points (activity and/or toxicity)

15.5 GENERAL TOXICOLOGICAL PROFILE

Single-dose toxicity studies are helpful for identifying the upper bounds of exposure or overdosage on target organs. When performed, they usually involve two species and the intended route of human administration. The generally accepted study design in rodents is a 28-day study with consecutive daily dosing, but it seldom uses nonrodent species. Usually, both genders are used in these studies, excluding nonhuman primates, unless the intended use is in only one gender of the human population. Multiple dose levels are used with high doses above the no observed adverse effect level dose to determine the dose–response relationship and the dose at which no immunotoxicity is observed.

15.5.1 ABSORPTION, DISPOSITION, AND CLEARANCE IN RELEVANT ANIMAL MODELS

Because the expected consequence of metabolism of biotechnologically derived pharmaceuticals is the degradation to small peptides and individual amino acids, the classical biotransformation studies as performed for pharmaceuticals are not needed.

15.5.2 SPECIFIC TOXICITY TESTS

15.5.2.1 Immunotoxicity studies

As per ICH guidelines, all new human pharmaceuticals should be evaluated for the potential to produce immunotoxicity using standard toxicity studies. Additional immunotoxicity studies as appropriate based on a weight-of-evidence review, including immune-related signals, should be completed before exposure of a large population of patients (eg, phase III). Immunogenicity may be related to either suppression or enhancement of immune response. Suppression can lead to decreased host resistance to infectious agents or tumor cells, whereas enhancement can exaggerate autoimmune diseases or hypersensitivity.

Additional testing may be based on: (1) findings from standard toxicity studies; (2) the pharmacological properties of the drug; (3) the intended patient population; (4) the disposition of the drug; and (5) clinical information.

Standard toxicity studies include: (1) hematological changes; (2) alternation in immune system organ weight and or histopathology; (3) changes in serum globulin; (4) increased incidence of infections; and (5) increased occurrence of tumors.

For immunotoxicity studies, the choice of an animal species depends on the ability to develop an immune response to the vaccine antigen. Most human vaccines are immunogenic to rodents or rabbits. In some cases, only nonhuman primates may show an adequate immune response.

The measurement of antibodies associated with administration of these types of products is performed in repeat-dose toxicity studies and immune response (eg, titer, number of responding animals, neutralizing or non-neutralizing) is correlated with any pharmacological and/or toxicological changes.

15.5.2.2 Development and reproduction toxicity

Development and reproduction toxicity studies are generally required for vaccines to determine the adverse effects on pregnancy/lactating female animals and development and growth of the embryo/fetus and the offspring. In such studies, the females must be exposed to the vaccine during the interval from implantation through closure of the hard palate and also at later stages of pregnancy. The offspring should be followed to weaning and observed for growth and development. In addition, immunological assessment may include the measurement of vaccine-induced antibody response to verify exposure to the embryo/fetus to maternal antibody.

15.5.2.3 Chronic studies

Chronic studies are usually not needed for biopharmaceuticals due to antibody formation, nature of the product (similar to endogenous peptide (protein)), and belief that the product would not be expected to constitute a real risk of carcinogenic potential.

15.5.2.4 Additional studies

Other toxicities studies (such as neurotoxicity) and any other studies needed due to unexpected toxicity that may be species-specific or due to frequency or findings related to immunogenicity may be undertaken.

15.6 CONCLUSION

Results of clinical experiences with biotechnology-derived products have shown that proteins, including endogenous protein, can induce a variety of toxic responses, but many times the toxicity is consistent with an exaggerated pharmacological response.

Biotechnology has provided not only the hope of potential new therapies but also the necessary tools to evaluate new therapies. Toxicology as a science has benefited from this experience in many ways. The case-by-case approach to preclinical safety evaluation should continue to provide for scientific advancement in toxicology and the infusement of quality research into safety assessment for the next generation of therapies. In the case of biologics, potential risks may be associated with host cell contaminants derived from bacteria, yeast, insect, plant, and mammalian cells that can result in allergic reactions and other immunological effects. For products derived from insects, plant and mammalian cells, or transgenic plants and animals, there may be additional risk of viral infections.

CHAPTER

16 Preclinical regulatory toxicology for biomaterials and medical devices

CHAPTER OUTLINE

16.1 INTRODUCTION

The term "medical device" covers a broad range of products, including needles, syringes, infusion pumps, endoscopes, examination gloves, dressings, and blood glucose meters, that are used every day in most healthcare settings. Materials and medical devices constitute an extremely diverse, heterogeneous category of items because the use of these products normally entails either direct or indirect contact

Fundamentals of Toxicology. DOI: http://dx.doi.org/10.1016/B978-0-12-805426-0.00016-0

with patients. Therefore, it is the obligation of the manufacturers to establish the safety of their products before they are marketed.

16.2 REGULATIONS

Until recently, the regulations for the manufacture and sale of these products varied greatly among countries. Since 1995, medical devices to be marketed in European Union (EU) have been required to comply with the EU Medical Devices Directive, which specifies requirements for safety assessment issues. The purpose is to promote a single European market for trade of medical devices while ensuring that users and patients are not exposed to unnecessary risks. Other international standards include the US FDA International Organization for Standardization: Biological Evaluation of Medical Devices (ISO 10993) and others. The details of other standards are beyond the scope of this chapter.

16.3 OBJECTIVES

The objective of the biological evaluation of these devices is to investigate the potential biological hazards by careful observations to determine any unexpected adverse reactions or events in humans during clinical use of the medical devices. The safety assessments of these devices are guided by toxicological and other studies recommended by the international standard protocol.

16.4 EXTRACT PREPARATIONS

Before testing of the material, an extract of the material is obtained using polar solvents such as physiological saline, water, liquid or culture media. Nonpolar solvents include freshly refined vegetable oil, such as cotton seed oil or sesame oil. Ethanol/water, ethanol/physiological saline, polyethylene glycol 400, and dimethyl sulfoxide may be used as an additional extracting media.

16.5 TEST PROTOCOLS

Testing protocols include both short-term and long-term tests. Safety evaluations of medical devices assess the risk of adverse health effects due to normal use and/or in the likelihood of their misuse. Because adverse effects could result from exposure to the materials from which a device is made, preclinical assessment of the toxic potential of such materials or components is needed to minimize the potential hazard to the patient. The range of potential biological hazards is wide and may include the following:

1. Short-term effects such as acute toxicity, irritation, sensitization, hemolysis, and thromogenicity
2. Long-term effects such as subchronic and chronic toxicity, sensitization, genotoxicity, carcinogenicity, and effects on reproduction and development

16.6 SHORT-TERM TESTS

16.6.1 ACUTE TOXICITY

For acute systemic toxicity, polar, nonpolar, or any other extracting media are injected in mice by either the intravenous (IV) or the intraperitoneal (IP) route. Observations of any signs of toxicity are made immediately and thereafter at 24-, 48-, and 72-h intervals.

16.6.2 PYROGENICITY

A program test is designed to limit the risk of febrile reaction to an acceptable level in the patient as a result of administration by injection of the extract of the product. The test involves measuring the increase in temperature of rabbits following the IV injection of a test solution. Temperature is subsequently recorded in 30-min intervals for 1 and 3 h to evaluate the increase in temperature, if any.

16.6.3 HEMOLYTIC PROPERTIES

The hemolytic properties test is used to assess the hemolytic potential of materials used in the fabrication of devices that will come in contact with the blood. The test specimens are exposed to rabbit blood under dynamic or static conditions and the change in plasma hemoglobin is measured. Comparisons are made with control materials under identical conditions.

16.6.4 INTRACUTANEOUS/INTRADERMAL REACTIVITY TEST

To test the potential of the material to produce irritation, the extract is injected intradermally. Polar and nonpolar extracts are injected on both sides of the rabbit. The observations are made immediately after the injection and thereafter at 24, 48, and 72 h. Then, tissue reactions are graded for erythema and edema.

16.6.5 SKIN IRRITATION

To test skin irritation, albino rabbits of either sex and a single strain are used. After close clipping of the fur on the dorsal side, the material is applied and covered with a nonocclusive dressing for 4 h. The skin is observed for erythema and edema at 24, 48, and 72 h to determine the primary irritation index.

16.7 LONG-TERM TESTS

16.7.1 DELAYED HYPERSENSITIVITY/SENSITIZATION TEST

There are several methods to determine skin sensitization in guinea pigs. The most commonly used methods are the maximization test for delayed hypersensitivity and the closed patch test for delayed hypersensitivity.

Maximization Test for Delayed Hypersensitivity: IV injections of test material and control extracts are administered to the guinea pig. Seven days after the intradermal injection, the induction phase begins. Fourteen days after the induction phase, the challenge phase with the test material begins. The animals are observed after 24, 48, and 72 h for sensitization potential of the test compound.

Closed Patch Test for Delayed Hypersensitivity: The extracts of the test material are applied on the clipped dorsal area of guinea pigs or rabbit. This procedure is repeated at weekly intervals for 3 weeks. Fourteen days after the last application, the animals are challenged with test material. The sites are examined after 24, 48, and 72 h for sensitization potential of the test compound.

16.7.2 IMPLANTATION

To test the biological safety of the material at the local site of the living tissue, the test material and the control material are implanted in living animals. The animals are examined for any abnormal response in the tissue.

Subcutaneous Tissue: Test material that is 10 mm to 12 mm in diameter and from 0.3 to 1 mm in thickness are implanted subcutaneously. Control material of the same size is also implanted subcutaneously. The animals are euthanized and examined for any reaction/response.

Implantation in Muscle: In this test, the test material and control specimens (1 to 3 mm in width and 10 mm in length) are implanted in the muscle. The following then occurs:

1. Appearance of muscle surrounding the implant is observed
2. Muscle sample is taken for the microscopic examination of sections of muscles
3. Assessment of tissues for necrosis, inflammation, eosinophils, plasma cell proliferation, fibro-endothelial proliferation, giant cell proliferation
4. Infection arising from the presence of sample, if any, is recorded

Implant in Bone: Implant sizes are based on the size of the test animal used/chosen. For rabbits, cylindrical implants 2 mm in diameter and 6 mm in length are implanted in the femur or fibia. The implantation is performed by low drilling speed and intermittent drilling with profuse irrigation using physiological saline and suction to avoid local tissue necrosis. After the implant of the test material and control material, the tissue response is observed.

16.7.3 GENOTOXICITY

To test the mutagenic potential, changes in chromosomal structure and gene mutations of the material are observed and mammalian cell culture or other techniques are used. The details of various tests are given in the chapter dealing with genotoxicity. The common genotoxicity tests used for medical devices are as follows:

In Vitro Tests: *Salmonella typhimurium*, reverse mutation assay; *Escherichia coli*, reverse mutation assay; in vitro mammalian cytogenic tests; in vitro mammalian cell gene mutation; and in vitro sister chromatid exchange.

In Vivo Tests: Micronucleus test; germ cell cytogenetic assay; chromosomal aberration analysis; mouse spot test; and mouse heritable translocation assay.

16.8 SUPPLEMENTARY TESTS

16.8.1 SUBCHRONIC TOXICITY

The animals are given repeated doses of the test extracts for part of their life span (not exceeding 10% of the life span). This test provides information about their effect on target organs, possibilities of accumulation, and an estimate of a no-effect level of exposure, which can be of use in selecting dose levels for further chronic studies and for establishing safety criteria for human exposure.

16.8.2 CHRONIC TOXICITY

These tests are used to determine the effects of either single or multiple exposures to devices, materials, and/or their extracts during the entire life span of the test animal (over 90 days in rats).

16.8.3 CARCINOGENICITY

These tests determine the effects of either single or multiple implants of devices or materials and/or exposure to their extracts over a period of the total life span of the test animal. The test examines both chronic toxicity (ie, long-term effects) and tumorigenicity.

16.8.4 DEVELOPMENTAL AND REPRODUCTIVE TOXICITY

Reproduction and development toxicity studies provide information about their effects on reproduction function, embryonic development (teratogenicity/malformations), and prenatal and early development toxicity of the fetus. These tests or bioassays should only be conducted when the device has the potential to affect the reproductive system.

16.9 CONCLUSION

Due to the diversity of medical devices, it has been recognized that not all the tests identified in a category will be necessary or practical for any given device. Testing for devices shall be considered on an individual merit basis. The ISO guidelines clearly state that the tests results should be reproducible by interlaboratory methods and repeatable by intralaboratory methods.

UNIT IV

CHAPTER

Toxic effects of pesticides (agrochemicals) 17

CHAPTER OUTLINE

17.1 INTRODUCTION

The term "agricultural chemicals" has largely been replaced by the term "pesticides." Approximately 1000 pesticides are available in various preparations such as dusting powder, emulsions, solutions, water dispensable powders, fumigants, and others. Pesticides are biocides capable of killing all forms of life. They are among the most widely used group of chemicals in the modern world and have provided immense benefits to humankind by enhancing food production and improving health via nutrition. However, their massive and indiscriminate use in crop protection, food preservation, and insect and pest control has led to acute or chronic poisoning incidents in humans, domestic animals, and wildlife, and has resulted in widespread ecological adverse effects.

A survey has indicated that insecticides are the most commonly used poisons consumed to commit suicide in India because they are easily available. Accidental poisoning as an occupational hazard is also common among those

Fundamentals of Toxicology. DOI: http://dx.doi.org/10.1016/B978-0-12-805426-0.00017-2

who spray insecticides on agricultural farms. Mass accidental food contamination due to pesticides is another cause of poisoning in India and other developing countries in the world. Homicide by these poisons is not possible because of the strong kerosene-like odor. Among insecticides, the organophosphorus (OP) group of compounds is used as nerve gas during warfare; these compounds are particularly potent because they cause death more rapidly and frequently than other insecticides. Among other pesticides, OP and carbamate (CM) insecticides, rodenticide (warfarin), and fumigant (aluminum phosphide) are the common causes of suicide poisonings in India because of their availability. Therefore, poisoning due to these pesticides has been dealt with in greater detail.

17.2 HISTORICAL BACKGROUND

Chemicals have been used to kill or control pests for centuries. The Chinese used arsenic to control insects, and the early Romans used common salt to control weeds and used sulfur to control insects. In the 1800s, pyrethrin (the flowers of the chrysanthemum, *Pyrethrum cineraefolium*) was found to have insecticidal properties. The roots of certain Derris plant species (*Derris elliptica* and *Lonchocarpus* spp.) have the active ingredient, rotenone, which was used for insect control. During the 1940s, a number of chemicals, such as chlorinated hydrocarbon insecticides (such as DDT) and phenoxy acid herbicides (such as 2,4-*D*), were introduced. Natural compounds such as red squill, derived from the bulbs of red squill (*Urginea* (*Scilla*) *maritima*) were effective in controlling rodents. Subsequently, a plethora of pesticides were synthesized and introduced on the market.

17.3 DEFINITION AND CLASSIFICATION

Pesticides are used to control, kill, or repel pests. They are also known as economic poisons, regulated by federal and state laws. Depending on what a compound is designed to do, pesticides have been subclassified into a number of categories:

1. *Insecticides*: Organochlorine (OC), OP, CM, pyrethrins and pyrethroids, formamidines, nicotinoids, and natural products (rotenone and nicotine)
2. *Fumigants*: Inorganic (aluminum phosphide, hydrogen cyanide, carbon disulfide, sulfur dioxide), organic (methyl bromide, ethylene dibromide, dibromochloropropane)
3. *Fungicides*: Inorganic (sulfur, metals), organic (organomercurial, chlorophenols, phathalimides, etc.)
4. *Herbicides*: Inorganic (arsenicals, chlorates), organic (chlorophenoxy and its derivatives, dinitrophenols, bipyridyls, ureas, and other herbicides)
5. *Rodenticide*: Warfarin

Table 17.1 WHO Classification of Pesticides Depending on LD_{50} (Rat) Body Weight (mg/kg)

Class		Color Represented	Oral Solid	Oral Liquid	Dermal Solid	Dermal liquid
I.	Extremely hazardous	Red	≤5	≤20	≤10	≤40
	Highly hazardous	Yellow	5–50	20–200	10–100	40–400
II.	Moderately hazardous	Blue	50–500	200–2000	1–1000	400–4000
III.	Slightly hazardous	Green	>500	>2000	>1000	>4000

In addition, there are other groups of pesticides such as nematicide, acaricide, algicides, bird repellents, and mammal repellents.

An important pesticide with widespread use and that is responsible for mass poisoning or have long-term effect have been dealt with in greater depth. A discussion of all groups of pesticides is beyond the scope of this book.

The US Environmental Protection Agency (EPA) has developed definitions of pesticides based on their toxicity. Category I pesticides are highly hazardous, are classified as restricted use, and have an oral LD_{50} ≤ 1 mg/kg of body weight. Category II pesticides are moderately toxic and have an oral LD_{50} ≤ 500 mg/kg. Category III pesticides are generally nontoxic and have an oral LD_{50} $\leq 15{,}000$ mg/kg. In addition, the US EPA has developed a "carcinogenicity categorization" to classify pesticides for carcinogenicity. The WHO classification of pesticides depending on LD_{50} (rat) in mg/kg has been summarized in Table 17.1.

17.4 INSECTICIDES

17.4.1 OC INSECTICIDES

The OC insecticides were introduced in the 1940s. Although DDT was synthesized in 1874, its insecticidal properties were not observed until 1939, when Dr. Paul Mueller, a Swiss chemist, discovered its effectiveness as an insecticide and was awarded a Nobel Prize for his work. During World War II, the United States used large quantities of DDT to control vector-borne diseases, such as typhus and malaria, to which US troops were exposed. After the war, DDT use became widespread in agriculture, public health, and

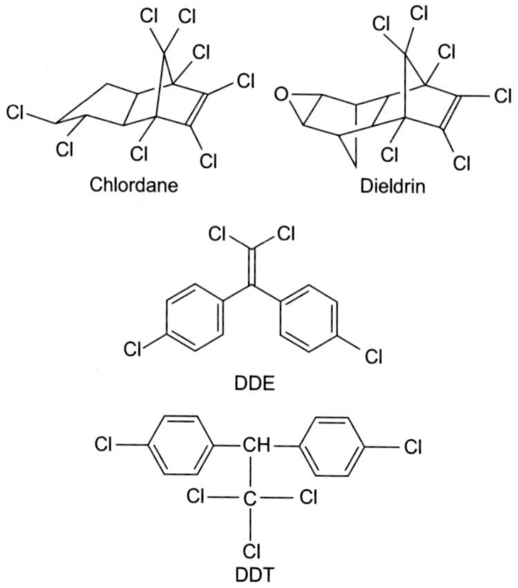

FIGURE 17.1

Structural formulae of selected organochlorine insecticides.

households. Its persistence, initially considered a desirable attribute, later became the basis for public concern. The publication of Rachel Carson's book *The Silent Spring* in 1962 stimulated this concern and eventually led to the ban of DDT and other chlorinated insecticides in the United States. Subsequently, cyclodiene and other groups of OC insecticides, such as methoxychlor, chlordane, heptachlor, aldrin, dieldrin, endrin, toxaphene, mirex, and lindane, were introduced and were used extensively. Some of them were removed from the market due to measurable residue levels penetrating into interiors and allegedly causing health problems. Residue levels of chlorinated insecticides continue to be found in the environment. The structural formulae of selected OC compounds are given in Fig. 17.1.

Mode of action Chlorinated hydrocarbons are neurotoxicants and cause acute effects by interfering with the transmission of nerve impulses.

Treatment OC insecticide toxicosis has no specific treatment. The treatment of acute poisoning should mainly be directed toward symptoms and control of convulsions. General measures should include gastric lavage. In case of skin contamination, the skin should be properly washed with soap and water. Cholestyramine 3–8 g four times daily and diazepam to control the convulsions should be administered.

17.4.2 OP AND CM COMPOUNDS

The first OP compound, tetraethyl pyrophosphate, was synthesized in 1854 by Philipe de Clermont. In 1932, one of the earliest OP insecticides synthesized by Schrader was parathion, which is still used worldwide. Prior to World War II (WWII), the German Ministry of Defense developed highly toxic OP compounds of the G series (tabun, sarin, and soman) and diisopropyl phosphorofluoridate. In the 1950s, OP compounds with supertoxicity of the V series, such as VX and VR, were synthesized in the United Kingdom and the Soviet Union. After WWII, thousands of OPs have been synthesized in the search for compounds with species selectivity (ie, more toxicity to insects and less toxicity to mammals). Malathion is an example. This compound has been used for more than half a century as the most popular insecticide. Today, more than 200 OPs are in use for a variety of purposes, such as protection of crops, grains, gardens, homes, and public health.

The first CM compound, physostigmine (serine alkaloid), was isolated from calabar beans (ordeal poison) of a perennial plant *Physostigma venenosum.* Approximately 50 years later, an aromatic ester of carbamic acid, neostigmine, was synthesized and used in the treatment of myasthenia gravis. Most of the CMs that are used as insecticides were synthesized in the 1960s and 1970s. Carbaryl was the first CM compound used as an insecticide. The most toxic compound of this class, aldicarb, was synthesized by mimicking the structure of acetylcholine (Ach). Like OPs, thousands of CMs have been synthesized, but less than two dozen compounds have been used practically. Today, CMs are preferred for pesticide use over OPs because some OPs have been found to be extremely toxic, whereas others cause delayed neuropathy in animals as well as in humans. Both OPs and CMs have broad applications in agriculture and veterinary medicine and, as a result of their indiscriminate use, acute poisonings has been very common in humans, animals, birds, fish, and wildlife.

They are used as insecticides, acaricides, soil nematicides, fungicides, herbicides, defoliants, rodenticides, insecticides synergists, insect repellents, chemosterilants, and warfare agents. The chemical structures of selected OP compounds used as insecticides are presented in Fig. 17.2. As insecticides, OPs comprise one of the major groups in use at present. As compared to OC and OP, CMs are much less environmentally persistent, much more biodegradable, less subject to biomagnifications, and usually unstable in the presence of sunlight, but they are much more acutely toxic to nontarget species. Several cases of poisoning frequently occur in humans, domestic animals, and wildlife.

17.4.2.1 OP Insecticides

As discussed previously, OP insecticides are often involved in serious fatal human poisoning incidences and are considered most dangerous orally or through the skin. Victims are usually children, farmers, and unskilled labor.

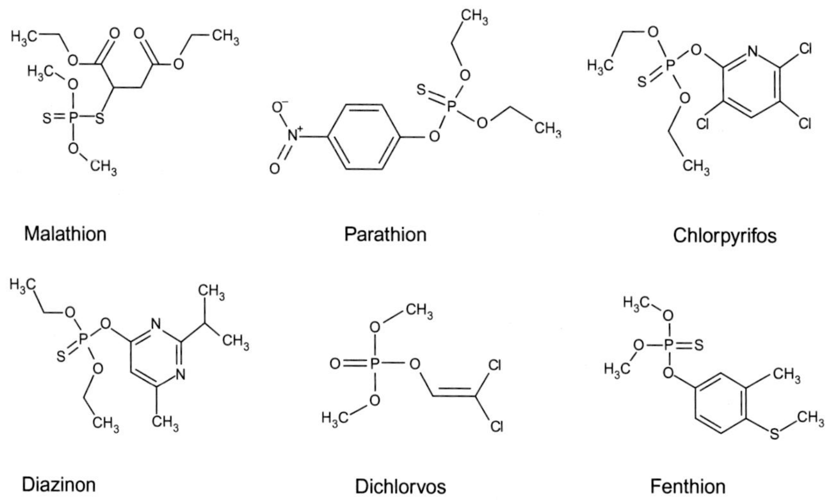

Malathion

Parathion

Chlorpyrifos

Diazinon

Dichlorvos

Fenthion

FIGURE 17.2

Structural formulae of organophosphorus compounds used as insecticides.

17.4.2.2 OP Nerve Agents/Gases

OP nerve agents include tabun (GA), sarin (GB), soman (GD), cyclosarin (GF), venom toxin (VX), and Russian VX (VR). The chemical structures of selected OP compounds used as nerve agents are presented in Fig. 17.3. These compounds are highly toxic and pose continuous threats for the lives of humans as well as animals, because they can be used as chemical weapons of mass destruction (WMD). So far, these agents have been used by dictators and terrorists. In some incidents, animals have been victims of military operations. These compounds produce toxicity by directly inhibiting AChE and are much more potent than OP insecticides because they cause lethality to animals in the micrograms range.

17.4.2.3 OP-Induced Intermediate Syndrome

OP-induced intermediate syndrome (IMS) was first reported in human patients in Sri Lanka in 1987. After exposure to methamidophos, fenthion, dimethoate, and monocrotophos, 10 patients within 24–96 h reported symptoms of acute cholinergic poisoning. This syndrome after exposure to methamidophos, fenthion, dimethoate, and monocrotophos was also reported in South Africa (1989), Turkey (1990), Belgium (1992), the United States (1992), Venezuela (1998), France (2000), and many other countries. To date, OPs that are known to cause IMS include bromophos, chlorpyrifos, diazinon, dicrotophos, dimethoate, disulfoton,

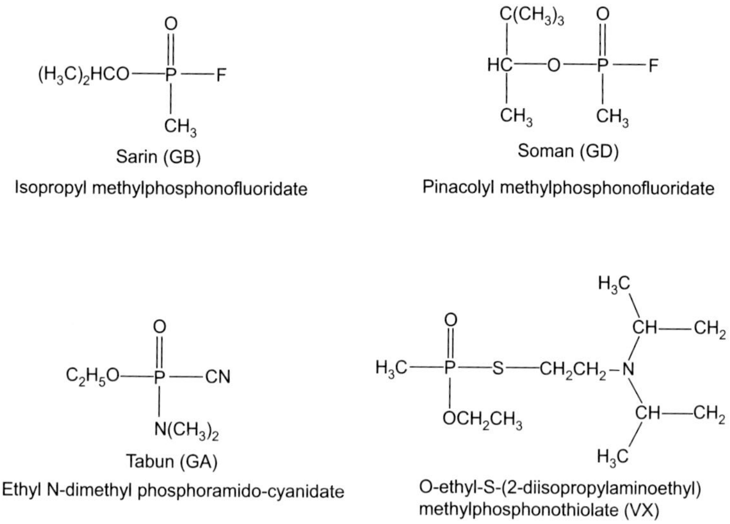

Sarin (GB)
Isopropyl methylphosphonofluoridate

Soman (GD)
Pinacolyl methylphosphonofluoridate

Tabun (GA)
Ethyl N-dimethyl phosphoramido-cyanidate

O-ethyl-S-(2-diisopropylaminoethyl) methylphosphonothiolate (VX)

FIGURE 17.3

Structural formulae of organophosphorus compounds used as warfare agents.

fenthion, malathion, methamidophos, methyl parathion, mo nocrotophos, omethoate, parathion, phosmet, and trichlorfon. IMS is usually observed in individuals who have ingested a massive dose of an OP insecticide either accidentally or in a suicide attempt.

In 2005, a CM insecticide, carbofuran, was also reported to cause IMS in patients accidentally or intentionally exposed to large doses of this insecticide. IMS is now known as a separate clinical entity from acute toxicity and delayed polyneuropathy caused by OPs and CMs. Clinically, this disease is characterized by acute paralysis and weakness in the areas of several cranial motor nerves, neck flexors, and facial, extraocular, palatal, proximal limb, and respiratory muscles. Generalized weakness, decreased deep tendon reflexes, ptosis, and diplopia are also evident. These symptoms may last for several days or weeks depending on the OP involved. A similar syndrome has also been observed in dogs and cats poisoned maliciously or accidentally with massive doses of certain OPs. It may be pertinent to mention that despite severe AChE inhibition, muscle fasciculations and muscarinic receptors associated with accumulation of Ach are absent. Although the exact mechanism involved in pathogenesis of IMS is unclear, studies involving rats suggest that decreases in AChE and nicotinic ACh receptor mRNA expression occur after oral poisoning with disulfoton. Currently, very little is known about the type of damage at the motor endplate or about risk factors contributing to its development.

17.4.3 CMs INSECTICIDES

The CM compounds are esters of carbamic acid and are used as insecticides. Unlike OPs, CM compounds are not structurally complex. Currently, the volume of CMs used exceeds OPs because they are relatively safer than OPs. The chemical structures of CMs are presented in Fig. 17.4.

The toxicity of CM compounds varies according to the phenol or alcohol group. One of the most widely used CM insecticides is carbaryl (1-napthyl methylcarbamate), a broad-spectrum insecticide. It is used widely in agriculture, including home gardens, where it generally is applied as a dust. Carbaryl is not considered to be a persistent compound because it is readily hydrolyzed. Based on its formulation, it carries a toxicity classification of II or III, with an oral LD_{50} of 250 mg/kg (rat) and a dermal LC_{50} of >2000 mg/kg. An example of an extremely toxic CM is aldicarb (2-methyl-2-(methylthio) propionaldehyde). Both oral and dermal routes are the primary portals of entry, and it has an oral LD_{50} of 1.0 mg/kg (rat) and a dermal LD_{50} of 20 mg/kg (rabbit).

Mode of action OP and CM insecticides share a common mode of toxicological action associated with their ability to inhibit the ChE enzyme within the nervous tissue and at the neuromuscular junction (NMJs). Both types of insecticides have a high affinity for binding to and inhibiting AChE, an enzyme specifically responsible for the hydrolysis of the neurotransmitter ACh. Thus, this leads to accumulation of Ach both at muscrinic and nicotinic receptors. Because the cholinergic

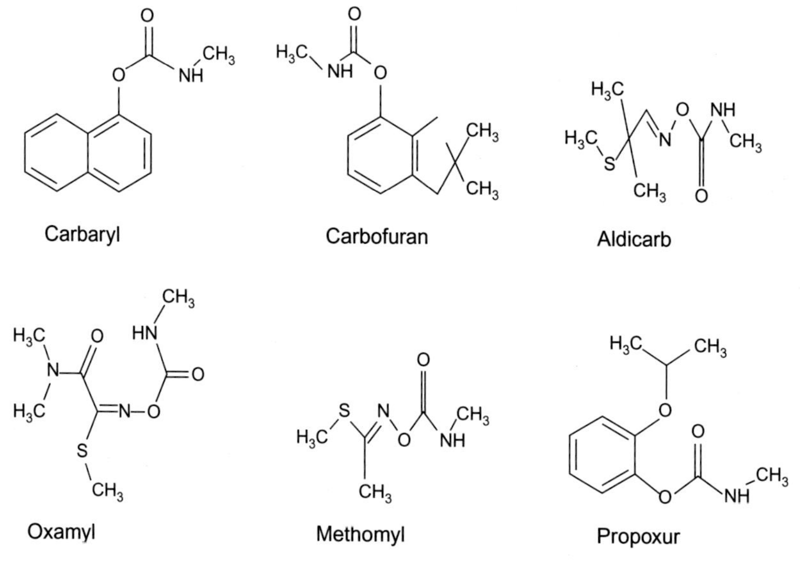

Carbaryl

Carbofuran

Aldicarb

Oxamyl

Methomyl

Propoxur

FIGURE 17.4

Structural formulae of selected carbamate compounds used as insecticides.

Table 17.2 Organophosphorus and Carbamate Insecticide-Induced Muscrinic and Nicotinic Signs of Toxicity

	Site of Action	Physiological Effects
Muscrinic (parasympathetic effects)	Sweat glands	Excessive sweating leads to hypothermia and electrolyte balance
	Pupil	Constricted
	Lacrimal glands	Lacrimation (red tears)
	Salivary gland	Excessive salivation
	Bronchial trees	Wheezing
	Gastrointestinal tract	Cramps, vomiting, diarrhea, tenesmus
	Cardiovascular	Bradycardia, decrease in BP
	Ciliary body bladder	Blurred vision
	Bladder	Urinary incontinence
Nicotinic effects	Striated muscles	Fasciculations, cramps, weakness, twitching, paralysis, respiratory distress, cyanosis/arrest
	Sympathetic ganglia	Tachycardia, BP raised
	Central nervous system effects	Anxiety, restlessness, ataxia, convulsions

system is widely distributed within both the central and peripheral nervous systems, chemicals that inhibit AChE are known to produce a broad range of well-characterized symptoms of Ach poisoning (both muscrinic and nicotinic types, Table 17.2). Important steps involved in the mechanisms of toxicity of OPs and CMs are shown in Fig. 17.5. In general, OPs and CMs are considered irreversible and reversible AChE inhibitors, respectively.

Like the OP compounds, the mode of action of the CM is AChE inhibition with the important difference that the inhibition is more rapidly reversed than with OP compounds.

Signs and symptoms

Acute Toxicity In acute poisoning, onset of clinical signs usually occurs within 15 min to 1 h, followed by signs of maximal severity. However, the timing of maximal severity signs tends to vary depending on the OP/CM compound and its dose and species. For example, onset of clinical signs is delayed with chlorpyrifos (Dursban) and dimethoate (Rogor). Clinical signs observed in individuals can be either local or systemic effects. The local effects involve the eyes and the lungs because of their exposure to vapors or droplets of the insecticides. These effects, however, are of significance when exposure is via spraying. The systemic effects are primarily on the brain, skeletal muscles, lungs, heart, and other organs. The clinical signs can be muscarinic, nicotinic, or central in origin.

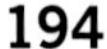

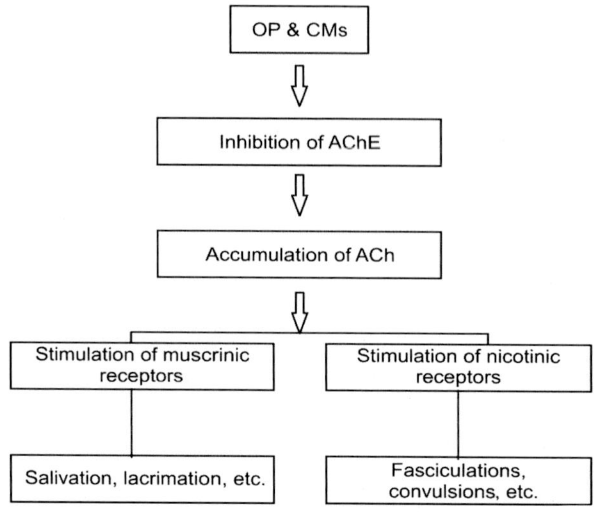

FIGURE 17.5

Important steps involved in mechanism of toxicity of organophosphorus (OP) and carbamate (CM) compounds.

Muscrinic and nicotinic effects produced by OP and CM insecticides are summarized in Table 17.2. Muscarinic receptor-associated effects are manifested by the following: vomiting; abdominal pain; salivation, lacrimation, urination, diarrhea (SLUD); miosis (pinpoint pupils); tracheobronchial secretion; lung edema; and cyanosis. The nicotinic receptor–associated effects are produced on autonomic ganglia and skeletal muscles, and the affected animals show twitching of muscles and tremors, followed by convulsions and seizures. This condition may lead to paralysis. The central effects include apprehension and stimulation, followed by depression, restlessness, ataxia, stiffness of the neck, and coma. Onset of death occurs due to respiratory failure and cardiac arrest. However, there are variations in clinical signs (as described) depending on the OP or CM compound and route of exposure. Poisoned individuals usually recover within 3 to 6 h with CMs and within 24 h with OPs; some individuals exposed to OP nerve agents may show signs of toxicity for days.

Chronic Toxicity Chronic toxicity is a major concern for those OP compounds that produce delayed neurotoxic effects. More than 40 years ago, tri-*o*-cresyl phosphate (TOCP) was known to produce delayed neurotoxic effects in humans and chickens, characterized by ataxia and weakness of the limbs, developing 10 to 14 days after exposure. This syndrome was called OP-induced delayed neuropathy (OPIDN). In recent literature, the syndrome has been renamed OP-induced delayed polyneuropathy (OPIDP). OPIDP is characterized by distal degeneration of long and large-diameter motor and sensory axons of peripheral nerves and the spinal cord. Among all animal species, the hen appears to be the most sensitive; therefore, it is used as an animal model. TOCP and certain other compounds have minimal or no anti-AChE properties; however, they cause phosphorylation and aging (dealkylation) of a protein in neurons called neuropathy target esterase (NTE) and subsequently lead to OPIDP. Today, many compounds, such as mipafox, tetraethyl pyrophosphate (TEPP), parathion, *o*-cresyl saligenin phosphate, and haloxon, are known to produce this syndrome. Some OPs as well as non-OP inhibitors (such as carbamates and sulfonyl fluorides) also covalently react with NTE but cannot undergo the aging reaction. As a result, these inhibitors do not cause OPIDP.

Diagnosis Poisoning cases of OP or CM are usually diagnosed based on clinical signs and quantified levels of AChE inhibition in blood. Inhibition of AChE activity is considered a positive case of poisoning. However, there is great species variability in normal values of AChE activity.

Treatment In acute poisoning, use of gastric lavage, cathartics, active charcoal, and other general treatment should be given. In case of dermal exposure, clothes should be removed and individuals should be washed thoroughly with water. Intravenous fluid therapy is always beneficial. In OP poisoning, antidotal treatment such as the combined use of atropine sulfate (2 mg in adults or 0.01–0.05 mg/kg in children, intravenous (IV) or intramuscular (IM), repeated after 15–60 min) and pyridine-2-aldoxime methochloride (2-PAM, 1–2 g in adults or 20–40 mg/kg in children, IV over 15–30 min, repeated in 1 h as required) should be administered. Atropine sulfate acts by blocking the muscarinic receptors from ACh. In OP and CM poisonings, the use of morphine, aminophyline, phenothiazine, and reserpine is to be avoided. However, use of respiratory support and correction of dehydration should be maintained. In CM poisoning, the use of oximes are contraindicated.

In the case of IMS, there is no specific treatment. The treatment is based on symptoms and therapy relies on atropine sulfate and 2-PAM. The administration of atropine sulfate and 2-PAM should be continued for a long period, even if the efficacy of these drugs in the development of IMS appears to be limited.

17.4.4 BOTANICAL INSECTICIDES

Extracts from plants have been used for centuries to control insects. Nicotine ((*S*)-3-(1-methyl-2-pyrrolidyl)pyridine) is an alkaloid occurring in a number of plants and was first used as an insecticide in 1763. Nicotine is quite toxic orally as well as dermally. The acute oral LD_{50} of nicotine sulfate for rats is 83 mg/kg, and the dermal LD_{50} is 285 mg/kg. Symptoms of acute nicotine poisoning occur rapidly, and death may occur within a few minutes. In serious poisoning cases, death results from respiratory failure due to paralysis of respiratory muscles. During therapy, attention is focused primarily on support of respiration. Pyrethrin is an extract from several types of chrysanthemum and is one of the oldest insecticides used by humans. There are six esters and acids associated with this botanical insecticide. Pyrethrin is applied at low doses and is considered to be nonpersistent. Mammalian toxicity to pyrethrins is quite low, apparently due to its rapid breakdown by liver microsomal enzymes and esterases. The acute LD_{50} for rats is approximately 1500 mg/kg. The most frequent reaction to pyrethrins is contact dermatitis and allergic respiratory reactions, probably as a result of other constituents in the formulation. Synthetic mimics of pyrethrins, known as the pyrethroids, were developed to overcome the lack of persistence. The toxicity of synthetic pyrethroid insecticides is discussed here.

17.4.5 PYRETHROID INSECTICIDES

As stated, pyrethrins are nonpersistent, which led pesticide chemists to develop compounds with a similar structure with insecticidal activity but that are more persistent. This class of insecticides, known as pyrethroids, has greater insecticidal activity and is more photostable than pyrethrins. There are two broad classes of pyrethroids depending on whether the structure contains a cyclopropane ring (eg, cypermethrin (($\pm$)-α-cyano-3-phenoxybenzyl ($\pm$)-*cis*,*trans*-3-(2,2-dichlorovinyl 2,2-dimethyl cyclopropanecarboxylate))) or whether this ring is absent in the molecule (eg, fenvalerate ((*RS*)-α-cyano-3-phenoxybenzyl(*RS*)-2-(4-chlorophenyl)-3-methylbutyrate)). They are generally applied at low doses (eg, 30 g/ha) and have low mammalian toxicities (eg, cypermethrin, oral (aqueous suspension), $LD_{50} = 4123$ mg/kg (rat) and dermal $LD_{50} > 2000$ mg/kg (rabbit)). Pyrethroids are used in both agricultural and urban settings (eg, termiticide). Pyrethrins affect nerve membranes by modifying the sodium and potassium channels, resulting in depolarization of the membranes. Formulations of these insecticides frequently contain the insecticide synergist piperonyl butoxide (5-(2-(2-butoxyethoxy) ethoxymethyl)-6-propyl-1,3-benzodioxole), which acts to increase the efficacy of the insecticide by inhibiting the cytochrome P450 enzymes responsible for the breakdown of the insecticide.

Signs and symptoms There are two types of pyrethroids, type I and type II. The signs of toxicity depend on the type of pyrethroid consumed. The usual signs of poising include restlessness, lack of coordination, sensory hyperactivity to external stimuli, fine tremors progressing to other parts of body, and hyperthermia.

Treatment There is no specific treatment. Treatment is based on symptoms and supportive; sedatives and central nervous system (CNS) muscle relaxants are recommended. Oils and fats should be avoided. Use of phenothiazine derivatives is contraindicated.

17.4.6 NEW INSECTICIDE CLASSES

There are new classes of insecticides that are applied at low dosages and are extremely effective but relatively nontoxic to humans. One such class is the fiproles, and one of these receiving major attention is fipronil ((5-amino-1-(2,6-dichloro-4-(trifluoromethyl) phenyl)-4-(1,*R*,*S*)-(trifluoromethyl)su-1-*H*-pyrasole-3-carbonitrile)). Although it is used on corn, it is becoming a popular termiticide because of its low application rate (approximately 0.01%) and long-term effectiveness. Another class of insecticides, the chloronicotinoids, is represented by imidacloprid (1-(6-chloro-3-pyridin-3-ylmethyl)-*N*-nitroimidazolidin-2-ylidenamine), which is also applied at low dose rates to soil and effectively controls a number of insect species, including termites (Fig. 17.6).

Treatment Most of these chemicals are nontoxic. In the case of toxicity, symptom-based treatment may be provided.

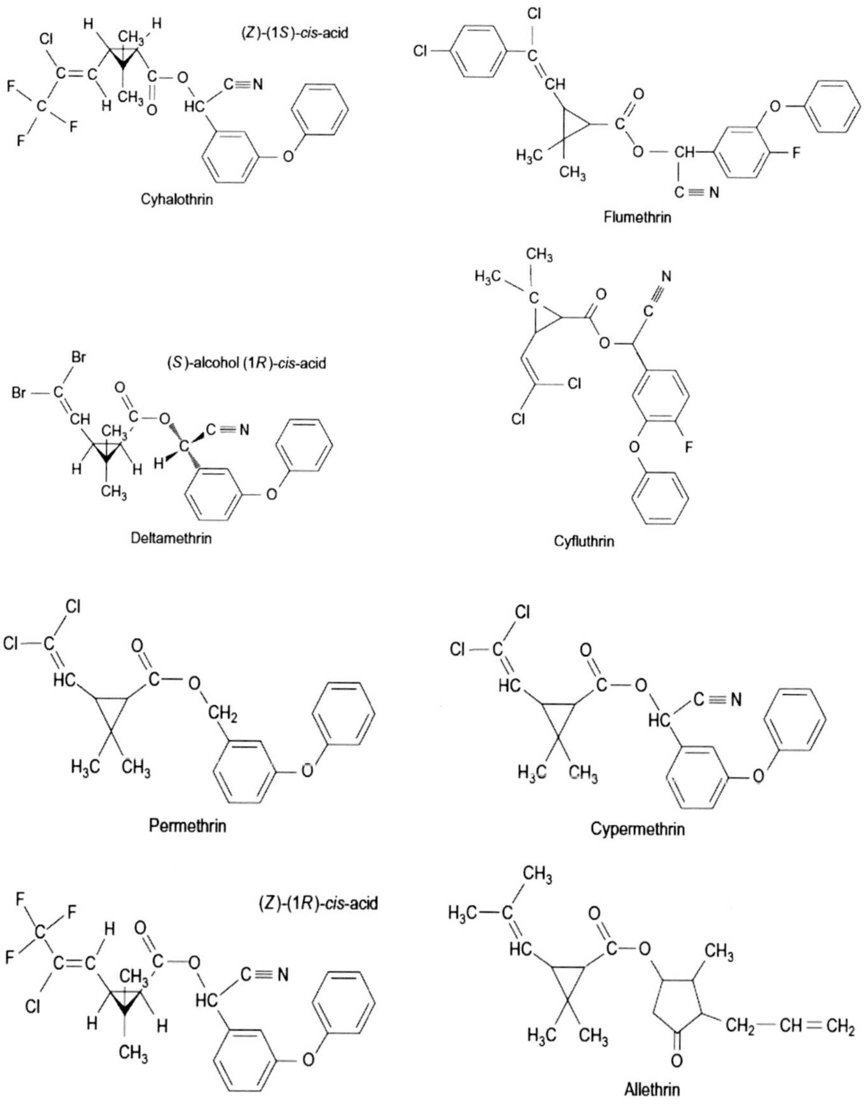

Cyhalothrin (*Z*)-(1*S*)-*cis*-acid

Flumethrin

Deltamethrin (*S*)-alcohol (1*R*)-*cis*-acid

Cyfluthrin

Permethrin

Cypermethrin

(*Z*)-(1*R*)-*cis*-acid

Allethrin

FIGURE 17.6

Structural formulae of selected pyrethroid insecticides.

17.5 HERBICIDES

Herbicides control weeds and are the most widely used class of pesticides. This class of pesticide can be applied to crops using many strategies to eliminate or reduce weed populations. These include preplant incorporation, pre-emergent applications, and postemergent applications. New families of herbicides continue to be developed; they are applied at low doses, relatively nonphytotoxic to beneficial plants, and environmentally friendly. The structural formulae of a few selected herbicides are given in Fig. 17.7.

Some of the newer families such as the imidazolinones inhibit the action of acetohydroxyacid synthase that produces branched-chain amino acids in plants. Because this enzyme is produced only in plants, these herbicides have low toxicities in mammals, fish, insects, and birds. The potential for environmental contamination continues to come from families of herbicides that have been used for years. The chlorophenoxy herbicides such as 2,4-*D* (2,4-dichlorophenoxy acetic acid) and 2,4,5-*T* (2,4,5-trichlorophenoxy-acetic acid) are systemic acting compounds to control broadleaf plants and have been in use since the 1940s. The oral toxicities of these compounds are low. A mixture of 2,4-*D* and 2,4,5-*T*, known as Agent Orange, was used by the US military as a defoliant during the Vietnam conflict, and much controversy has arisen over claims by military personnel of long-term health effects. The chemical of major toxicological concern was identified as a contaminant, TCDD (2,3,7,8-tetrachlorodibenzo-*p*dioxin), that was formed during the manufacturing process. TCDD is one of the most toxic

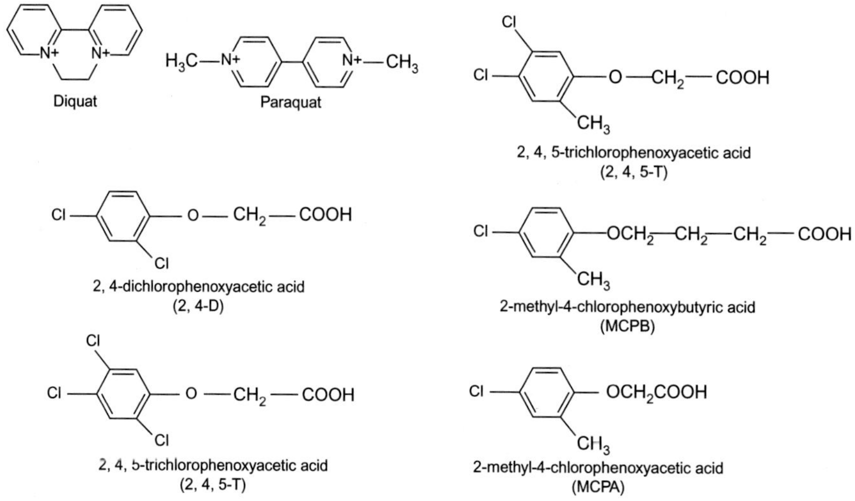

Diquat

Paraquat

2, 4, 5-trichlorophenoxyacetic acid (2, 4, 5-T)

2, 4-dichlorophenoxyacetic acid (2, 4-D)

2-methyl-4-chlorophenoxybutyric acid (MCPB)

2, 4, 5-trichlorophenoxyacetic acid (2, 4, 5-T)

2-methyl-4-chlorophenoxyacetic acid (MCPA)

FIGURE 17.7

Structural formulae of selected herbicides.

synthetic substances known in laboratory animals. In addition, it is toxic to developing embryos in pregnant rats and has been shown to cause birth defects. TCDD is a proven carcinogen in both mice and rats, with the liver being the primary target. This chemical has also been shown to alter the immune system and enhance susceptibility in exposed animals. Another family of herbicides, the triazines, continues to cause concern for environmentalists and toxicologists because of the contamination of surface and groundwater supplies that become public drinking water. The major concern with these types of compounds is their carcinogenic effects. A member of the bipyridylium family of herbicides is the compound paraquat (1,1-dimethyl-4,4-bipyridinium ion as the chloride salt). It is a very water-soluble contact herbicide that is active against a broad range of plants and is used as a defoliant on many crops. The compound binds tightly to soil particles following application and becomes inactivated. However, this compound is classified as a class I toxicant with an oral LD_{50} of 150 mg/kg (rat).

Mode of action The bipyridinium compounds are caustic and irritant agents that cause ulceration and necrosis of the skin and mucous membranes. They also cause progressive irreversible pulmonary fibrosis. Paraquat (Fig. 17.7) is actively taken up by the alveolar cells via a diamine or polyamine transport system, where it undergoes NADPH-dependent reduction. These are easily reduced to the radical ions, which generates superoxide radicals that react with unsaturated membrane lipids. The excess of superoxide anion radical O_2^- and H_2O_2 cause damage to the cellular membrane in lungs, which reduces the functional integrity of lung cells, affects efficient gas transport and exchange, and results in respiratory impairment. Diquat (Fig. 17.7) is also a very reactive compound and exerts its action in a similar manner, but it affects liver and kidney and does not cause pulmonary edema or alter lung function. Signs of CNS excitement and renal impairment occur in severely affected patients.

Signs and symptoms Most poisoning cases, which are often fatal, are due to accidental or deliberate ingestion of paraquat. Toxicity results from lung injury from the preferential uptake of paraquat by the lungs and the redox cycling mechanism.

Treatment There is no specific treatment for paraquat or diquat poisoning. Treatment is supportive and based on symptoms. Oxygen therapy is contraindicated because it will act as a ready source for the formation of more superoxides.

17.6 FUNGICIDES

The fungicide chlorothalonil (tetrachloroisophthalonitrile) is a broad-spectrum fungicide that is used widely in urban environments. It is relatively cheap and controls approximately 140 species of organisms. As a result of the popularity of this compound, it is found routinely in surface waters entering public drinking water supplies. In the formulation that can be purchased by the general

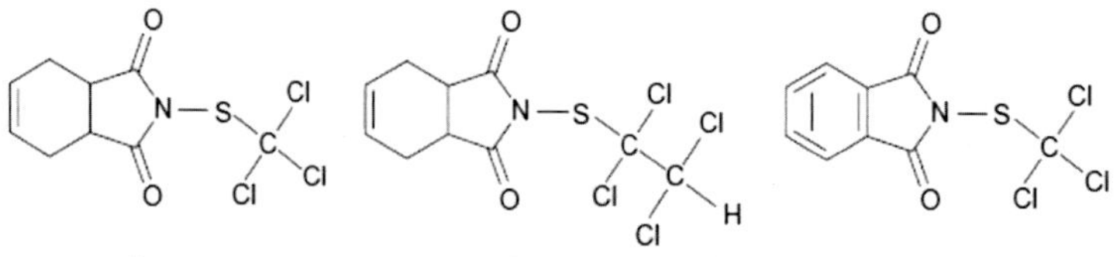

Captan Captafol Folpet

FIGURE 17.8

Structural formulae of selected fungicides.

public, it is relatively nontoxic. Other fungicides such as captan, captafol, folpet, dithiocarbamates, sulfur derivatives of dithiocarbamic acid, and metallic dimethyldithiocarbamates are commonly used. The latter group includes mancozeb (a coordination product of zinc ion and manganese ethylene bisdithiocarbamate), maneb (manganese ethylenebisdithiocarbamate), and zineb (zinc ethylenebisdithiocarbamate). All are effective fungicides and are used on a variety of crops, including grapes, sugar beets, and ornamental plants. Although relatively nontoxic, they do hydrolyze and produce known carcinogens such as ethylthiourea (ETU). The structural formulae of captan, captafol, and folpet are summarized in Fig. 17.8.

Treatment In most cases there is no specific treatment. Treatment is based on symptoms and supportive.

17.7 RODENTICIDES

This class of compounds is used to control rodents that cause yearly losses of 20% to 30% in grain and other food storage facilities. These pests harbor diseases in the form of fleas that carry bacteria and other organisms. A number of the rodenticides have been used for years and include warfarin (3-(α-acetonylbenzyl)-4-hydroxycoumarin), an anticoagulant. This is a potent toxicant with an oral LD_{50} of 3.0 mg/kg (rat). As the rats navigate through narrow passages, they bruise themselves, developing small hemorrhages. Anticoagulants prevent the blood from clotting, and the patients bleed to death in approximately 1 week. Other rodenticides poison the animal, and many times they are applied along with an attractant such as peanut butter to overcome bait shyness. Fluoroacetamide is a fast-acting poison with an oral LD_{50} (rat) of 15 mg/kg. This material is supplied as bait pellets or grains. ANTU (α-naphthylthiourea), strychnine, thallium salts, zinc phosphide, and others are also fast-acting poisons that have been on the market for many years. Most of the rodenticides are classified as restricted use and are applied only by licensed pest control operators. Human poisonings associated with rodenticides usually result from accidental or suicidal ingestion of the compounds. For details of toxicity, the reader may refer to individual compounds in others chapters of this book. The toxicity due to warfarin rodenticide has been discussed.

Mode of action Warfarin interferes with the normal function of vitamin K and causes coagulation defects characterized by decreased blood concentrations of coagulation protein factors. The decreased coagulation factors lead to massive internal hemorrhages and the affected individuals die due to tissue hypoxia.

Signs and symptoms After ingestion, the affected individuals show signs of hemorrhaging of gums, epistaxis, and massive internal bleeding, followed by shock and death.

Treatment In acute toxicity with warfarin, vitamin K_1 (phytonadione), if the poisoning is severe, and blood transfusions, if necessary, should be used. For poisoning due to other rodenticides, the treatment is supportive and based on symptoms.

17.8 FUMIGANTS

Fumigants are extremely toxic gases used to protect stored products, especially grains, and to kill soil nematodes. These materials are applied to storage warehouses, freight cars, and houses infested with insects such as powder post beetles. They present a special hazard due to inhalation exposure and rapid diffusion into pulmonary blood; therefore, extreme care must be taken when handling and applying this class of pesticides. All fumigants are classified as restricted use compounds and require licensed applicators to handle them. The most effective fumigants are aluminum phosphide and methyl bromide. Methyl bromide essentially sterilizes soil when applied because it kills insects, nematodes, and weed seed, but it is also used to fumigate warehouses. Overexposure to this compound causes respiratory distress, cardiac arrest, and central nervous effects. The inhalation LC_{50} is 0.06 mg/L (15 min) of air (rat) and 7900 ppm (1.5 h) (human). Methyl bromide has been classified as an ozone depleter under the Clean Air Act and is due to be phased out of use by 2005. Chloropicrin (trichloronitromethane) is another soil/space fumigant that has been used for many years. It has an inhalation LC_{50} of 150 ppm (15 min). Thus, it is highly toxic by inhalation, can injure the heart, and can cause severe eye damage. For details of toxicity due to hydrogen cyanide and carbon disulfide and other individual fumigants, the reader is referred to other chapters in this book.

Treatment The treatment is supportive and based on symptoms. In case of poisoning by methyl bromide antacids and sodium bicarbonate, therapy is given to control acidosis. Convulsions can be controlled by barbiturates. In case of dermal exposure, removal of clothes and washing of the skin may be useful.

17.8.1 ALUMINUM PHOSPHIDE

Aluminum phosphide is a solid fumigant pesticide widely used as a grain preservative in India. It is marketed as grayish green tablets (trade names: Alphos, Celphos, Chemfume, Delicia, Fumigrain, Phosphume, Quickphos, Synfume, etc.). It is used as suicidal and homicidal poisoning.

Mode of action On exposure to air or moisture, it liberates phosphine and can produce multiorgan damage.

Signs and symptoms Signs and symptoms include metallic taste; garlicky odor; nausea; pain in gullet, stomach, or abdomen; vomiting; diarrhea; cough dyspnea; respiratory failure; headache; anxiety; hypotension tachycardia/bradycardia; myocarditis; hepatosplenomegaly; renal failure; coma; and others. The fatal dose is 5 g and the fatal period is up to 24 h.

Treatment Symptom-based treatment should include removal of clothing and washing of the contaminated skin with water. Ematics, gastric lavage with 3 to 5% $NaHCO_3$, and general supportive measures along with vitamin K therapy may be useful.

17.8.2 NAPHTHALENE (MOTHBALLS)

Naphthalene is used as a household insecticide. It is a solid volatile substance obtained from the middle fraction of coal tar distillation and has chemical properties similar to benzene. It occurs as large, lustrous, crystalline plates with a characteristic odor. It is soluble in water and dissolves freely in ether, chloroform, alcohol, and oils. Accidental poisoning in children is common and humans may use it for the purpose of suicide.

Mode of action Naphthalene is an irritant, nephrotoxic, hemolytic, and hepatotoxic.

Signs and symptoms Signs of toxicity such as nausea, vomiting, abdominal pain, strangury, hemoglobinuria, nephritis, jaundice, and hemolytic anemia may be common, followed by optic neuritis, profuse perspiration, cyanosis, convulsions, and coma. The fatal dose is 2 g and the fatal period is uncertain.

Postmortem findings Skin and gastrointestinal mucosa are yellowish, congested, or inflamed. Liver and kidney may show severe damage. The respiratory tract show signs of irritation and other organs are congested.

Treatment General measures such as blood transfusion and stomach wash should be used. Magnesium sulfate and sodium bicarbonate orally may be useful to alkalinize the urine. A dose of 25 g hydrocortisone hemisuccinate and IV glucose may also be useful.

CHAPTER

Toxic effects of metals 18

CHAPTER OUTLINE

18.1 INTRODUCTION

Metals are certainly one of the oldest toxicants known to humans due to their very early use. For instance, human use of lead probably started before 2000 BC, when abundant supplies were obtained from ores as a by-product of smelting silver. The first description of abdominal colic in a man who extracted metals is credited to Hippocrates in 370 BC. Arsenic and mercury are discussed by Theophrastus of Erebus (370–287 BC), and by Pliny and Elder (AD 23–79). Arsenic was used for decorating Egyptian tombs and as a "secret poison." These metals have also been used to make utensils, machinery, and other products. These activities have increased environmental levels of metals. More recently metals have found a number of uses in industry, agriculture, and medicine. These activities have increased exposure not only to metal-related occupational workers but also to the environment. Contamination to the public is prevalent. Despite the wide range of metal toxicity and toxic properties, there are a number of toxicological features that are common to many metals. A few these metals that are important are discussed here.

18.2 ARSENIC (SANKHYAL, SOMALKAR)

Arsenic is a heavy, metallic, inorganic, irritant poison. Metallic arsenic is not poisonous because it is insoluble in water and cannot be absorbed from the gastrointestinal (GI) tract. However, arsenious oxide or arsenic trioxide (sankhyal or somalker) is poisonous. Two organic nontoxic arsenic variants mostly present in food regularly consumed by humans are arsenobetaine and arsenocholine.

Fundamentals of Toxicology. DOI: http://dx.doi.org/10.1016/B978-0-12-805426-0.00018-4

They are found in shellfish, cod, and haddock. Sources of poisoning include soil, well water, shellfish, and arsenic compounds. Absorption is possible through all routes.

Mode of action Arsenic compounds act by inactivating the sulfhydral enzymes, which in turn interfere with the cellular metabolism in the liver, lungs, intestinal wall, and spleen. Arsenic can replace phosphorus in the bones, where it may remain for years. It also gets deposited in the hair. Studies of arsenic in drinking water suggest that arsenic can cause skin, lung, liver, kidney, and bladder cancer in 1 in 1000 cases. The fatal dose is 100 to 200 mg of arsenious oxide and the fatal period is usually 2 to 3 days. The toxicity rating is 5 for all arsenic salts, except arsenic trioxide.

Signs and symptoms Arsenic poisoning clinically manifests in three forms: (1) acute (fulminating); (2) subacute (gastroenteritis type); and (3) chronic.

Acute Poisoning (Fulminating Type) In acute poisoning, symptoms appear within half an hour, especially when heavy doses of arsenic are consumed (3–5 g). The acute fulminating type occurs due to inhibition of the sulphydryl enzyme system, which is necessary for cellular metabolism, and also due to its potential capillary poisoning action. It causes marked dilatation of capillaries and myocardial failure, resulting in decrease of blood pressure, shock, and instantaneous death.

Subacute Poisoning (Gastroenteritis Type) Subacute poisoning occurs when small doses of arsenic are administered at repeated intervals. It resembles cases of cholera or food poisoning. The first symptoms are dyspepsia, cough, and tingling in the throat, followed by vomiting, purging with abdomen pain, and tenesmus. At first, the stool is watery, but later it becomes bloody. However, the difference between arsenic poison and cholera may be enumerated as follows:

- In arsenic poisoning, vomiting precedes purging (stools are watery initially and later are blood-stained), there is pain in the throat, the voice remains unaffected, conjunctiva becomes inflamed, and vomit contains mucous, bile, and streaks of blood. Arsenic can be detected on chemical examination.
- In cholera, purging precedes vomiting (stools are watery throughout and passed in a continuous involuntary jet), there is no pain in the throat, the voice becomes rough and whistling, conjunctiva is normal, and vomit is watery. *Cholera vibrio* can be detected on microscopic examination.

Chronic Poisoning Chronic poisoning occurs in occupational workers engaged in smeltering or refining ore or long-term exposure to arsenic compounds. Chronic poisoning with arsenic presents with a sequence of five different manifestations:

- *Gastrointestinal:* The victim shows gradual weight loss, malnutrition, fatigue, loss of appetite, cirrhosis of liver, nausea, and vomiting.
- *Catarrhal changes:* Symptoms include runny nose, headache, conjunctivitis, and bronchial inflammation.

- *Raindrop pigmentation:* This is known to produce a "milk and roses" complexion initially, followed by patchy brown pigmentation of the skin (especially face), which resembles raindrops. It might also show hyperkeratosis of the skin of the palm and soles, which is prone to change into basal cell carcinoma at a later stage. The scalp may also show alopecia (baldness).
- *Meese's lines:* The victim's nails manifest with whitish lines 1 to 2 mm across the nails of the fingers and toes, representing the deposition of the poison as a result of high sulfhydral content of the keratin.
- *Arsenical neuritis:* The victim presents with polyneuritis, optic neuritis, anesthesias, paresthesias, and atrophy of extensors resulting in wrist and foot drop.

Diagnosis A urinary level >100 mg/24 h is suggestive of arsenic toxicity. Blood and hair levels are not reliable.

Postmortem findings Postmortem findings include dehydrated body, pigmented (or rarely jaundiced) skin, cyanosed hands and feet, and Mee's lines on the nails. Rigor mortis takes unusually longer. Stomach is velvety red or brown, patchy areas with small ulcerations are seen on the stomach mucosa, and gastric contents emit a garlicky odor. Heart shows subendocardial hemorrhage. Other viscera may show fatty degeneration of liver, kidney, and heart. Brain may show acute encephalitis with hemorrhagic spots.

Treatment Symptomatic treatment including hemodialysis is the first-line choice in massive arsenic poisoning. Gastric lavage is performed with warm water or with freshly prepared hydrated ferric oxide solution. Butter and other greasy substances that act as demulcents are given to prevent further absorption of the poison.

Specific antidotes are BAL—chelation therapy in the dose of 400–800 mg on the first day, followed by 200–400 mg on the next 2 days, and then the dose is tapered slowly. DMSA (Dimercapto succinic acid) or DMPS (Dimercapto propane sulfonate) penicillamine, calcium disodium versnate, and others may also be useful. Injection of vitamin B_1 helps with peripheral neuritis.

18.3 MERCURY (QUICK SILVER, LIQUID METAL, PARA, PADARASA)

Mercury is a liquid metal and a metallic, inorganic, irritant poison. It is available in inorganic, organic, and metallic forms. Metallic mercury is a heavy, silvery liquid; it is not poisonous. However, it volatilizes at room temperature, and the inhalation of vapors is toxic. A potential source of elemental mercury is at home, which includes mercury switches and mercury-containing devices such as thermometers, thermostats, and barometers. Other sources include laboratories, dental amalgam filling, cosmetics, calomel teething powder, and industrial sources. Absorption is possible through all routes. The pure metallic form is nontoxic. However, mercurial compounds can act by inactivating sulfhydral enzymes, thus interfering with cellular metabolism. A classic example of environmental contamination due to mercury

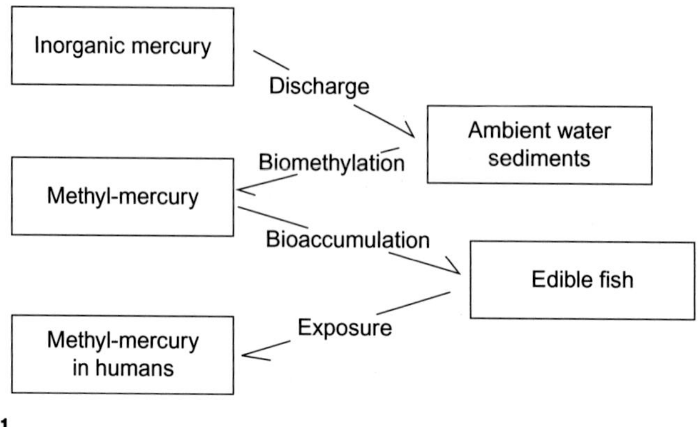

FIGURE 18.1

Environmental cycling and conversion of inorganic mercury to methyl-mercury.

and its health implications is the Minamata Bay disaster in Japan in the 1950s, which consisted of a devastating epidemic of mercury poisoning.

Environmental cycling The discharge of mercury led to large-scale human methyl mercury exposure and toxicity during the 1950s and 1960s. Less toxic inorganic mercury gets converted through biomethylation to a more toxic form of mercury. The schematic representation of mercury's environmental cycling, biomethylation, and food chain transfer is shown in Fig. 18.1.

Toxicity Although the metallic form of mercury is nontoxic, its vapors as well as finely divided small particles can be toxic. The health effects depend on its chemical form, route of exposure, and duration of exposure. The clinical manifestations of toxicity involve multiple organ systems with variable features and intensity. Vapors from elemental mercury and methyl mercury are more easily absorbed than inorganic mercury salts and are more harmful. Elemental mercury volatilizes and inhalation of vapors potentially causes adverse health effects because it is easily absorbed. This discharge caused large-scale human methyl mercury exposure and toxicity during the 1950s and 1960s and led to our present-day appreciation of mercury's environmental cycling, biomethylation, and food chain transfer (Fig. 18.1). In general, the target system of various forms of mercury is as follows:

- *Elemental Mercury*: the vapors target the respiratory system.
- *Inorganic Mercury*: mainly affects kidneys and the GI tract.
- *Organic Mercury*: mainly affects the central nervous system.

There is convincing evidence that shows inorganic and organic mercury are associated with genotoxicity, teratogenicity, and embryotoxicity. There are several inorganic mercurial compounds that are toxic. A fatal dose of mercuric chloride is 100–400 mg, and the fatal period is a few hours to 1 to 2 weeks. Table 18.1 summarizes the manifestations of mercury toxicity.

Table 18.1 Summary of Mercury Toxicity

Organ or System Affected	Manifestations
Brain	Memory loss, attention deficit, ataxia, impairment of hearing and vision, sensory disturbances, fatigue, autism in children
Motor system	Disruption of motor function, decreased muscular strength, late walking in children
Kidney	Increased plasma creatinine level
Heart	Alteration of normal cardiovascular homeostasis
Immune system	Decreased immunity, multiple sclerosis, autoimmune thyroiditis
Reproductive system	Decreased fertility rate, abnormal offspring

Acute Poisoning Symptoms usually commence within half an hour after swallowing mercuric chloride:

- Initially, there is an acrid, metallic taste; constriction of the throat; hoarse voice; and difficulty in breathing. The tongue and mouth get corroded, followed by a burning sensation extending down the abdomen. Vomiting of grayish slimy material with bloody streaks occurs, followed by blood-stained diarrhea and tenesmus. Oral consumption can lead to glossitis, ulcerative gingivitis, and necrosis of the jaw.
- Nephrotoxicity leads to albuminuria, uremia, and acidosis. Urine is scanty and contains blood and albumin. Toxic mercury compounds are considered nephrotoxic poisons and cause renal tubular and glomerular necrosis.
- Inhalation of mercury fumes can lead to metallic taste, salvation, gingivitis, and loosening of teeth, along with fetid teeth.
- Strong concentrations may cause ataxia, paresis, and delirium.
- Locally, mercury salts have corrosive action.
- Blood peripheral smear can show leukocytosis, whereas leucopenia occurs with organic mercurial poisoning.

Chronic Poisoning (Hydrargyrism/Mercurialism) The word hydrargyrism is from the Latin word *hydragyrus*, which means mercury. Chronic poisoning occurs when the victim is exposed to mercury fumes in factories or when an excessive dose of mercurial compound is used for a prolonged period. Symptoms begin to appear at blood levels of 100 nanogram % of mercury. The main manifestations are:

- Excessive salivation (ptyalism/sialorrhea), with swollen and painful salivary glands, metallic taste in the mouth, glossitis, ulcerative gingivitis, and necrosis of the jaw.
- A blue line on the gums called the Burtonian line is a common clinical finding of chronic poisoning.

- Nausea, colicky pain, vomiting, and diarrhea are other gastrointestinal manifestations.
- Evidence of nephritis and uremia may be seen.
- *Mercuria lentis* develops; it is due to a brownish deposit of mercury through the cornea on the anterior lens capsule and can be observed as a brown reflex on slit-lamp examination.
- *Mercurial tremors* can be detected during early stages with a change in handwriting of the person because they first affect the muscles of the finger, followed by muscles of the tongue, causing stammering and slurring speech; finally, they affect the muscles of the face, arms, and legs. This was referred to as Hatter's shake among the workers in the hat industry, in which mercury was used extensively to give a peculiar kinking shape to felt hats. Other drugs and poisons that produce tremors are alcohol, phenothiazines, caffeine, theophylline, tricyclic antidepressants, carbon monoxide, and phosphorus.
- *Mercurial erethism* comprises personality change, resulting in an abnormally high degree of irritability, sensitivity, or excitability, shyness, amnesia, insomnia, delusions, and hallucination, leading to insanity.

Postmortem findings Apparently, there are no specific postmortem findings. The mucous membranes of the lips, mouth, and pharynx show a diffuse, grayish white, escharotic appearance. Stomach and intestine show severe irritation and corrosion with ulceration and softening. Intestines, especially the cecum, colon, and rectum, are inflamed, ulcerated, or even gangrenous when the patient survives for some days. The kidneys show findings of toxic nephritis. The liver shows fatty degeneration. The heart shows subendocardial hemorrhages and fatty degeneration.

Treatment Treatment is symptom-based. Gastric lavage with a 5% solution of sodium formaldehyde sulfoxylate is often used. Approximately 100 mL of the same may be left in the stomach after the lavage. Administration of demulcents like egg albumin, medicinal charcoal, with magnesium sulfate, is of great use.

Specific antidotes are BAL (dimercaprol at a dose of 3–4 mg/kg body weight, every 4 h), penicillamine at a dose of 250 mg to 2 g orally, or sodium formaldehyde sulphoxylate as a chemical antidote.

18.4 LEAD (SHISHA)

Lead is a metallic, inorganic, irritant poison. According to Health and Human Services Department USA, lead poisoning is the most important environmental problem for young children. Blood levels once thought to be safe have been shown to be associated with IQ deficits, behavior disorders, slow growth, and impaired hearing. Studies of population blood–lead concentrations have shown a decrease by up to 80% in the past 20 years, but cases of lead poisoning continue to occur. Poisoning is more common from chronic occupational exposure among lead smelters, battery manufacturers, painters, and decorators. Chronic exposure may also occur at home from paint, pottery, and drinking water contaminated by lead pipes used for the city water supply. Absorption is possible through all routes.

Mode of action Pure metallic forms of lead are nontoxic, as is the steel gray metal. However, lead compounds can act by producing spasms of the capillaries and arterioles or by fixation of the poison in tissues such as brain and bones. It can also combine with sulfhydryl enzymes and interfere with their action. Lead can decrease the synthesis of heme, leading to anemia, and it can bring about hemolysis as well as release immature red blood cells (RBCs) into circulation (reticulocytosis and basophilic stippling of RBCs). Lead can destroy nerve cells and myelin sheaths in central nervous system, and it can also produce cerebral edema. It also exerts toxic effects on kidneys (nephritis) and the reproductive system (infertility). Common toxic compounds are lead acetate, lead carbonate, lead chromates, lead oleate, lead oxide, lead sulfide, lead tetroxide, and tertraethyl lead. The fatal dose depends on the toxic compound (20 g of lead acetate). The fatal period is 1 to 2 days.

Signs and symptoms

Acute Poisoning Acute poisoning usually occurs with a high dosage of lead acetate. It starts with burning and dryness in the throat, salivation, and intense thirst. Vomiting occurs within 24 h, with colicky pain and a tender abdomen. Constipation is a common feature and urine is scanty. Finally, there may be peripheral circulatory collapse, headache, insomnia, paresthesia, depression, convulsions, exhaustion, and coma leading to death.

Subacute Poisoning Subacute poisoning occurs from repeated small doses of lead acetate. A blue line is seen on the gums, along with GI symptoms. Urine is scanty and deep red in color. During the later stages, nervous symptoms become prominent, with numbness, cramps, and flaccid paralysis of the lower limbs. Death is rare, but it may occur after convulsions and coma.

Chronic Poisoning (Plumbism, Saturnism) Chronic poisoning with lead compounds may lead to the following:

Facial Pallor: Pallor that is seen especially around the mouth. It is also known as circum oral pallor and is due to the vasospasm of the capillaries and arterioles around the mouth.

- *Anemia*: Hypochromic, microcytic anemia with reticulocytosis and punctuate basophilia with the presence of marked basophilic stippling in the RBCs. Platelet count decreases. Anemia is probably due to decreased survival time of RBCs and inhibition of heme synthesis by interference with the incorporation of iron into protoporphyrin.
- *Burtonian line (lead line)*: A stippled blue line seen at the junction of the gums, usually nearer to tooth caries, especially in the upper jaw. This is due to the deposition of lead sulfide formed by the action of the combination of lead sulfide formed by the action of the combination of lead with hydrogen sulfide, which evolved from the decomposed food debris in the caries tooth.

- *Lead colic and constipation*: The victim will report severe colicky pain in the abdomen relieved by pressure and bowel irregularities. Abdominal muscles become tense and retracted.
- *Lead palsy*: A typical paralysis affecting the extensor muscles of the fingers and wrist causing wrist drop and claw-shaped hand. Similarly, paralysis may extend to the extensor muscles of the foot, leading to foot drop.
- *Lead encephalopathy*: Mostly seen in infants presenting with severe ataxia, vomiting, lethargy, stupor, convulsion, and coma; cerebral psychic effects may be present.
- *Cardiorenal manifestations*: Elevated blood pressure and arteriosclerotic changes are observed. Urine contains albumin and an abnormal quantity of lead, coproporphyrin III, and delta amino laevulinic acid. Interstitial nephritis may occur.
- *Sterility/infertility*: Both may be observed.
- *General manifestations*: These include weakness, anorexia, metallic taste in the mouth, dyspepsia, and foul breath.

Diagnosis

- Urine lead levels of more than 0.08 mg/L collected in 24 h
- Blood lead level more than 0.8 mg/L
- Increased coproporphyrin level in urine
- Increased urine and plasma delta-amino laevulinic acid
- X-ray evidence of increased density or radio-opaque bands or lines at the metaphyseal ends of long bones in children; this is also referred to as lead lines
- Presence of lead as radio-opaque material on X-ray of stomach and intestines may be seen in children, particularly those with a history of pica (abnormal craving for non-nutritive substances)

Postmortem findings In acute poisoning, stomach–gastric mucosa is congested, eroded, and patchy in appearance with grayish white deposits. Large intestine may show black fecal matter. There may be evidence of renal tubular degeneration.

In chronic poisoning, a blue line on the gums is seen. Muscles are flaccid and show fatty degeneration. Intestines are contracted and thickened. Liver and kidneys are hard and contracted. Heart is hypertrophied. Renal tubular necrosis is usually noticed.

Treatment For acute poisoning, supportive therapy such as emetics, stomach wash with 1% magnesium or sodium sulfate solution, 25 g of magnesium sulfate orally with demulcent drinks, calcium gluconate 1 g to relieve colic, and intravenous fluids may be useful.

- Potassium or sodium iodine for eliminating lead through the kidney
- Large dose of sodium bicarbonate: 20 to 30 g per day in divided doses increases the output of lead because of the transformation of the insoluble tribasic lead phosphate into the soluble dibasic lead phosphate through the liberated carbonic acid

- Calcium gluconate or calcium chloride to relieve colic
- Specific treatment like EDTA, Bal, penicillamine, and calcium disodium versanate may be useful as chelating agents

18.5 COPPER (THAMBE, BLUE VITRIOL)

Copper, an inorganic metallic irritant, is not poisonous in the metallic state, but some of its salts are poisonous, such as copper sulfate (blue vitriol) and copper subacetate (verdigris).

Copper Sulfate: Copper sulfate is a blue crystalline salt and a metallic taste. In a small dose of 0.5 g, it acts as an emetic; however, in large doses it acts as an irritant poison. Poisoning is usually accidental or suicidal. Homicidal use is rare because of its metallic taste and striking blue color.

Copper Subacetate or Verdigris: Copper subacetate is a bluish green salt. It is formed by the action of vegetable acids while cooking in copper utensils that have been not properly tin-lined. Thus, accidental verdigris poisoning from contamination of food cooked in such utensils is often reported.

Chronic poisoning is common among industrial workers working with copper and copper salts or its alloys because of inhalation of copper dust or fumes. Copper welders may develop metal fume fever. Chronic copper poisoning is also observed among those who consume contaminated food with verdigris obtained from dirty copper vessels for a long period. Airborne dust of inorganic copper salts has been reported to produce low toxicity. Hystiocytic granulomatous lung and liver disease have been observed among individuals who were exposed to copper sulfate spray for 2 to 15 years.

Signs and symptoms

Acute Poisoning Renal failure and death may follow ingestion of as little as 1 g of copper sulfate. However, fatal poisoning by copper is very rare. Symptoms of poisoning commence within 15 to 30 min after swallowing the poison. There is a metallic taste in the mouth. Salivation and thirst are present. The mucosa of the mouth has a blue discoloration. There is pain in the mouth, esophagus, and stomach. Vomiting and diarrhea occur. Vomit is blue or green in color. Stool is brownish or bloody. Oligurea, hematuria, and uremia may develop in some individuals. There may also be low urinary output, with casts and albumin in the urine. Jaundice occurs in severe cases due to centrilobular necrosis and biliary stasis. Later, muscular spasms cramps, coma, and circulatory collapse precede death.

Intravenous copper intoxication leads to symptoms of nausea, vomiting, abdominal pain, diarrhea, anxiety, and depression. Copper released from copper tubing during hemodialysis was noticed among patients undergoing hemodialysis.

Chronic Poisoning The symptom complex of chronic poisoning is called by several names, such as hemochromatosis, bronzed diabetes, and pigment cirrhosis. It presents with a green or purple line on the gums, coppery taste in the mouth, nausea, headache, colicky pain, vomiting, diarrhea, and anemia. Atrophy of the muscles may be the other symptom observed. Skin is jaundiced and urine and perspiration become green.

A fatal dose of copper sulfate is 30 g, and that of verdigris is 15 g.

Postmortem findings In acute poisoning, externally, the mucosa of the mouth and tongue may show a bluish or greenish blue tinge. Internally, the same tinge is observed on the mucous membranes of the esophagus and stomach. Stomach mucosa is congested, desquamated, and hemorrhagic. The upper part of the small intestine may also show mild to moderate irritation. The chief findings are fatty degeneration of the liver and degeneration of the epithelial cells of the kidney.

In chronic poisoning, the gums appear unhealthy and have a bluish lining. There is mucosal atrophy. Liver and kidneys show varying degrees of degeneration. Poisoning due to inhalation of vapors can chronically present with findings of chronic pneumonitis. The blood picture may show premature cells in the peripheral smear of the victim. Skin may be yellow due to jaundice. The mucosa of the mouth, esophagus, and stomach has a greenish-blue discoloration and may show areas of corrosion and congestion. The colon and rectum may show large ulcerations or perforations. The liver may be enlarged and show fatty degeneration. Copper is one of those poisons that can be detected by its characteristic color. The kidneys are congested and may show focal necrosis of proximal tubules.

Treatment General management should include removal of the cause and prevent further exposure. The following should be performed:

- Provide fresh air, give massage and warm bath, provide proper diet; copper vessels, if used for cooking, should be tinned and regularly kept scrupulously clean
- Stomach washes with warm water
- Egg albumin acts as an antidote by forming an insoluble and innocuous copper albuminate

Stomach wash with potassium ferrocyanide 1% solution in water also acts as an antidote by forming cupric ferrocyanide. Calcium EDTA or BAL is the recommended antidote. Maintain electrolyte and fluid balance.

18.6 IRON

Iron is an inorganic metallic irritant. Most exposures involve children younger than age 6 years who have ingested pediatric multivitamin preparations. Most of these patients remain asymptomatic or develop minimal toxicity. Concentrated iron supplement overdoses more often result in serious poisoning. However, if the patient does not develop any symptoms within 6 h of ingestion, it is unlikely that iron toxicity will develop.

Iron salts are used for treatment of prophylaxis from iron deficiency anemia. There are several iron preparations containing different amounts of elemental iron. Usually, iron salts poisoning incidences are reported in children due to consumption of an adult dose by mistake or due to IV injection. Ferrous sulfate and ferric chloride are some of the toxic compounds.

Mode of action The early features of iron poisoning are due to corrosive effects of iron, whereas later effects are largely due to the disruption of the cellular process. Iron tablets may adhere to the stomach and duodenum, causing irritation in some cases and causing hemorrhagic necrosis and perforation in severe cases. Absorbed iron is rapidly cleared from extracellular spaces by uptake into parenchymal cells, particularly in the liver. It causes mitochondrial damage and cellular dysfunction, resulting in metabolic acidosis and necrosis. Eventually, widespread organ damage becomes apparent, and hepatic failure with hypoglycemia and coagulopathy may develop. This is often fatal.

Signs and symptoms The clinical course of iron poisoning occurs in four phases:

Phase 1: During the first few hours (from 30 min to several hours) after ingestion, there is vomiting, abdominal pain, and hemorrhagic gastroenteritis with black or gray vomit and stool with a metallic odor. In severe cases, gastrointestinal hemorrhage can result with circulatory collapse, and coma may supervene.

Phase 2: During the second stage, 6–24 h after ingestion, the patient shows improvement and the clinical symptoms abate. The patient either recovers or moves on to the next phase. In severe cases, this may not appear or a latent phase occurs and is deceptively reassuring.

Phase 3: The third stage occurs 12 to 48 h after ingestion and is characterized by severe lethargy, coma, convulsions, gastrointestinal hemorrhage, shock, cardiovascular collapse, metabolic acidosis, hepatic failure with hepatocellular necrosis, jaundice, hypoglycemia, coagulopathy, pulmonary edema, and renal failure.

Phase 4: This is a late phase, with complications such as formation of gastric strictures and pyloric stenosis occurring after 2–5 weeks.

A fatal dose is 20–40 g of ferrous sulfate or >150 mg of elemental iron. The fatal period is uncertain.

Diagnosis X-ray of the abdomen shows iron tablets. Serum iron level is >150 microgram %.

Treatment

Nonspecific Nonspecific treatment includes gastric lavage with a dilute solution of sodium bicarbonate (2%). Demulcent drinks like milk or egg albumin are useful. Whole-bowel irrigation in acute poisoning is found to be safe and effective. However, there is no report in controlled studies that confirm this finding. Electrolyte correction and intravenous (IV) glucose may be useful.

Antidote Deferoxamine (Desferrioxamine) is the specific antidote. A solution of 2 g in 1 L of water can be used for gastric lavage, followed by 2 g in 10 mL of sterile water that should be left in the stomach; 2 g of this is then administered intramuscular (IM) or by a slow IV infusion at the rate of 15 mg/kg body weight per hour to a maximum of 80 mg/kg in 24 h.

CHAPTER

Toxic effects of nonmetallics 19

CHAPTER OUTLINE

19.1 INTRODUCTION

Nonmetallic chemicals such as phosphorus, chlorine, bromine, iodine, formaldehyde, methyl aldehyde, and methylene oxide act as irritant poisons and produce inflammation on the site of contact, especially in the gastrointestinal (GI) tract, respiratory tract, and the skin. When a poison has a systemic effect and death occurs, then it is classified as a cerebral poison or a spinal poison. Irritant poisons should be differentiated from certain natural diseases of the GI tract such as cholera, acute gastritis, acute gastroenteritis, perforated gastric ulcer, peritonitis, and colic. In general, after ingestion, irritant poisons will manifest (within 30–60 min).

19.2 TOXICITY OF NONMETALLICS

In general, the following signs and symptoms of nonmetallic toxicity may be observed.

GI Symptoms: GI symptoms include burning pain in the mouth, throat, esophagus, and stomach that radiates all over the abdomen, intense thirst, and dysphasia due to painful deglutition. The individual cannot ingest water or food, which leads to dehydration and starvation with continuous painful vomiting. Initially the vomit shows normal contents, but later it turns bilious or contains altered blood. The patient will have continuous severe diarrhea and tenesmus. Stools initially will be soft and loose, but later they are mixed with mucus and blood.

Collapse due to shock with rapid, feeble pulse; pale, anxious face; cold, clammy skin; sighing respiration; and cramps in leg muscles may develop.

Fundamentals of Toxicology. DOI: http://dx.doi.org/10.1016/B978-0-12-805426-0.00019-6

Convulsions, loss of consciousness, extreme exhaustion, and death can also occur when not treated properly. If the person survives, then stricture may develop in the esophagus later, which can contribute to dysphagia and lead to starvation.

Respiratory Symptoms: Respiratory symptoms include cough, feeling of constriction of the chest, breathlessness, suffocation, pulmonary edema, and hemoptysis.

Dermal Symptoms: Dermal symptoms are (as in the case of radioactive substances, insect and snake bites, etc.) pain, irritation, itching, redness, vesication, and blisters.

19.3 PHOSPHORUS

Phosphorus is a nonmetallic, inorganic, hepatotoxic, protoplasmic irritant poison. It exists in two forms—white or yellow and red phosphorus. Derivatives of phosphorus include aluminum phosphide, zinc phosphide, and phosphine gas.

Mode of action Phosphorus acts as a protoplasmic poison that causes normal metabolism to be disturbed and cellular oxidation to be severely affected, resulting in specific changes in liver, bone, kidneys (acute renal failure), and lungs.

Liver: Liver changes include necrobiosis, which resembles ischemia, prevents cellular metabolism, and inhibits glycogen deposition with excess fat deposition, resulting in extensive fatty degeneration and acute hepatic necrosis. Thus, phosphorus is a hepatotoxic substance.

Bone: The observed bone change is called Phossy jaw. Phossy jaw is a type of osteomyelitis of the jaw observed in chronic cases of phosphorus poisoning. Bone formation under the epiphyseal cartilage, haversian canal, and marrow canal increases. This results in a decrease in blood circulation to bone, resulting in necrosis and sequestration of bone.

Lung: Phosphene gas (PH_3) reduces oxyhemoglobin in the blood and may be fatal if more than 20 parts of phosphene is present in 100,000 parts of air. It can also induce respiratory inflammation and pulmonary symptoms.

Kidneys: Kidney changes constitute renal damage with acute renal failure.

Signs and symptoms Massive intake of phosphorus (more than 1 g) results in fulminating poisoning. The chief clinical feature is peripheral vascular collapse and death in 12–48 h.

Acute Poisoning is observed in three phases: (1) primary phase, due to the local irritant action on the gastrointestinal tract; (2) dormant or silent secondary phase; and (3) tertiary phase, which is due to action of the absorbed poison.

Primary phase: occurs within 2–6 h of ingestion and may last up to 3 days. Occasionally, the onset may be immediate. The initial features include garlicky taste and severe burning sensation in the mouth, throat, retrosternal area, and epigastrium, followed by nausea, vomiting, and diarrhea. Breath and vomit have a garlicky odor. The vomit and stools are luminous and dark. There may be hemetemesis. The stools may give rise to faint fumes constituting smoky stool syndrome.

Secondary Phase: is a symptom-free phase. The patient feels well enough, and this may last for 2–6 days or even more after the subsidence of the primary phase.

Tertiary Phase: is due to systemic effects of the absorbed poison. The original symptoms of the primary phase will reappear with increased severity, along with manifestations of hepatic damage. There will be tender hepatomegaly, jaundice, pruritus, and bleeding from multiple sites and anemia. Finally, hepatic encephalopathy develops, leading to stupor and coma. Oliguria, hematuria, albuminuria, and acute renal failure leading to death also occur.

Chronic Poisoning is usually observed in industrial workers due to long-term (2–5 years) occupational exposure to phosphorus fumes, resulting in a condition known as Phossy jaw. The fatal dose is 60–120 mg (1–2 mg/kg body weight) and the fatal period is 4–8 days.

Postmortem findings The affected individuals show signs of jaundice and hemorrhages under the skin and from various natural body orifices. The body is emaciated and may emit a garlicky smell. Phossy jaw may be observed in chronic cases. A garlicky odor is emitted if the abdomen is opened, and if putrefaction has not taken place. Inflammation and erosion of GI mucosa (yellowish or greenish-white, softened, thickened, inflamed, eroded, and occasionally perforated) may be observed.

Liver shows necrobiotic changes (enlarged but sometimes shrunken, doughy, yellow, soft, greasy liver with necrosis and fatty degeneration). In acute poisoning, there is atrophy of the liver, with a greasy, leathery, and dirty yellow appearance. The capsule is wrinkled and cells containing leucin and tyrosin crystals are necrosed.

Other viscera like the kidneys, heart, and muscles may also show fatty degeneration.

The preservative used for viscera is a saturated solution of sodium chloride (never use rectified spirit because phosphorus is soluble in it).

Treatment Treatment includes general management with symptomatic and specific therapy such as early gastric lavage with a 1 in 5000 solution of potassium permanganate or dilute solution of copper sulfate (0.2%) and bowel evacuation. Avoid oral administration of oil, fat, and eggs because phosphorus is soluble in these agents and would enhance its absorption. Intravenous saline is helpful for combating shock. Administer IV dextrose to protect the liver; vitamin K (65 mg slow IV drip) can help with hypoprothrombinemia. Use vitamin B complex and C, if required. Administer IV calcium gluconate (5–10 mL of 10% solution) to maintain the serum calcium level.

In *chronic poisoning*, avoid further exposure. Proper care of dental should be followed.

19.4 CHLORINE

Chlorine is a halogen that is an inorganic, nonmetallic irritant poison. It is a yellowish green gas with an irritating pungent odor. Chlorine acts as a direct irritant of the mucous membrane of the respiratory tract by locally forming hydrochloric acid when it comes in contact with moisture.

Signs and symptoms The main symptoms after inhalation are choking, suffocation, and a feeling of tightness in the chest with laryngeal spasm. Headache, nausea, sore throat, lacrimation, rhinorrhea, and cough are also common. Breathlessness is due to the collection of secretions inside the respiratory passage. Death occurs due to laryngeal or pulmonary edema.

The fatal dose is >400 ppm for a few minutes (inhalation) or 1 part chlorine in 1000 parts air and exposure for 5 min. The fatal period is 24 h from inhalation of pure chlorine gas.

Postmortem findings Characteristic odor, massive pulmonary edema, and respiratory epithelium denudation are commonly observed.

Treatment Treatment includes inhalation of humidified oxygen. Administer bronchodilators (aminophylline/salbutamol). Wash the affected eye with saline water and provide other symptomatic treatment.

19.5 BROMINE

Bromine is a reddish brown liquid that volatilizes to red fumes at room temperature and emits an unpleasant odor. Bromides are more often in use as medicine and act as a sedative and cough elixir.

Signs and symptoms If ingested in liquid form, bromine acts as a corrosive poison. Intense burning pain throughout the gastrointestinal tract, dysphagia, vomiting, eructation of offensive vapors, and purging are due to the corrosive action of bromine liquid on the GI tract.

If inhaled in its gaseous form, then bromine causes violent catarrhal inflammation of the respiratory tract. Symptoms include cough, feeling of constriction of the chest, pulmonary edema, hemoptysis, edema of the glottis and larynx, and death from suffocation.

Bromide poisoning is usually chronic, and it is also known as "Bromism." It occurs due to repeated administration of bromides of ammonium, sodium, and potassium as sedatives in medical doses over a prolonged period. Clinically, bromism manifests with:

- Skin rashes in the form of red papules (Bromine rash), similar to acne vulgaris, which may transform into a pustular lesion/uncerate at the hair roots (Bromoderma) and on the face, neck, and upper part of chest
- Problems with memory, muscular weakness, and coordination
- Delusions, hallucinations, and personality changes in severe cases
- The fatal dose and fatal period are uncertain. The maximum permissible level of vapor in the air is 0.1 ppm.

Postmortem findings In cases of oral ingestion of bromine in liquid form, there is inflammation of the esophagus and stomach, which present with a leathery, parchment-like appearance. Occasionally, perforation may be found. Pulmonary edema and edema of glottis are common when bromine is inhaled.

Treatment Treatment includes withdrawal of the bromide-containing product, followed by a symptom-based line of treatment such as stomach wash, use of oral starch, diuretics, caffeine to combat respiratory failure, and hemodialysis.

19.6 IODINE

Iodine is a type of halogen that is an inorganic, nonmetallic irritant poison. It is a volatile crystalline substance with a purple glistening color, a characteristic odor, and an acrid taste. It emits violet fumes/vapors at room temperature, acts as an antiseptic, and is a powerful irritant and vesicant.

Signs and symptoms

Acute Poisoning

- Burning pain from the mouth to the epigastrium, intense thirst, excessive salivation, vomiting, purging, giddiness, cramps, convulsions, and fainting
- Lips and mouth are stained brownish
- Vomit and stool are dark yellow/bluish, show the presence of blood, and emit iodine odor
- Urine is suppressed, is reddish-brown in color, and shows the presence of albumin
- Pulse is low and weak
- Skin is cold and clammy; the patient passes into a state of uremia and collapse, but consciousness is retained until death

Chronic Poisoning Chronic iodine poisoning is also known as "iodism." The problem occurs in patients who take large doses of potassium iodine continuously as medication. Symptoms include erythema, urticaria, acne, inflammation of all mucous membranes, parotitis, lymphadenopathy, anorexia, and insomnia.

The fatal dose is 2–4 g of iodine or 30–60 mL (1–2 ounces) of tincture iodine. The fatal period is approximately 24 h.

Postmortem findings Brownish stains of skin and mucosa, characteristic iodine odor, and congestion of all the viscera are common postmortem findings. Stomach may show blue contents if starchy food is present. The heart and liver may show fatty degeneration and the kidneys show glomeruler/tubular necrosis.

Treatment

- Evacuation of stomach: administer starch/flour solution 30 g/L of water; milk is helpful
- Sodium thiosulphate solution (1–5%) orally
- Symptomatic treatment with intravenous fluids to treat dehydration and shock

In iodism, a liberal intake of sodium chloride or bicarbonate of sodium is useful.

19.7 FORMALDEHYDE (FORMALIN, METHYL ALDEHYDE, METHYLENE OXIDE)

Formaldehyde is an irritant poison. It is a colorless gas with a pungent odor. However, commercially, it is available as formalin, which is a 40% aqueous solution of formaldehyde gas.

Formalin is a disinfectant, antiseptic, deodorant, tissue fixative, and embalming and agent. It also has an irritant action and can act by all routes of absorption.

Signs and symptoms

Acute Poisoning Inhalation of vapors can induce irritation of the respiratory tract, resulting in headache, rhinitis, dyspnea, lacrimation, and cough.

Oral ingestion can result in corrosion of the GI tract, with painful abdomen, nausea, vomiting, and diarrhea. Pupils will be constricted and the face is flushed. It can cause severe acidosis that results from rapid conversion of formaldehyde to formic acid. Coma, hypotension, and renal failure are the usual complications in severe ingestion cases.

Chronic Poisoning It is known to be a carcinogenic in animal experiments, but its relationship to occupational cancer is uncertain. Repeated exposure to formaldehyde may cause some individuals to become sensitized to it in few days to months, or even after first exposure, and this can result in an asthmatic reaction at levels that are too low to create any symptoms in other people.

The fatal dose is 30–90 mL and the fatal period ranges from 24 to 48 h.

Postmortem findings On opening of the body, there is the typical smell of the compound. Stomach mucosa may be red, inflamed, and eroded; extravasation of blood may make it hard and tough like leather. Intestines and lungs are congested. The liver may show fatty degeneration and the kidneys are inflamed.

Treatment Symptom-based and supportive lines of treatment include:

1. Milk or water is used in alert patients as a first aid measure. This may reduce its local effects.
2. Gastric lavage with 0.1% solution of ammonia is used because it reacts with formaldehyde to form harmless methanamide.
3. Hemodialysis is life-saving in severe cases.

CHAPTER

Neurotoxic agents

20

CHAPTER OUTLINE

20.1 INTRODUCTION

Chemicals that act on any part of the nervous system, such as cerebral cortex, spinal cord, or peripheral nerves, are classified as neurotoxic agents. Thus, these chemicals are grouped as cerebral, spinal, and peripheral neurotoxic agents. Some of them are therapeutically used to produce analgesia and sleep (eg, opium and its derivatives, pethidine, etc.). The classification of neurotoxic agents is summarized in Table 20.1.

Fundamentals of Toxicology. DOI: http://dx.doi.org/10.1016/B978-0-12-805426-0.00020-2

Table 20.1 Classification of Neurotoxic Agents

Groups	Site of Action	Main Toxic Action	Examples
Cerebral neurotoxins	Central nervous system	Analgesic, initial stimulation, followed by depression/ sleep, narcosis	Opium and its derivatives, pethidine, etc.; alcohols (ethyl alcohol, methyl alcohol, ethylene glycol, etc.); chloroform, ether, chloral hydrate; barbiturates, datura, belladonna, hyoscyamus, cannabis, cocaineBenzodiazepines (diazepam, flurazepam, etc.); halogenated compounds (diesel oil, petrol, kerosene, benzene, carbon tetrachloride); organophosphorus compounds, carbamates and organochloro compound (insecticides)
Spinal neurotoxins	Spinal cord	Stimulation, convulsion	Nux-vomica and its alkaloids, gelsemium
Peripheral neurotoxins	Peripheral end plates of the motor nerve terminals	Paralysis	Hemlock, curare, conium, etc.

20.2 OPIUM (AFIM) DERIVATIVES

The common name is white poppy plant or opium (afim) plant (Fig. 20.1). Opium is a gray mass with a bitter taste that is obtained on drying the milky latex of the unripe seed capsule of the poppy plant, *Papaver somniferum*. Opium is usually collected after all the flower petals have fallen off the capsule by making slits along its circumference, allowing the milky latex to ooze out and harden. After the plastic gummy opium is removed, it can be refined into heroin, morphine, and codeine.

Opium is used extensively as a sedative and painkiller. The various derivatives are also habit-forming narcotics. Seeds inside are nonpoisonous and called khaskhas, which constitute a condiment in Indian cooking.

Active Principle: The milky latex juice of the poppy plant has opium alkaloids. An alkaloid is a complex substance with a nitrogenous base that behaves like an alkali and unites with acid-forming salts. The crude opium has approximately 25 alkaloids that belong to two groups, phenanthrine derivatives and benzyl isoquinoline derivatives. Phenanthrine derivatives generally have alkaloids with sedative and analgesic properties, whereas the benzyl isoquinoline derivatives have alkaloids with antitussive and smooth muscle relaxant effects. The most commonly available natural, semi-synthetic, and synthetic analogs of opiates and opioids are summarized in Table 20.2.

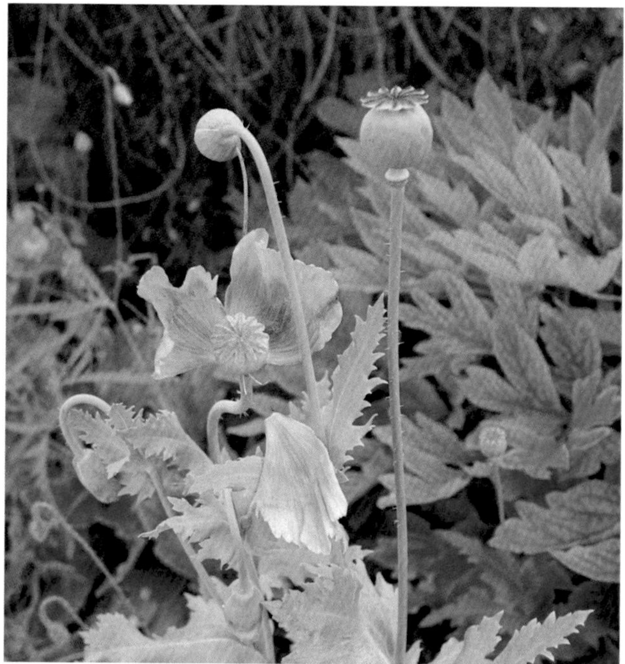

FIGURE 20.1

Opium plant leaves and seeds.

Source: Wikimedia Commons. Available at: https://en.wikipedia.org/wiki/Papaver_somniferum.

Table 20.2 Selective List of Natural, Semi-Synthetic, and Synthetic Opiates and Opioids

Natural Opium Derivatives	Semi-synthetic Analogs	Synthetic Analogs
Phenanthrine derivatives: morphine, codeine, and the baine *Benzyl-isoquinoline derivatives*: papaverine, narcotine, noscapine	Heroin, hydromorphine (dilaudid), oxycodone (in percodone), oxymorphone (numorphan)	Alphaprodein (nisentil), anileridine (laritine), butarphanol (stadol), dextromethorphan, diphenoxylate (lomotil), fentanyl (in sublimaze), levorphanol (levo-dromoran), meperidine (pethidine, demerol), methadone (dolophine), nulbuphine (nubain), pentazocine (talwin), propoxyphene (darvon, darvocet)

20.2.1 OPIOID POISONING

Acute Toxicity: On the basis of its action on the central nervous system (CNS), the effects of opioids are traditionally divided into three stages. It acts by a combination of stimulation and depression of CNS, producing a stage of excitement, followed by a stage of depression or stupor, and then merges into a third and final stage of narcosis. Common signs and symptoms are summarized in Table 20.3.

Central Nervous System Stage of Excitement: This stage is chiefly due to the initial stimulation of CNS and includes a sense of euphoria, pleasurable feelings, hallucinations, and convulsions, especially in children.

Stage of Depression (Stupor): In this stage, the victim presents with weariness, weakness, headache, giddiness, heaviness in the limbs, urge to sleep, itchy skin, and constricted pupils (pinpoint pupils).

Stage of Narcosis: As time passes, the victim of the stupor stage goes into the stage of narcosis/deep sleep and convulsions, followed by death.

CVS: Patients may show orthostatic hypotension and syncope when trying to assume the supine to sitting position.

Gastrointestinal (GI) Tract: Opiates in toxic doses can produce a decrease in gastric motility and an increase in antral muscle tone and proximal duodenal muscle tone. An increase in segmental contractibility and decreased longitudinal propulsive peristaltic movement of the small intestine and colon may create spasms. Increase in ileocecal valve and anal sphincter tone can result in anti-diarrheal action. Side effects of opiates, such as intestinal cramps, atony, and fecal impaction, may be observed. Nausea and vomiting may be due to the stimulation of the chemoreceptor trigger zone in the area postrema of the medulla.

A fatal dose of crude opium is 200–900 mg (in a nonaddicted adult). A fatal dose of morphine is 180–480 mg (addiction is known with morphine).

The fatal period is 45 min to 12 h, and the maximum is 2–3 days.

Chronic Toxicity (Synonym: Opium/Opiate Addiction, Morphinomania, Morphinism, Opioid Dependence, Opioid Abuse) The major complications of chronic opiate administration are development of tolerance, psychological dependence, and physical dependence; therefore, opium is a drug of addiction. Regular use of opium for painful conditions results in addiction. The condition is also called morphinomania or morphinism.

Table 20.3 Toxic Effects of Acute Opiate Intoxication

Severe Overdose	Less Severe Overdosage
Apnea	Central nervous system depression: coma, convulsions, urinary retention
Circulatory: collapse	Miosis: pinpoint pupils, may be dilated when hypoxia is severe
Cardiovascular: arrest	Respiratory depression: bradycardia, cyanosis
Death	Noncardiogenic: pulmonary edema
	Cardiovascular depression: hypotension

Abrupt cessation of opiate intake can cause withdrawal syndrome (abstinence syndrome, cold turkey). Generally, withdrawal syndrome symptoms develop at the time when the next dose would have been administered. The intensity and character of withdrawal symptoms are directly related to the daily amount of opiate used and the state of increased excitability of the bodily functions that have been depressed by the opiate.

Treatment

Acute Poisoning Emetics may be useful only in cases examined immediately after taking the poison, because later the vomiting center also becomes depressed. Gastric lavage with 1:1000 $KMnO_4$ (useful for even parenteral poisoning cases because the morphine absorbed is resecreted by the gastric glands into the stomach). Use of caffeine and maintenance of body warmth are useful.

Specific antidotes such as oxymorphone derivatives, naloxone, naltrexone, and nelmefene are useful.

Chronic Poisoning Gradual withdrawal of opiates should be initiated. Substitute therapy with methadone should be started at 30–40 mg/day and then gradually tapered off.

A beta adrenergic blocker like propanolol is useful. Clonidine can be used alternatively, which ameliorates symptoms of opioid withdrawal syndrome. Bone and muscle pain, insomnia, and cravings for euphoric effects of opioids are not relieved by clonidine.

Nitrous oxide has shown promising results; however, it is not recommended because of uncertain results. Antispasmodics may help abdominal cramps, vomiting, and diarrhea.

1. Sedation by tranquilizers at bedtime may be necessary.
2. Psychiatric counseling is mandatory.

20.3 PETHIDINE (MEPERIDINE)

Classification Pethidine is an opioid (narcotic analgesic drug that is a synthetic derivative of opium).

Signs and symptoms An overdose leads to cerebral excitation, flushing of the face, dilated pupils, disturbances of vision, dry mouth, tachycardia, increase in body temperature, vomiting, excitement, tremors, and convulsions. These may be followed by drowsiness, coma, and death from respiratory depression.

The fatal dose is 1–2 g; however, even a much smaller dose can be fatal. The fatal period is 24 h.

20.3.1 PETHIDINE ADDICTION

This is quite severe and difficult to treat, and it has a high mortality rate. Pethidine is often used for its analgesic, sedative, and tranquilizing effects and may lead to tolerance. Common victims of addiction are doctors, nurses, or other paramedical professionals to whom the drug is easily available. Continued use can lead to addiction, which is characterized by euphoria, dullness of intelligence, and impairment of memory. Withdrawal symptoms occur when the drug is withheld.

Larger doses can result in a confused state with hallucinations, illusions, and personality changes; this occurs more rapidly than with morphine. Accidental poisoning with therapeutic doses has also been reported.

Postmortem findings Postmortem appearances are those of asphyxia.

Treatment Symptom-based and supportive treatment such as gastric lavage and intravenous (IV) administration of coramine are useful.

20.4 ALCOHOL

In a pure form, alcohol is a transparent, colorless, volatile liquid with a spirit-like odor and burning taste. It is both water-soluble and lipid-soluble. It is an inebriant cerebral neurotoxic poison and has been classified as a sedative and hypnotic. Alcohol in general refers to an aqueous solution containing 95% ethyl alcohol; it is one of the oldest intoxicants ever known to humans. Consumption of alcoholic beverages is increasing in every part of the world. Many countries have tried prohibition, but with little success. Illegal imports, illicit manufacture, consumption of dangerous substitutes like methylated spirits, production and consumption of cheap and dangerous imitations, and forgery of liquor permits are some of the consequent problems of prohibition. Recently, it has been observed that crimes involving alcohol, directly or indirectly, are also increasing significantly.

Routinely, three categories of alcohols (monohydoxy alcohols, dihydroxy alcohols, and trihydroxy alcohols) are used. Ethyl alcohol is also known as alcohol, ethanol, or grain alcohol.

Mode of action Ethyl alcohol mainly acts as a CNS depressant. The initial apparent stimulation seen during the early stage is due to the depression of the higher inhibitory/evolutional centers (such as centers regulating conduct, judgment, and self-criticism), which normally control human behavioral attitudes, resulting in behavioral changes followed by depression of the vital centers of medulla, producing cardiorespiratory failure, alcoholic coma, and death. It also acts as a hypnotic, diaphoretic, and, in small doses, as an appetizer. A little brandy has a carminative effect. Diuresis with alcohol intake is usually due to the inhibition of release of antidiuretic hormones from the posterior pituitary. It is believed to be an aphrodisiac, but actually it is not.

Signs of intoxication Clinically, alcohol poisoning presents in two forms, acute and chronic. However, these are more often referred to as alcohol intoxication and alcohol addiction, respectively.

Acute (Alcoholic Intoxication/Alcohol Overdose) Consumption of any preparation containing alcohol, either in small doses at short intervals or in one large dose, beyond a person's capacity resulting in a blood alcohol concentration exceeding 150 mg/100 mL constitutes acute alcohol poisoning. In general, deliberate heavy drinking is the cause of acute poisoning. Rarely, poisoning can occur accidentally due to continuous inhalation of alcoholic vapors.

Intoxication leads to depression of the CNS (both higher and vital centers). Initially, there may be a stage of excitement, followed by lack of coordination and coma.

Stage of Excitement: This stage develops with a blood alcohol concentration (BAC) of 0.05 or 0.15% (ie, 50–150 mg/100 mL of blood). In a nonaddicted person, there is a sense of well being or euphoria due to the depression of inhibition-controlling capacity of higher evolutionary centers. There is a change in behavior and the person becomes free in action, speech, and emotions.

Stage of Lack of Coordination: This is due to further depression of higher centers of the brain. The individual may become morose, happy, irritable, excitable, quarrelsome, or sleepy depending on the dominant impulses released. Memories of recent events are impaired. This is followed by lack of coordination, inability to perform skilled movements, and altered speech. There will be excessive sweating and loss of body heat, resulting in a decrease in body temperature (subnormal temperature), which may be due to the depression of the temperature regulation center.

Stage of Coma: Higher blood alcohol concentration (BAC) leads to the stage of coma (>0.25%, ie, >250 mg/100 mL of blood). This occurs when both motor and sensory cells are deeply affected, resulting in thick, slurred speech. The victim may become giddy, may stagger, and may fall because coordination is markedly affected. Ultimately, the person may go into the stage of coma with stertorous breathing, rapid and barely perceptible pulse, and subnormal temperature.

Chronic (Synonyms: Alcohol Addiction, Alcoholism, Ethanolism) Consumption of heavy doses of ethyl alcohol beverages for a long period, regularly, and characterized by a morbid desire to drink alcohol, blackout episodes with intoxication, and withdrawal symptoms on stopping alcohol consumption. The chronic alcoholic patient will suffer from a set of manifestations involving various systems and organs of the body. These comprise the GI tract and CNS symptoms.

Treatment

Acute Intoxication The single most important factor in the treatment of the acutely alcohol-intoxicated patient is to provide respiratory support. Gastric lavage, induction of emesis, and activated charcoal are usually not indicated in cases of acute alcohol intoxication, but they may be indicated when concomitant drug ingestion is suspected. However, gastric lavage and bowel evacuation with an alkaline solution (5% sodium bicarbonate in warm water) are effective when administered to the patient within 2 h of ingestion. The patient should be kept warm. Vitamin B_6 accelerates the metabolism of alcohol, and IV administration in a dose of 5–100 mg may lead to rapid recovery. Coramine 3–5 mL by slow

IV may render amazing results. Other general management should include the following:

- Isotonic saline with 5% glucose (preferably fructose) may be required to deal with symptoms of hypogylcemia, if present.
- Increased intracranial pressure may be treated with saline purges and IV hypertonic glucose solution.
- Artificial respiration with oxygen is essential when severe respiratory depression ensues.
- Acidosis (common with methyl alcohol poisoning), if present, will require oral administration of sodium bicarbonate in a dose of 2 g in 250 mL water every 2 h. When oral therapy is not possible, 50 g of sodium bicarbonate dissolved in 1 L of 5% dextrose solution can be given intravenously, along with 10–15 units of insulin.
- An alcohol-intoxicated person may become belligerent and require special precautions and attentions to protecting self and others.
- Hemodialysis or peritoneal dialysis may be life-saving measures in very serious cases.

Chronic Poisoning Use of antiabuse therapy (disulfiram, metronidazole) causes nausea and vomiting if alcohol is ingested, which makes the alcoholic want to give up alcohol. Use of hypnosis and psychotherapy may also be helpful.

Withdrawal symptoms in chronic alcoholics Sudden stopping of alcohol intake in a chronic alcoholic can provoke a withdrawal syndrome/reaction, which can lead to one or more of the following:

1. Common abstinence syndrome
2. Alcoholic hallucinosis
3. Alcohol seizures (rum fits)
4. Alcohol ketoacidosis
5. Delirium tremens (DTs)
6. Wernicke-Korsakoff syndrome

Common Abstinence Syndrome The syndrome complex comprises manifestations such as tremors in the hands, legs, and trunk. The patient will present with a mental state of extreme emotional disturbance (agitation), sweating, nausea, headache, and insomnia. All these events come into sight within 6–8 h of stopping the alcohol intake.

Treatment: Clonidine 0.2 mg orally administered several times daily over a 4-day period is effective for some of the adrenergic manifestations of alcohol withdrawal. Other drugs suggested to be of potential use are dexamethasone, phenobarbital chlormethiazole, and beta-blockers (for mild symptoms); subanalgesic doses of nitrous oxide, clorazepate, haloperidol, and hydroxybutyric acid can also ameliorate some of the symptoms associated with alcohol withdrawal.

Alcoholic Hallucinosis The person starts seeing objects with distorted shapes and their shadows moving. The patient will report hearing someone shouting at him or music. All these events occur within 24–36 h of stopping alcohol intake.

Treatment: Administration of phenothiazines (eg, chlorpromazines 100 mg/8 h) is useful.

Alcohol Seizures (Rum Fits) These comprise clonic–tonic movements with or without loss of consciousness. These manifestations appear within 6–48 h of either cessation or precipitous decline of alcohol intake. True alcohol seizures will usually manifest prior to the onset of DTs.

Treatment: The seizures do not require any long-term anticonvulsant therapy because the seizers are self-limited.

Alcohol Ketoacidosis This problem develops due to sudden withdrawal of alcohol and results in gastritis or pancreatitis. This results in mobilization of fat from adipose tissues as an alternate source of energy. Fatty acids are oxidized, which leads to ketoacidosis.

Treatment: Infusion of normal saline with dextrose, potassium supplementation, and thiamine (50–100 mg) is recommended.

Delirium Tremens Delirium tremens is a medicolegally important toxicological problem because it has an element of unsoundness of mind due to acute insanity associated with chronic alcoholism. It is the most dangerous complication of alcoholism.

Treatment: Initially, treatment comprises IV diazepam 10 mg, followed by 5 mg IV every 5 min until full control. Later, switch to 5–10 mg orally three times per day to control the feeling of fear/agitation. Administration of thiamine, control of dehydration, and correction of electrolyte imbalance are important.

Wernicke-Korsakoff Syndrome This is a rare form of withdrawal syndrome, which is a combination of Wernicke encephalopathy and Korsakoff psychosis. Wernicke encephalopathy is an acute form characterized by drowsiness, amnesia, ataxia, peripheral neuropathy, horizontal nystagmus, and external ocular palsies. When the recovery from this is incomplete, a chronic amnesic syndrome develops called Korsakoff psychosis, which is characterized by impairment of memory and confabulations (falsification of memory).

Treatment: Wernicke encephalopathy can be treated with thiamine 50–100 mg IV daily, infused slowly in 500 mL of fluid for 5–7 days, accompanied by fluid replacement.

20.5 ETHYLENE GLYCOL

Ethylene glycol is a colorless, nonvolatile liquid with a bittersweet taste. It is an inebriant neurotoxic substance. Toxic action is mainly due to metabolites such as glycolic acid, lactic acid, and oxalic acid.

Signs and symptoms Mild intoxication (first stage) leads to nausea, vomiting, convulsions, and coma (CNS stage); cardiorespiratory symptoms like tachycardia, tachypnea, and congestive heart failure develop in 12–14 h (CVS stage). Death may supervene within a day or so because of renal failure due to crystals of calcium oxalate in the kidney tubules and interstitial tissues, resulting in tubular necrosis within 24–72 h. Liver damage may also occur. This may be followed by cerebral edema and other abnormalities of a serious nature.

The fatal dose is 100–200 mL. The fatal period is approximately 24 h.

Treatment Symptom-based and supportive treatment such as gastric lavage and hemodialysis/peritoneal dialysis followed by administration of ethyl alcohol should be used. Administration of pyridoxine (50 mg) and thiamine (100 mg) intramuscular will hasten metabolism and excretion of ethylene glycol.

20.6 CHLOROFORM

Chloroform is a heavy, colorless, volatile liquid with a strong odor and a sweet, burning taste. It is an inebriant cerebral poison with anesthetic properties and prominent respiratory symptoms.

Signs and symptoms After oral ingestion, symptoms are similar to alcohol. However, there may be burning pain in the mouth, throat, and stomach, leading to vomiting. Within 10 min, unconsciousness and coma with slow, stertorous breathing occurs. Pupils are dilated and pulse is feeble, rapid, and irregular.

Inhalation of vapors causes analgesia, excitement, anesthesia, and paralysis. The muscles are relaxed, pupils are dilated, and reflexes are lost completely. Body temperature is subnormal. Death is due to cardiac or respiratory failure.

The fatal dose is 30 mL by mouth ($>0.04\%$ in blood). The fatal period is approximately 30 min.

Treatment After oral ingestion, gastric lavage, demulcent drinks, stimulants, and symptomatic measures are useful. After inhalation, provide artificial respiration, oxygen, and cardiac stimulants. Maintain body warmth if necessary.

20.7 ETHER

Ether is a colorless, volatile, highly inflammable liquid with a penetrating ethereal odor and sweet, pungent taste. It is an inebriant cerebral poison that acts as an anesthetic and respiratory depressant.

Signs and symptoms Oral ingestion leads to burning of the throat, esophagus, and stomach, nausea, and vomiting, followed by inebriation, as is seen in alcohol poisoning.

Inhalation of vapors causes analgesia, excitement, anesthesia, and paralysis. The muscles are relaxed, pupils are dilated, and reflexes are lost completely. Body temperature is subnormal. Death is due to cardiac or respiratory failure.

The fatal dose is 30 mL by mouth. The fatal period may be immediate due to syncope during anesthesia.

Treatment Supportive and maintenance therapy including gastric lavage, demulcents, stimulants, and anticonvulsants should be initiated immediately.

20.8 CHLORAL HYDRATE (TRICHLOROACETALDEHYDE)

Chloral hydrate is a sedative and hypnotic (induces sleep). A small dose is hypnotic (0.3–1.2 g), and a large/toxic dose can paralyze the vital centers, including the CNS. It is well absorbed from the GI tract.

Signs and symptoms

Acute Poisoning Ingestion of fatal doses can result in a burning sensation in the throat, followed by nausea and vomiting, drowsiness, unconsciousness with loss of reflexes, and muscular relaxation, followed by depression of medullary centers, and resulting in a decrease of blood pressure (BP) and respiratory rate, convulsions, and, ultimately, death. Pupils are usually constricted and "pinpoint." Because chloral hydrate is radio-opaque, radiographs can help in the diagnosis of acute oral poisoning.

Chronic Poisoning (Chloral Hydrate Addiction) Frequent consumption of the drug over a long period can lead to digestive symptoms such as epigastric pain, nausea, vomiting, and severe gastritis. Skin erythematous rashes, nervous manifestations such as neuralgia, tremors, and convulsions are commonly observed. The fatal dose is 5–10 g. However, recoveries have been reported even with large doses. The fatal period ranges from 8 to 12 h, but it may be delayed for 2–3 days.

Treatment General treatment should include gastric lavage with water containing an alkali that can decompose unabsorbed chloral hydrate. Symptomatic treatment to maintain cardiac and respiratory systems should be initiated immediately.

20.9 BARBITURATES

The slang names of barbiturates are barbs, goofballs, downers, yellow jackets, red devils, reds and blues, rainbows, pinks, blockbusters, and Christmas trees.

Barbiturates are derived from barbituric acid, which was discovered by Adolph von Baeyer in 1864. Barbitone was discovered by Joseph von Mering and Emil Fisher in 1892, and phenobarbitone was synthesized in 1912. Even though this group of drugs has been used extensively in the past, benzodiazepines have replaced the use of many of the barbiturates, but they are still available and abused. Using barbiturates in conjunction with alcohol is especially dangerous; alcohol is a CNS depressant, so the harmful effects of both are multiplied.

Table 20.4 Classification of Barbiturates

Ultra-short-acting (duration of action <15–20 min)	Thiopentone sodium, methohexitone, pentothal sodium, hexobarbital sodium, kemithal sodium, thiamylal sodium, etc.
Short-acting (duration of action <3 h)	Cyclobarbitone, pentobarbitone, amobarbitone, aprobarbitone, butobarbitone, hexabarbitone, etc.
Intermediate-acting (duration of action 3–6 h)	Amylobarbitone, butobarbitone, probarbitone sodium, amobarbitone, aprobarbital, vinbarbital, allobarbitone, etc.
Long-acting (duration of action 6–12 h)	Barbitone, phenobarbital, mephobarbitone, methyl phenobarbital, diallylbarbituric acid, etc.

Overdose deaths are more frequent when alcohol and barbiturates are mixed, whether accidentally or deliberately. One feature remains that is common to all barbiturates: there is only a slight difference between a dose that produces sedation and a dose that may cause death.

20.9.1 CLASSIFICATION

Barbiturates are sedatives, which are a hypnotic type of cerebral poison used in medical practice as sedatives, hypnotics, anesthetics, and antiepileptics, or in strychnine poisoning cases. Barbiturates are functionally grouped into two groups: long-acting and short-acting agents. The latter further consists of three types: ultrashort-, short-, and intermediate-acting agents (Table 20.4). Barbiturates are classified into four types depending on their time of onset and duration of action.

Long-acting: barbiturates act within 2 h. The duration of action lasts for 6–12 h (eg, barbitone, phenobarbital, mephobarbitone, methyl phenobarbital, diallylbarbiuric acid, etc.).

Intermediate-acting: barbiturates act within 30 min to 1 h. The duration of action lasts for 3–6 h (eg, amylobarbitone, butobarbitone, probarbitone sodium, amobarbitone, aprobarbital, vinbarbital, allobarbitone, etc.).

Short-acting: barbiturates act within minutes. The duration of action lasts <3 h (eg, cyclobarbitone, pentobarbitone, amobarbitone, aprobarbitone, butobarbitone, hexabarbitone, seconal, ortal, etc.).

Ultrashort acting: barbiturates act immediately. The duration of action lasts for <15–20 min. Because they act immediately and the action passes within a short time, they are basically used as anesthetic agent (eg, thiopentone sodium, methohexitone, pentothal sodium, hexobarbital sodium, kemithal sodium, thiamylal sodium, etc.). Barbiturates used as sedative hypnotics are administered orally. IV administration is usually reserved for management of status epilepticus or induction/maintenance of general anesthesia. Barbiturates are absorbed from the GI tract, including the rectum, and from the subcutaneous (SC) tissues. After absorption, they are distributed widely in the body fluids. Metabolism of barbiturates occurs by oxidation in the liver, resulting in the formation of alcohols, ketones, phenols, or carboxylic acids, which are excreted in urine as such or in the form of glucuronic acid conjugates. Approximately 25% of phenobarbitone is excreted unchanged in urine.

Mode of action Barbiturates act as a depressant at all levels of the CNS. However, depending on the dose, the degree of depression can be altered from tranquility to deep coma. It can also act synergistically with analgesics and other drugs (eg, with alcohol, it increases the action of alcohol). The drug also has cumulative effects because its metabolism and excretion are very slow (cumulative poison). Therefore, barbiturates are not indicated in cases of hepatic and renal damage.

Barbiturates bind to specific sites on gamma-aminobutyric acid (GABA)-sensitive ion channels found in the CNS, which is the major inhibitory neurotransmitter in the CNS. Barbiturates also block glutamate (excitatory neurotransmitter) receptors in the CNS.

Compared to long-acting agents, short-acting agents are more lipid-soluble, more protein-bound, have a higher pKa, have a more rapid onset, have a shorter duration of action, and are metabolized almost entirely in the liver to inactive metabolites (which are excreted as glucuronides in the urine). Long-acting agents, which are less fat (lipid)-soluble, accumulate more slowly in tissues and are excreted more readily by the kidney as an active drug. For instance, urinary excretion accounts for 20–30% of phenobarbital and for 15–42% of primidone (both long-acting agents).

Short-acting agents have an elimination half-life less than 40 h compared to long-acting agents, which have an elimination half-life longer than 40 h.

Barbiturates stimulate the hepatic cytochrome P-450 mixed function oxidase microsomal enzyme system; thus, barbiturates affect the drug levels of medications that are dependent on this system.

CNS Effects: Barbiturates mainly act on the CNS and, as a consequence, affect other organ systems. Direct effects include sedation and hypnosis at lower dosages. The lipophilic barbiturates, such as thiopental, cause rapid anesthesia because of their tendency to penetrate brain tissue quickly. Barbiturates all have anticonvulsant activity because they hyperpolarize cell membranes; therefore, they are effective adjuncts in the treatment of epilepsy.

Pulmonary Effects: Barbiturates can cause a depression of the medullary respiratory center and induce respiratory depression. Patients with underlying chronic obstructive pulmonary disease (COPD) are more susceptible to these effects, even at doses that would be considered therapeutic in healthy individuals. Barbiturate overdose fatality is usually secondary to respiratory depression. Pulmonary embolism has also been reported following barbiturate overdosage.

CVS Effects: Cardiovascular depression may occur following depression of the medullary vasomotor centers; patients with underlying congestive heart failure (CHF) are more susceptible to these effects. At higher doses, cardiac contractility and vascular tone are compromised, which may cause cardiovascular collapse.

Pregnancy: Barbiturates freely cross the placenta and can have adverse effects on the fetus, such as decrease in fetal intelligence, possible addiction, and possible withdrawal. Overactivity, visible tremors, hypertonicity, hyperphagia, and vasomotor instability characterize neonatal withdrawal syndrome. Withdrawal begins 4–7 days after birth and may last up to 4 months.

Signs and symptoms

Acute Intoxication Acute intoxication will lead to giddiness, ataxia, and slurred speech, followed by stupor. The limbs become flaccid, reflexes are lost, pupil reaction varies, and there may be diplopia. Pupils may show hippus. As the poisoning advances, the face tends to become progressively cyanotic. Respiration becomes slow, sighing, and periodic (Cheyne-Stokes), soon turning rapid and shallow. There will be a decrease in blood pressure. Body temperature will be subnormal. Oliguria may develop, with urine containing albumin and sugar, followed by coma and death (respiratory failure may be edema of lungs, bronchopneumonia, and cardiac failure, etc., all of which may occur suddenly and unexpectedly).

Occasionally, patients may recover gradually from coma. On recovery, patients will have physical weakness, low blood pressure, and anemia.

Barbiturate Automatism: Using barbiturate tablets repeatedly to sleep ultimately results in acute toxicity and is called barbiturate automatism.

Chronic Intoxication (Barbiturate Addiction) Barbiturates are some of the most addictive drugs. They are often a substitute for alcohol (because similar effects are produced). People use barbiturates to get a sense of euphoria and relaxation. It is illegal to use barbiturates without a prescription and without the supervision of a doctor.

Chronic intoxication will lead to apathy, loss of power to concentrate, somnolence, vertigo, tremors, ataxia, thick speech, delirium, hallucinations (visual), emotional instability, and general mental disorientation. Urine will show albumin, sugar, and casts microscopically.

The fatal dose depends on different barbiturates: long-acting, 3–4 g; intermediate-acting, 2–3 g; and short-acting, 1–2 g. The fatal period varies from 24 to 48 h; however, patients may be in a coma for several days before death occurs.

Treatment Supportive treatment should be initiated. Ipecac-induced emesis is not recommended. The same treatments as those suggested for drug addiction may be followed.

20.10 BENZODIAZEPINES

Acute overdose toxicity has been associated with short-acting benzodiazepines such as midazolam and triazolam and intermediate-acting flunitrazepam than with diazepam, lorazepam, and nitrazepam. However, benzodiazepines are the most commonly used drugs in clinical practice as sedatives, hypnotics, anxiolytics, muscle relaxants, and anticonvulsants. Death due to benzodiazepines is common.

Mode of action It acts as a CNS depressant and can bring about anxiety relief. It also acts as a muscle relaxant and is used to control convulsions.

Signs and symptoms Benzodiazepines are considered safe. However, sometimes symptoms of acute poisoning and/or chronic poisoning due to repeated administration of benzodiazepines may be observed.

Acute Poisoning Acute poisoning may be mild or moderate to severe. In the mild form, drowsiness, sedation, somnolence, diplopia, ataxia, amnesia, and weakness are the common symptoms of poisoning. In the moderate to severe form, vertigo, slurred speech, nystagmus, partial ptosis, lethargy, and coma have been observed.

Chronic Poisoning Continuous use of benzodiazepines is associated with development of tolerance associated with mild withdrawal reactions. It is characterized by fits and psychosis, anxiety, insomnia, headache, spastic muscles, anorexia, vomiting, tremor, weakness, convulsions, and psychiatric disturbances (rarely) such as disordered perception (which comprises feelings of unreality), abnormal bodily sensations, and hypersensitivity to stimuli.

Significant depression is seen in neonates with floppy baby syndrome, which is characterized by hypotonia, lethargy, respiratory depression, hypothermia, and poor reflexes. Seizures prolonging hypotonia and prolonging respiratory depression are seen in newborns from mothers receiving treatment with lorazepam. In some newborn babies, dysmorphic features such as craniofacial abnormalities, including low nasal bridge, short palpebral fissures, epicanthic folds, a short upturned nose, slightly malformed and/or low-set ears, and hypoplastic mandible, were reported for those born from mothers receiving benzodiazepines during early pregnancy.

Treatment

Acute Poisoning General management of poisoning and use of symptom-based treatment may be followed. Use of antidotes such as doxapram (100 mg IV) or any physostigmine may be given. Specific antidotes such as imidazodiazepine can block the central effects of benzodiazepines. It is given slowly in an IV dose of 0.1 mg/min as an infusion to a total of 1 mg. If resedation occurs in 20–120 min, then the dose can be repeated until a cumulative dose of 3.5 mg is reached.

Chronic Poisoning Phenobarbitone substitution technique is recommended for benzodiazepines withdrawal. It uses propranolol for acute somatic symptoms, whereas phenobarbitone is used for detoxification. However, the most frequently used method among clinicians is the replacement of a short half-life benzodiazepine (such as alprazolam) with a long half-life benzodiazepine (such as clonazepam) before initiating a taper and final discontinuation.

20.11 HYDROCARBONS

For details of toxicity dealing with hydrocarbon types such as aliphatic (eg, diesel oil, petrol, kerosene, etc.), aromatic (eg, benzene), and halogenated (eg, carbon tetrachloride), please refer to individual compounds in this book.

20.12 INSECTICIDES

Toxic effects of insecticides such as organophosphorus (OPs), carbamates (CMs), and organochloro (OC) compounds are discussed in Chapter 17, Toxic Effects of Pesticides (Agrochemicals).

20.13 DATURA

The common names of datura are thorn apple, stinkweed, angel's trumpet, and Jamestown weed. It is a vegetable and deliriant type of cerebral poison. The botanical name is *Datura stromanium.* Commonly, there are two varieties of plants: *Datura alba* (with white flowers) and *Datura nigra* (with blackish or purple flowers). A view of the plant along with its fruits and seeds is shown in Fig. 20.2.

The active principles are alkaloids such as hyoscine (scopolamine), hyoscyamine, and atropine.

Mode of action Poisoning occurs only if seeds are masticated and swallowed. It has a bitter taste and can initially lead to stimulation of higher centers of brain. Later, the vital centers are depressed, followed by death due to respiratory paralysis.

Signs and symptoms It produces characteristic manifestations of anticholinergic poisoning (remember as six Ds):

1. Dryness of mouth, nausea, vomiting
2. Dysphagia
3. Dysarthria (1–3 are due to inhibition of salivation)
4. Diplopia (due to dilated pupil)
5. Dry, hot (due to inhibition of sweat secretion), and red (due to the dilation of cutaneous blood vessels) skin, especially in the face/chest
6. Drowsiness leading to coma

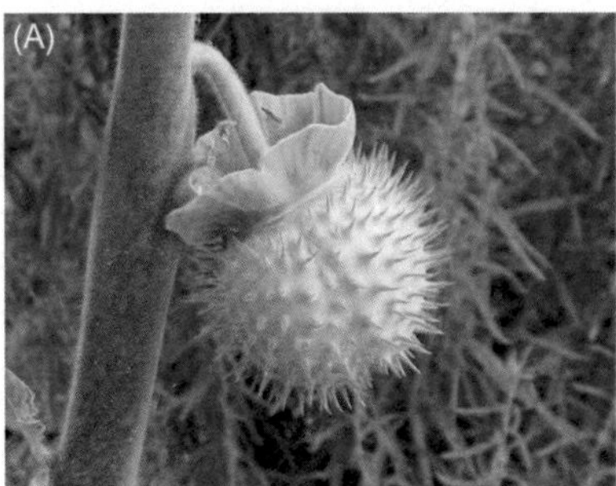

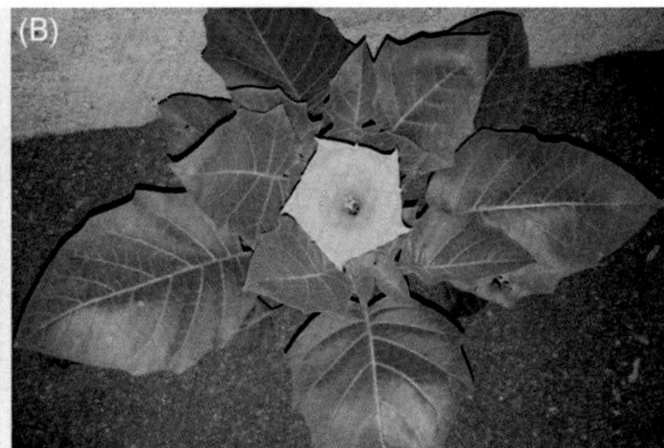

FIGURE 20.2

Datura plant fruit (A), and flower (B).

Source: Wikimedia Commons. Available at: https://en.wikipedia.org/wiki/Datura.

Other symptoms are include confusion (ie, deliriant or muttering delirium), hallucinating, and exhibiting typical pill rolling movements or movements like pulling imaginary threads from fingertips. There may be urinary retention or dysuria. Death is usually due to respiratory failure or cardiac arrhythmias.

In summary, the clinical features of datura poisoning in their classic phase are described as blind as bat, hot as a hare, dry as a bone, red as a beet, and mad as a hen.

The fatal dose is 50–75 seeds (0.6–1 g). The fatal period is between 4 and 24 h.

Treatment Treatment consists of supportive care and GI decontamination by gastric lavage with potassium permanganate ($KMnO_4$) 1:5000 solution. Due to decreased GI motility, a lavage may be useful even during the late stage of poisoning. Activated charcoal in multiple doses is useful for reducing the absorption of toxins from the gut. The following treatment should be given: prostigmine 0.5 mg SC injection; pilocarpine nitrate; and chloraldehyde or a slow-acting barbiturate (do not give morphine). Physostigmine should be reserved for severe hallucinations and agitation cases only. Inject 2 mg IV slowly over a few minutes. Repeat the dose every 10 min until the cessation of the life-threatening condition. However, do not exceed the dose of 4 mg in 30 min.

20.14 CANNABIS

Cannabis is classified as a delirium cerebral neurotic plant poison. It is also classified as a mild hallucinogen, sedative, or narcotic. In fact, the drug is believed to produce all these effects in various individuals in a different way. It can be absorbed through both GI and respiratory tracts. However, presently, it is considered as the *most abused drug* worldwide. Slang terms for cannabis include hash, grass, pot, ganja, spliff, and reefer.

Cannabis is a collective term used for psychoactive compounds derived from the plant *Cannabis sativa* or *hemp plant*. It belongs to the botanical family Cannabinaceae and is a tall weed growing up to 15 feet in height (Fig. 20.3).

Cannabis is often referred to as *Indian hemp* (in India), *Dagga* (in South and Central Africa), *Hashish* (in Egypt), and *Marijuana* (in the United States). It grows all over the globe, especially in India, Africa, Egypt, and the United States. The whole plant is poisonous. Its active principal is usually a fat-soluble oleoresin called *cannabinol* (ie, delta tetrahydrocannabinol (THC)).

Cannabis is usually dried and either smoked or eaten. The cannabis preparations usually emit a peculiar odor that is described as that of *burned rope*. It is used in three forms.

Ganja: The resinous mass that contains approximately 25% of the active principle. It is usually mixed with tobacco and smoked in a pipe (*chilam*). The drug is commonly consumed by Indian *Sadhus* and *Fakirs*. A person under the

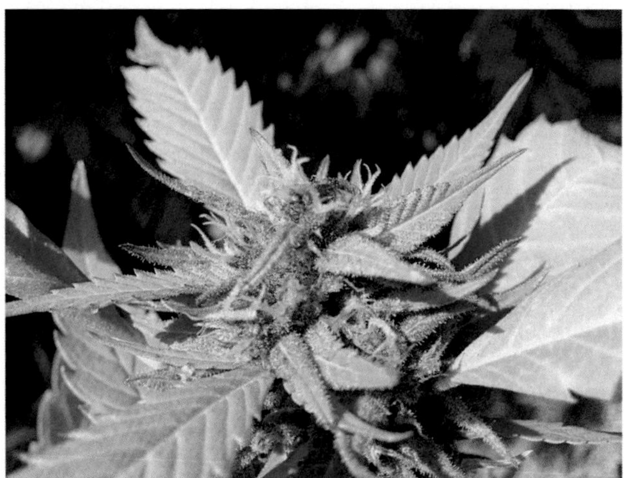

FIGURE 20.3

Cannabis plant flowers.

Source: Grow Weed Easy. Available at: http://www.growweedeasy.com/advanced-breeding-techniques.

effect of ganja smoking is able to perform ordinary duties, feels lazy, and indulges in day dreaming. It is believed that the compound helps to provide courage before performing an act of violence or any crime such as homicide.

Charas: Also called *hashish*, it is the purest form of cannabis. It comprises the dried resinous exudates from the flower tops. It is dark green or brown in color and contains 25–40% of the active principle. This is also mixed with tobacco and used to smoke in a pipe or hookah.

Bhang: Also called siddhi, patti, or sabji, it is the crudest form of cannabis. It is prepared as a decoction of dried mature leaves and flower stems and contains 15% of the active principle. It is usually consumed in the form of a beverage. It has a very mild form and produces a feeling of exhilaration for approximately 3–4 h, followed by sleep. Other forms of cannabis used elsewhere are as follows.

Marijuana (pot, grass, tea, Mary Jane, etc.): is the most common illicit drug used in the United States. It refers to any part of the cannabis plants or its extract that is used to induce psychotomimetic or therapeutic effects. It is eaten alone or as a part of a confection, drank in beers or some other beverages, or smoked in pipes or after being rolled into cigarettes. After consumption, one can recall things that had been long since forgotten.

Sinsemilla: is the unpollinated or seedless female plant. It accounts for approximately 85% of the domestic production (in California, United States) and contains approximately 5% of the active principle.

Signs and symptoms The clinical effects experienced by an individual depend on their mood, personality, environment, and the dose taken. With smoking, the onset of effects is observed in 10–30 min, and on ingestion the onset occurs in 1–3 h. The effects may last for approximately 4–8 h. However, a crude extract of cannabis may also be injected intravenously and cause nausea, vomiting, diarrhea, abdominal pain, fever, hypotension, pulmonary edema, acute renal failure, disseminated intravascular coagulation, and death.

In *acute* poisoning, the clinical features vary with the dose consumed. With a low dose, there is initial *euphoria* associated with over-talkativeness, perceptual alterations followed by relaxation, drowsiness, hypertension, tachycardia, slurred speech, ataxia, excessive appetite, and eating food with great pleasure.

At a higher dose, there is conjunctival congestion and miosis, acute paranoid psychosis, anxiety, depersonalization, confusion, hallucinations (especially of sexual character; therefore, cannabis is considered an aphrodisiac), and disorientation regarding time and space. This may be followed by giddiness, confusion, drowsiness, dilated pupils, tingling and numbness in the extremities, and generalized anesthesia (may be seen in severe cases). The victim will then go into a deep sleep and can be awoken soon without depression, nausea, or any hangover effects. Rarely, the victim may have paralysis of muscles, loss of reflexes, coma, and death. However, a few individuals may turn *violent* and "run amok."

20.14.1 CANNABIS ADDICTION

Cannabis addiction is a chronic poisoning state that results from continued use of the drug in any form and is characterized by anorexia, loss of weight, weakness, tremors, impotence, and moral deterioration. The victim might become lethargic, apathetic, and disinterested in work. Poor concentration (*amotivational syndrome*) may also result.

A cannabis addict is often found to suffer from mental disorders such as hallucinations and delusions of a persecution nature, presentation with an irresistible desire to destroy life and property willfully, or commit homicide out of jealousy; however, there will be no recollection afterwards. A condition called "run amok" is rarely reported with continued use or sudden consumption of cannabis; it is characterized by a frenzied desire to commit murders. After the intake of the drug, the person may kill a number of individuals, with the first few being those against whom the patient has some enmity (real or imaginary), followed by others who are just in the way, until the homicidal tendencies end. The person may finally commit suicide or surrender himself or herself to the police.

The fatal dose is 2000 mg of *charas*, 8000 mg of *ganja*, and 10,000 mg/kg body weight of *bhang*. For nonaddicts, one can experience effects with 1–5 g of *Cannabis indiaca* (equivalent to three reefer cigarettes). After a lethal dose, the fatal period is usually within 12 h.

Treatment

Acute Poisoning Symptom-based treatment with supportive therapy such as the use of gastric lavage with warm water/emesis is recommended. Use of activated charcoal orally is effective in cases reported within 1 h of ingestion. Caffeine and artificial respiration, if necessary, may be provided. Saline purgatives may be helpful. Haloperidol is to be given to control psychotic manifestation, if any.

Chronic Poisoning Management of chronic poisoning consists of gradual withdrawal of the drug, administration of diazepam for the control of sedation, and use of haloperidol for the control of psychotic reactions. Use of psychotherapy is also helpful.

20.15 COCAINE

Cocaine is a cerebral neurotoxic deliriant. It is obtained from the dried leaves of the coca plant (*Erythroxylon coca*). The coca plant (Fig. 20.4), however, should not be confused for the cocoa plant, which contains caffeine rather than cocaline.

The slang names for cocaine are snuff, rock, crack, coke, snow, Cadillac, and white lady.

Cocaine hydrochloride is a white, colorless, crystalline substance that has a bitter numbing taste. It is slightly soluble in water but freely soluble in alcohol, chloroform, and glycerin. After oral consumption it gives a feeling of numbness in the tongue and mucosa of the mouth. It has synthetic substitutes, namely,

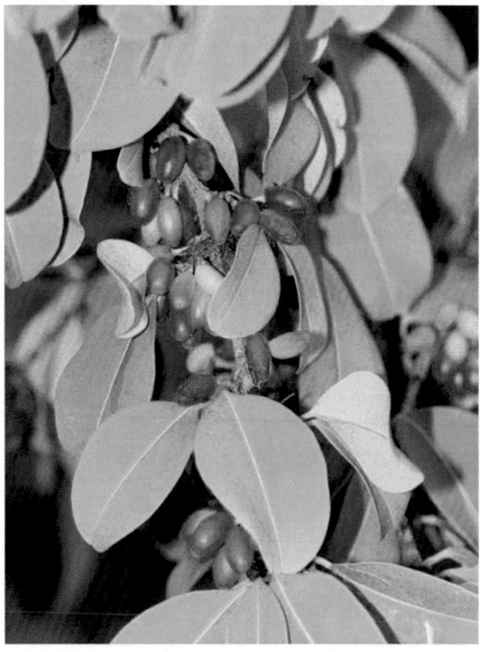

FIGURE 20.4

Coca plant leaves and flowers.

Source: Entheology.com. Available at: http://entheology.com/plants/erthroxylum-coca-coca-bush/.

novocaine and nupercaine, which are used frequently as local anesthetics. It cannot be used for smoking because it decomposes during heating. Crack cocaine is a cocaine preparation that has been separated from its hydrochloride base (free base) by adding baking soda and water, followed by heating and then drying. It can be mixed with tobacco and smoked. The name *crack* arises from the noise made when it is being prepared, as well as the *fissured* appearance of heated cocaine. Chronic consumption can lead to an addiction to cocaine.

Signs and symptoms Adverse effects of cocaine depend on the chronic use of cocaine and may affect the CNS, lungs, heart, and other organs, as shown in Fig. 20.5.

With small doses, the peak "high" effect appears and weans off after some time. In most cases, the effects of cocaine resolve in approximately 20 min, except when used intravenously. However, in fatal cases, onset and progression of symptoms are accelerated and death may occur in minute. It has a stage of initial stimulation of the CNS, followed by depression.

There will be a sense of physical and mental energy and an increase in sexual desire. Bruxism (teeth grinding), nausea, vomiting, pallor, dizziness, headache, cold sweats, tremors, twitching, and dryness of the mouth with a bitter taste are other findings in mild to moderate cases.

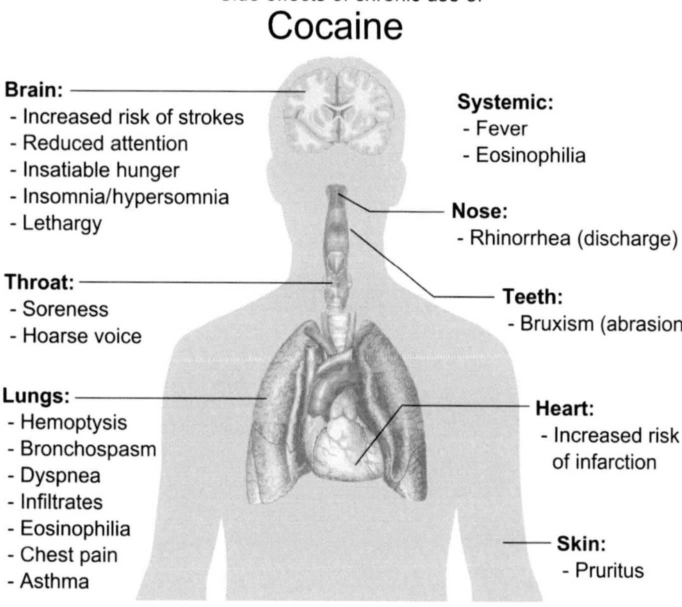

FIGURE 20.5

Effects of chronic use of cocaine.

Source: Häggström, Mikael. Medical gallery of Mikael Häggström 2014. Wikiversity Journal of Medicine 1 (2). Available at: https://commons.wikimedia.org/wiki/File:Side_effects_of_chronic_use_of_Cocaine.png.

Higher doses result in stimulation of the motor cortex, leading to restlessness, excitement, and delirium. Brief stimulation of the medullary centers result in face flushes and dilated pupils with blurring of vision. The victim may have tachycardia, hallucinations (tactile, auditory, olfactory), ventricular ectopics, hypertension, and an increase in respiratory rate and body temperature (cocaine fever). Severe hypertension may cause hemorrhagic stroke. The coronary artery may suffer spasms, resulting in myocardial ischemia or infarction even in patients with normal coronary arteries. It may also lead to hypotension, cyanosis, cardiac arrhythmias, and renal failure. As the stimulation spreads down to lower centers, lack of coordination, muscular twitches, and convulsions may develop. This is followed by depression of the CNS characterized by loss of reflexes, muscle paralysis, pulmonary edema, feeble respiration, and circulatory and respiratory failure, followed by death.

Complications of acute cocaine poisoning include:

1. Stroke, including subarachnoid and intracerebral hemorrhage and cerebral infarcts
2. Cardiovascular complications such as myocardial infarction, ventricular arrhythmias, and cardiac arrest
3. Intestinal ischemia

Treatment Treatment depends on the route of administration:

- *If applied to mucosa*: Wash with warm water or normal saline
- *If swallowed*: Perform gastric lavage with a dilute solution of potassium permanganate or tannic acid or medicinal charcoal. Give activated charcoal (adult, 50 g; child, 1 g/kg) if it is within the first hour of oral ingestion.

Additional treatment is purely supportive care, such as monitoring of BP, heart rate, ECG, and body temperature.

- Use diazepam (0.1–0.2 mg/kg body weight) to control excitement, agitation, or psychotic patients. This also reduces central stimulation, which in turn can decrease tachycardia, hypertension, and pyrexia. However, for controlling psychotic reactions, it is better to avoid the use of phenothiazines/haloperidol because they can lower the threshold for convulsions.
- Cardiorespiratory stimulants and artificial respiration may be provided if necessary. Because cocaine-induced myocardial infarction is due to spasm rather than thrombus, it is better to avoid thrombolytics. Further administration of thrombolytics may be fatal, resulting in intracranial hemorrhages. However, if the patient suffers from *cocaine-induced angina*, then hospitalization may be necessary to provide necessary coronary care of the patient.

20.15.1 COCAINISM

Cocainism is also known as chronic cocaine poisoning (cocainophagia, cocainomania, cocaine addiction, cocainism). For the euphoric effects of cocaine, addicts usually take cocaine by SC injection, eat it wrapped in *paan*, or inhale it as snuff.

Signs and symptoms Victims usually have an unstable nervous system or initial psychopathic tendencies, such as:

- Anorexia, weight loss, weakness, tremors, impotence, moral deterioration, insanity, increased erotic tension, etc.
- Occasionally, sexual perversion
- Cocaine insanity may present with characteristic delusions of persecution and hallucinations that are chiefly tactile (Magnan symptom) or of visual origin.

Magnan symptom (cocaine bugs)

- Magnan symptom is type of tactile hallucination that makes addicts feel as if insects (bugs) are crawling under their skin. One may even report the presence of sand grains under the skin. In chronic users, the teeth and tongue are black.

Treatment The treatment of withdrawal symptoms is usually successful with the cooperation of the patient.

20.16 STRYCHNINE

Strychnine is a spinal poison caused by *Strychnos nuxvomica* (kuchila plant) (Fig. 20.6). It contains alkaloids such as strychnine, brucine, and loganine.

Mode of action For the onset of action, the seeds (bitter in taste) must be chewed and swallowed, and the site of action is the anterior horn cells of the spinal cord. It acts by competitive antagonism of inhibitory neurotransmitter glycine at the postsynaptic motor neurons of the spinal cord.

Signs and symptoms After ingestion of seeds, within 15 min to 1 h it produces epigastric pain followed by stiffness in the muscles and typical strychnine convulsions, which are initially clonic (intermittent), followed by tonic (sustained),

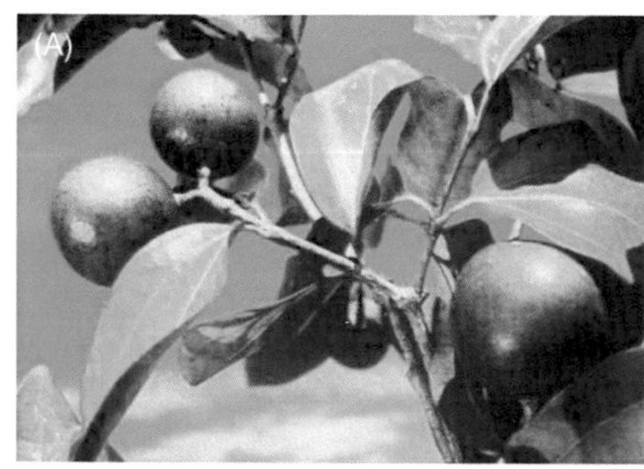

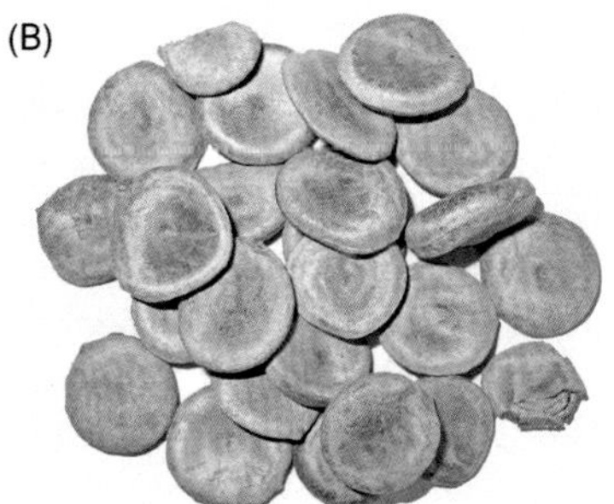

FIGURE 20.6

Strychnine plant along with fruits (A), and seeds (B).

Source: (A) The Poison Diaries. Available at: http://thepoisondiaries.tumblr.com/post/36597628648/strychnos-nux-vomica; (B) Wikimedia Commons. Available at: https://en.wikipedia.org/wiki/Strychnos_nux-vomica.

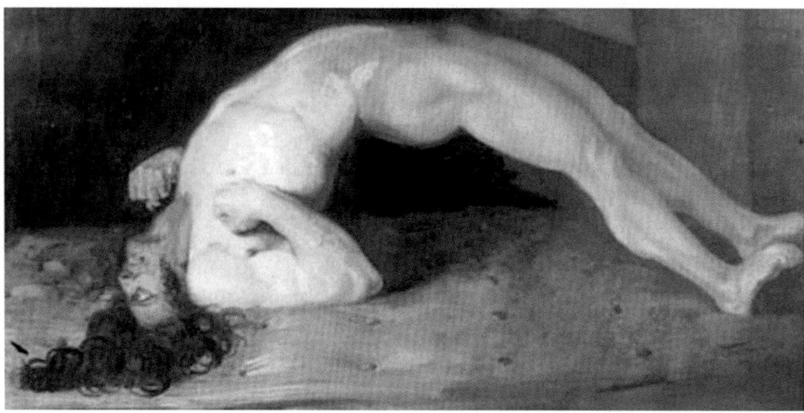

FIGURE 20.7

Uncontrolled muscle contractions and seizures are symptoms of strychnine poisoning.

Source: Adnan, A., 2015. Treating Strychnine Poisoning, Part 1. In: Prodding Physiology. Available at: http://www.proddingphysiology.com/?p=182.

affecting both the flexor and extensor muscles of the body simultaneously. The clinical picture after strychnine poisoning is shown in Fig. 20.7.

1. Facial muscles become fixed in a "grin" (clinically called *Risus sardonicus*) and there is prolonged spasm of the jaw muscles producing "lock-jaw" (called *trismus*).
2. Other muscles of the body may contract and become fixed in one of the following postures:
   a. *Opisthotonus*: the body is bent backwards (hyperextension of spine), making it rest on the occiput and heels like a bow
   b. *Emprosthotonus*: the body is bent forward
   c. *Pleurothotonos*: the body is bent laterally (to left/right).

Other symptoms are cyanosis, dilated pupils, frothy salivation, and respiratory distress and failure, leading to death. Consciousness is retained, resulting in an agonizing death.

The fatal dose is one or two crushed seeds. The fatal period is 1–2 h.

Treatment To control convulsions, administer IV diazepam or barbiturates. If these are not effective, then administer general anesthesia or neuromuscular blockade and oxygen (artificial respiration). Administration of IV succinylcholine chloride 50 mg is useful for controlling of convulsions.

CHAPTER

Toxic effects of cardiac poisons

21

CHAPTER OUTLINE

21.1 INTRODUCTION

Cardiac poisons act mainly on the heart, either directly or through the nerves. Although there may be several cardiac poisonous plants, three are important: (1) oleanders (nerium and cerbera); (2) aconite; and (3) nicotine.

21.2 OLEANDERS

Oleanders are widely cultivated in various parts of the world for their ornamental flowers (Fig. 21.1).

There are three types of oleanders.

1. *Nerium odourum*: Common names are white/pink oleander and kaner. Nerium odourum has nerin, which contains the following cardiac glycosides: (1) neriodorin; (2) neriodorein; (3) karabin; (4) oleandrin; (5) folinerin; and (6) rosagerin.
2. *Cerbera thevetia*: Common names are yellow oleander, peela kaner, exile, and bastard oleander. Cerbera thevetia has three glycosides: (1) thevetin (one-eighth as potent as ouabain, which is similar in action to digitalis); (2) thevitoxin, which is less toxic than thevetin; (3) nerifolin, which is more potent than thevetin; (4) peruvoside; (5) ruvoside; and (6) cerberin.
3. *Cerbera odollum*: Common names are dabur, dhakur, and pilikibir. All parts of the plant are poisonous, especially the fruit with its kernels or seeds and the nectar from the flowers, which yields poisonous honey. In cerbera thevetia, the milky juice that exudes when cutting any part of the plant yields the toxic principles. Cerbera odollum contains glyciside and cerberin.

Fundamentals of Toxicology. DOI: http://dx.doi.org/10.1016/B978-0-12-805426-0.00021-4

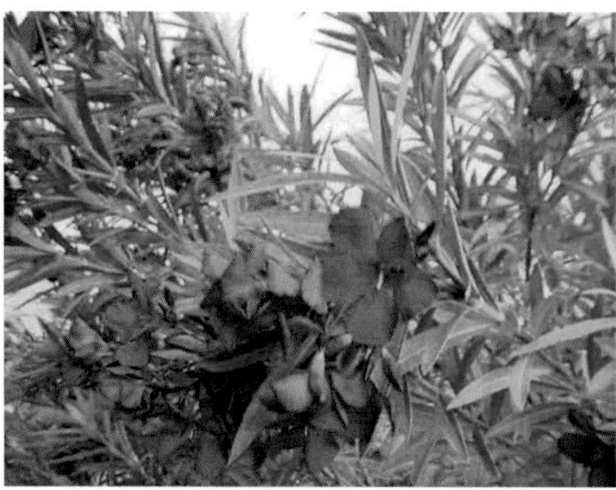

FIGURE 21.1

Oleander plant.

Source: Isaacs, T.M. A brief history of the oleander plant. Available at: http://www.tbyil.com/oleander3.htm.

Mode of action Oleanders act like digitalis; toxic doses can produce malignant dysrhythmias and cardiac failure, cardiac arrest, and convulsions. Oleanders are absorbed easily via skin and the gastrointestinal (GI) route.

Signs and symptoms In general, oleander poisoning closely resembles digitoxin poisoning with predominantly GI and cardiac symptoms. Severe toxic effects result from cardiotoxicity, and specifically from ventricular ectopy and cardiovascular collapse. Digitalis toxicity is characterized by increased ectopy and conduction delay, which may persist for 3–6 days (eg, supraventricular tachycardia with atrioventricular block).

Nerium Odourum: Poisoning leads to nausea, vomiting, abdominal pain, restlessness, and slow and weak pulse followed by fast respiration. Victims may experience dysphagia and lock jaw, followed by tonic convulsions, leading to exhaustion, drowsiness, coma, heart failure, and death.

Cerbera Thevetia: Poisoning leads to a burning sensation in mouth, tingling of the tongue, dryness of the throat, vomiting, diarrhea, headache, dilated pupils, and irregular action of the heart, followed by drowsiness, coma, collapse, and death.

Cerbera odollum: Poisoning shows symptoms similar to those seen with cerbera thevetia.

The fatal dose of *Nerium odourum* is 15 g of root, of *Cerbera thevetia* is 10 seeds, and of *Cerbera odollum* is the kernel of one fruit.

The fatal period for *Nerium odourum* is 24–36 h. For *Cerbera thevetia*, if powdered and fed to a child mixed with milk, the fatal period is 3 h. In the case of Cerbera odollum, the fatal period is 1–2 days.

Postmortem findings *Nerium Odourum*: Nonspecific petechial hemorrhages of the heart are important. The poison is heat-resistant and can be detected even in the ashes of a burned dead body (another such poison is arsenic).

Cerbera Thevetia: GI irritation, congestion of viscera, generalized venous engorgement, and subendocardial hemorrhage are common. The poison restricts putrefaction and can be detected even on exhumation.

Treatment Treatment is mainly supportive and symptom-based, such as gastric lavage, fluid administration, use of atropine, isoproterenol, antiarrhythmics, and early administration of activated charcoal.

Hemodynamic decompensation may require temporary use of a cardiac pacemaker and digoxin-spcific Fab antidote fragments. Doses of 200 mg and 480 mg IV have been useful in life-threatening oleander intoxication.

21.3 ACONITE

Aconite is a plant (Fig. 21.2) that is grown in gardens. Common names are monkshood, blue rocket, Wolf bane, mithazaha/mitha vish (meaning "sweet poison" in Hindi). The whole plant is poisonous; however, roots are highly toxic and used commonly.

Toxic Principle: The toxic principles are deterpene alkaloids known as aconitine, misaconitine, and hypaconitine. These alkaloids are sparingly soluble in water and considered the most virulent poison with a sweetish taste. Other alkaloids that are present in small quantities in the plant are picraconitine, pseudoaconitine, and aconine.

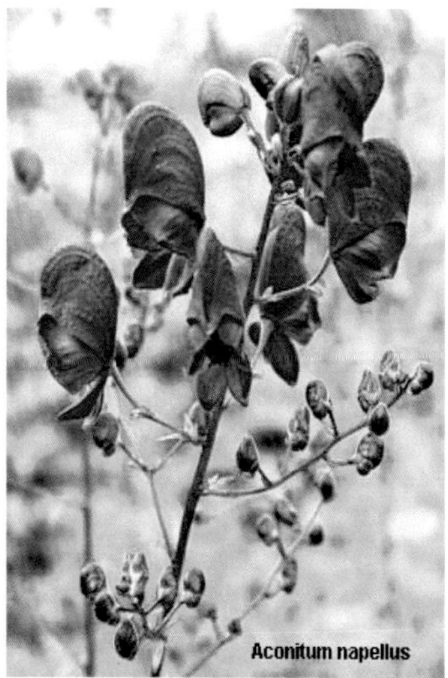

FIGURE 21.2

Aconite plant with leaves and flowers.

Source: Antosh, G., 2012. Aconite Plant: How To Grow Monkshood Plants. Plant-Care.com. Available at: http://www.plant-care.com/aconite-plant.html.

Mode of action Deterpene alkaloids are neurotoxins that can cause conduction block and paralysis through their action on voltage-sensitive sodium channels in the axons, resulting in initial neurological stimulation, followed by depression of myocardium, smooth muscles, skeletal muscles, the central nervous system (CNS), and the peripheral nervous system. Aconite is absorbed via the skin and orally. Symptoms generally appear within 30–90 min after ingestion of the poison and last up to approximately 30 h.

Signs and symptoms Some of the typical features of poisoning are:

Cardiovascular: Palpitation, hypertension, and ventricular ectopics/arrhythmias.

GI Tract: Nausea, salivation, pain in stomach, vomiting, and diarrhea.

Neurological: Paresthesia and tingling and numbness in the lips, mouth, tongue, and pharynx. It may extend to all parts of body, followed by profuse sweating, weakness, impending paralysis of the extremities, and/seizures. Typical symptoms in the forehead include band-like, sudden, violent bursting (Fig. 21.3). Deep tendon reflexes may be absent.

Eye: There may be difficulty in vision due to hippus. Hippus means that, initially, there is alternate dilatation and constriction of pupils, followed by complete dilation.

In general, there may be acidosis and hypokalemia, and the conscious state of the victim may be reduced. The patient experiences hypertension, followed by sustained ventricular tachyarrhythmia, convulsions, respiratory paralysis, and death.

The fatal dose is 1 g of root, 250 mg of root extract, 20 drops of tincture extract, and 3 to 5 mg (average 4 mg) of the alkaloid aconitine.

The fatal period is 3–24 h (average, 6 h).

Postmortem findings Root pieces may be detected in stomach contents; lesions, as seen in asphyxia, may be observed. Aconite is highly unstable and excreted in

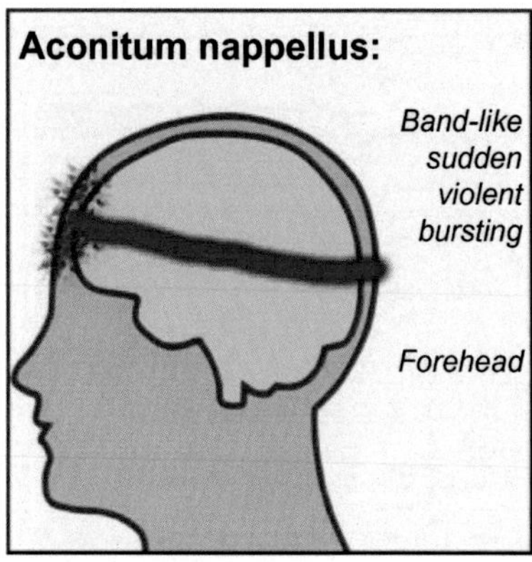

FIGURE 21.3

Effects of aconite nappellus on forehead.

Source: Bisciotti, K., 2014. 9 Homeopathic Remedies for 9 Common Headaches. Musings of a Modern Hippie. Available at: http://musingsofamodernhippie.com/2014/02/homeopathyforheadaches.html.

urine and body fluids. The toxins are destroyed quickly and may not be detected on chemical analysis; therefore, acetic acid is added to the rectified spirit to preserve the vomit to be sent for chemical examination.

Treatment Treatment is symptom-based, such as gastric lavage with warm water and/or weak solution of iodine in potassium iodide or tannic acid to precipitate the alkaloid; animal charcoal is another treatment. Artificial respiration (oxygen) and use of atropine to prevent vagal inhibition of the heart and 0.1% novocaine 50 mL to control the cardiac arrhythmias are recommended.

21.4 NICOTINE (TOBACCO)

Nicotine grows in all tropical regions of the world. The common name is tobacco and the botanical name is *Nicotiana tobacum* (Fig. 21.4). Dried leaves and stems of *Nicotiana species* include *N. tobacum* (cultivated tobacco), *N. attenuate* (wild tobacco,), *N. glauca* (tree tobacco), and *N. trigonophylla* (dessert tobacco). Lobeline is the chief constituent of Indian tobacco and is obtained from the leaves and tops of *Lobelia inflatea*, an alkaloid similar to nicotine but less potent. It is used in antismoking tablets and lozenges.

Nicotine contains an alkaloid known as nicotine, which is a colorless liquid that turns amber on exposure to light. More recently, nicotine sulfate has been used as a dog-controlling agent (at approximately 285 mg of nicotine/mL). It is also used in animal tranquilizer darts (with a strength of 240 mg of nicotine/mL). However, its use as an insecticide has been drastically reduced.

Most criminal use of nicotine in developing countries is to induce infanticide, either by applying the nicotine extract over the nipples of the nursing mother or by feeding it to the child mixed with milk. Another form of criminal use is

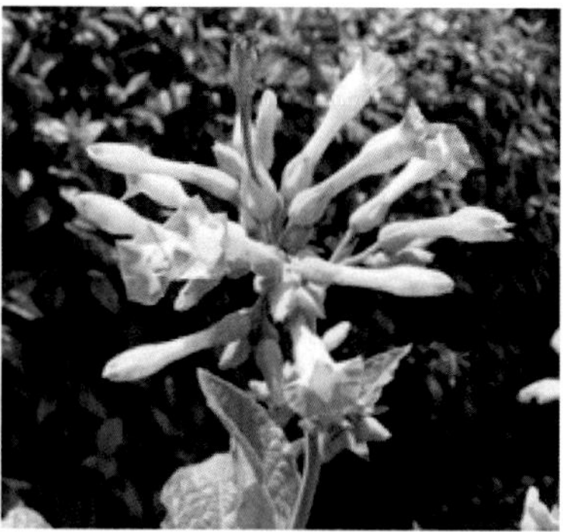

FIGURE 21.4

Nicotine plant with flowers.

Source: GeoChemBio.com. Available at: http://www.geochembio.com/biology/organisms/tobacco/#top.

keeping the tobacco leaves in the arm pits for a few minutes, which brings about a local increase in temperature, resulting in fever and sickness.

Mode of action Nicotine is absorbed via intact skin, oral mucosa, the GI tract, and the respiratory system. It is detoxified mainly in the liver, but also in the kidneys and lungs. The major metabolic product of nicotine is cotinine. Cotinine, along with a nonmetabolized form of nicotine, is excreted in urine. Elimination is complete in 16 h; however, acidic urine increases urinary excretion. Nicotine is also excreted in the milk of lactating woman.

Signs and symptoms In general, nicotine affects a wide range systems such as the CNS, heart, lungs, GI tract, muscles, joints, and endocrine system. Side effects induced by nicotine are shown in Fig. 21.5.

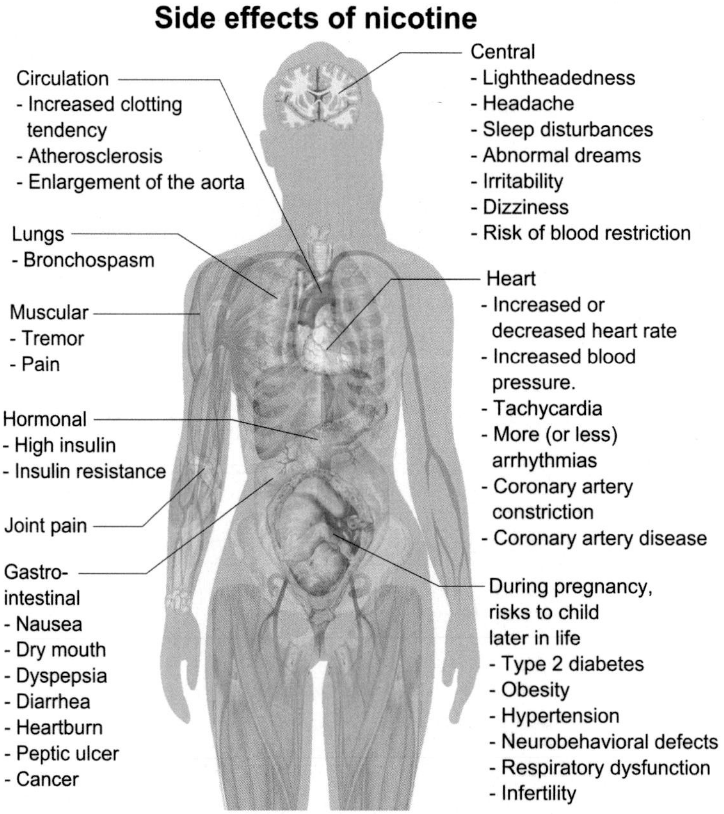

FIGURE 21.5

Toxic potential of nicotine on various systems of body.

Source: Häggström, M., 2014. Medical gallery of Mikael Häggström. Wikiversity Journal of Medicine 1 (2). Available at: https://commons.wikimedia.org/wiki/File:Side_effects_of_nicotine.png.

Brain symptoms include stimulation and depression, followed by paralysis of cells of the peripheral autonomic ganglia, midbrain, spinal cord, and muscles. Mild poisoning frequently occurs by chewing the dried leaves, producing dizziness, nausea, vomiting, headache, perspiration, weakness, and cardiac irregularities. The victim usually returns to normal in a few hours.

Acute Poisoning Acute poisoning occurs chiefly due to central/peripheral stimulations. Manifestations include all the signs of toxicity as observed in mild poisoning and other symptoms of poisoning, such as burning in the mouth, throat, and stomach and prostration, followed by convulsions, cardiac irregularities, and sometimes even cardiac arrest and death. Virtually all toxicity from nicotine is reported from cigarettes. More than 90% of toxic exposure from cigarettes in the United States is reported in children younger than 5 years of age. In Germany, reports of such incidences have been reported among infants as young as 7 months of age.

The available evidence indicates that nicotine is a highly addictive substance.

Chronic Poisoning Chronic poisoning is known as nicotine addiction, and it is common among nicotine insecticide sprayers, tobacco chewers, and cigarette smokers. Continuous use of tobacco can lead to tobacco heart, lung cancer, and spontaneous abortion.

Victims may show chronic cough, bronchitis, laryngitis, pharyngitis, dermatitis, angiospasms, tremors, amblyopia, narrowing of field of vision, and blurry vision. The effect of nicotine on the heart is called "tobacco heart," which is characterized by extrasystole and angina. Chronic cases may also frequently manifest with thromboangitis obliterans (TAO) of extremities.

The fatal dose is 2 g of tobacco or 60 mg of nicotine.

The fatal period varies from a few minutes to a few hours.

Postmortem findings The stomach emits a typical tobacco smell with brownish discoloration of the stomach wall. Brownish stains may be seen on skin, mucosa may show signs of irritation, and lungs show pulmonary edema.

Treatment Gastric lavage, activated animal charcoal, purgative, and atropine 1.5 mg (if there is salivation) are useful treatments. Use cardiorespiratory stimulants along with symptom-based treatment. Stopping smoking altogether is recommended.

CHAPTER

Toxic effects of asphyxiants 22

CHAPTER OUTLINE

22.1 DEFINITION

Asphyxiants are gaseous poisons that produce respiratory distress, leading to asphyxia.

22.2 CLASSIFICATION

Gaseous poisons comprise four basic types:

1. Chemical asphyxiants
2. Simple asphyxiants
3. Respiratory/pulmonary irritant asphyxiants
4. Systemic asphyxiants

Fundamentals of Toxicology. DOI: http://dx.doi.org/10.1016/B978-0-12-805426-0.00022-6

22.2.1 CHEMICAL ASPHYXIANTS

Chemical asphyxiants reduce the body's ability to absorb, transport, or utilize inhaled oxygen. In other words, by their specific toxic action they render the body incapable of utilizing the supply of adequate oxygen to the tissues.

22.2.2 SIMPLE ASPHYXIANTS

Simple asphyxiants are inert gases that deprive tissues of oxygen by their ability to displace oxygen. Thus, these asphyxiants displace the oxygen from the inspired gas mixture, creating diminished uptake. Examples include carbon dioxide, helium, nitrogen, nitrous oxide, aliphatic hydrocarbon gases such as butane, ethane, methane, and propane, and noble gases such as argon, helium, neon, and radon.

22.2.3 RESPIRATORY/PULMONARY IRRITANT ASPHYXIANTS

Respiratory or pulmonary asphyxiants are gases that can damage the respiratory tract by destroying the integrity of the mucosal barrier and produce noncardiogenic pulmonary edema, which impairs the oxygen diffusion across the alveolar membrane. Examples include ammonia, chlorine, formaldehyde, hydrogen sulfide, and methyl isocyanate, and oxides of nitrogen, ozone, phosgene, and sulfur dioxide.

22.2.4 SYSTEMIC ASPHYXIANTS

These are gases that produce significant systemic toxicity by specialized mechanisms. Examples include carbon monoxide, cyanide, and smoke.

Carbon monoxide, carbon dioxide, war gases, hydrogen sulfide, cyanides, and ammonia are discussed in great detail here.

22.3 CARBON MONOXIDE

Carbon monoxide (CO) is a colorless, tasteless, odorless nonirritant gas produced whenever there is incomplete combustion of carbon. It is water-soluble and burns with a blue flame. This gas accounts for many deaths in developed countries, such as the United States and Europe, through suicide attempts and accidental poisoning.

The most important source of CO is the incomplete combustion of fuel such as wood, charcoal, gas, and kerosene. Other sources include automobile exhaust, fire, and tobacco smoke. Endogenous CO resulting from heme degradation constitutes another source of CO. Thus, CO is an end product of normal metabolism and is formed during the conversion of heme into biliverdin. However, this can

Table 22.1 Severity of Toxicity in Relation to Carboxyhemoglobin (COHb) (%) in Carbon Monoxide Poisoning

Saturation of COHb (%)	Severity of Poisoning
10–30%	Mild
30–40%	Moderate
>40%	Severe

never reach toxic levels. The normal CO level in plasma is 1–5%, and this may increase up to 7–8% in chronic smokers. City dwellers and smokers may show a carboxyhemoglobin (COHb) level of 3.5% in their blood; however, these levels vary with the CO contamination of the atmosphere. Severity of toxicity in relation to saturation of COHb (%) in carbon monoxide poisoning is summarized in Table 22.1.

CO is commonly used to commit suicide in the West (United States); attempts include inhaling motor vehicle exhaust or putting one's head in a gas oven (United Kingdom). Another major cause of poisoning is an accidental cooking gas leakage in a home kitchen. At times mass deaths are observed, such as when a large building catches fire; the cause of death is inhalation of smoke containing CO.

Mode of action CO has 200- to 300-times more affinity for hemoglobin (Hb) than oxygen (O_2), forming COHb, which is quite stable. This renders hemoglobin incapable of carrying oxygen, resulting in tissue anoxia. As long as CO is in the atmosphere, it continues accumulating and becomes fixed in blood, leading to acute chemical asphyxia. The CO absorbed by the lung rapidly combines with hemoglobin (85%). Elimination occurs exclusively through the lungs.

Signs and symptoms

Acute Poisoning The severity of poisoning usually depends on the percentage of COHb. Thus, the signs and severity depend on the degree of saturation of CO in the blood. Table 22.1 highlights the signs and symptoms of acute poisoning depending on an increase in the percentage of COHb in the blood. Formation of COHb can lead to anoxemia, resulting in weakening of the vascular walls, degeneration of nerve elements, weakening of the heart due to lack of nutrition, and, ultimately, death due to deprivation of O_2.

Fatality with CO poisoning is rapid (if the victim is asleep in an ill-ventilated room). Kerosene or other hydrocarbons are often the culprits.

Chronic Poisoning Chronic poisoning is observed due to frequent exposure to CO. This type of poisoning is observed in individuals working in gas houses, automobile workers, traffic police, people living in houses and shops adjacent to roads with heavy traffic.

The common signs of toxicity include nausea, upset digestion, frontal headache, palpitation and aggravation of angina, anemia, visual disturbance, and loss of sensation in the fingers. There may be symptoms of atrial fibrillations, bundle branch blocks, atrioventricular block, abnormal left ventricular function, decreased cognitive ability, loss of memory, mental retardation, psychosis, Parkinsonism, and incontinence. Coma is accompanied by degenerative changes in the brain and capillaries. Neurological symptoms include blindness and decerebrate rigidity.

Postmortem findings There is cherry red discoloration of the skin, mucosa, blood, and viscera. If the blood is placed in a test tube and diluted with water and then held against a light or a white background, then the pink color will be observed.

Treatment Treatment should include providing the patient with fresh air. Use of artificial respiration and providing 100% oxygen using a tight-fitting mask or endotracheal tube until COHb decreases to 15–20%. Provide gastric lavage during the early stage to help prevent aspiration pneumonia.

1. Monitor the cardiac and respiratory status. Keep the patient completely at rest for a minimum of 48 h.
2. Prevent cerebral edema by hyperventilation (PCO 25–30 mm Hg), head elevation, and infusion of mannitol (0.25–1 g/kg of 20% solution for 30 min). Avoid administering steroids.

To control convulsions, use diazepam or phenytoin; to prevent lung infection, antibiotics should be administered prophylactically. A whole-blood transfusion is useful.

Antidote: Administration of hyperbaric oxygen (HBO) is considered a specific antidote and may be helpful in reducing neuropsychiatric symptoms. However, giving HBO has its own risks, such as cerebral gas embolism, rupture of tympanic membrane, visual deficits, and oxygen toxicity such as convulsions and pulmonary edema. Any patient with COHb level >25% should be administered HBO with carbon dioxide (CO_2).

22.4 CARBON DIOXIDE

CO_2 is a heavy, odorless, poisonous gas produced by complete combustion of carbon-containing compounds. It is also formed during respiration, combustion, fermentation, and decomposition of organic matter, mine explosions, and when refrigerating plants. In solid form it is called dry ice. Atmospheric air usually contains 0.4% CO_2.

Accidents usually occur among workers involved with deep well cleaners, unloading of wet grains from cargo ships (fermented CO_2), or in any ill-ventilated room containing a crowd of people.

Signs and symptoms The symptoms of toxicity vary with the concentration of gas. The pure CO_2 leads to vagal inhibition and spasm of glottis, followed by death. All other symptoms are chiefly due to lack of oxygen.

The fatal concentration minimum is 25–30% and the maximum is 60–80%. The fatal period is instant collapse and death.

Postmortem findings The findings include cyanosis, marked capillary and venous congestion, petechial hemorrhages, and froth at the nostrils and mouth. The blood is dark and fluid-like, and there is deep congestion of viscera.

Treatment Treatment is supportive, such as providing the patient with fresh air, maintenance of body warmth, and use of artificial respiration plus O_2 therapy. The use of cardiac stimulants such as amphetamine sulfate (long-term exposure can lead to irreversible brain changes) is useful.

22.5 CYANIDE (PRUSSIC ACID, CYANOGEN)

Cyanide may be a gas, liquid, or solid. In a gaseous state, it is referred to as hydrogen cyanide (HCN); in liquid form, it is called hydrocyanic acid or prussic acid or cyanogens. It is a solution of either 2% or 4% of HCN in water. Pure acid is a colorless, transparent, volatile liquid with a penetrating odor of bitter almonds. However, approximately 20–40% of the population cannot smell the gas, and the ability to detect the smell is a sex-linked recessive trait. On exposure to light it rapidly decomposes. Cyanide salts occur as solids, and these cyanides of sodium/potassium are white powders. Cyanides are also considered a cardiac poison.

HCN is the normal constituent of the human body (15–30 micrograms). Cyanides are present as harmless glucoside amygdalin in fruits and leaves such as the following: bitter almond, apricot, cherry, peach, and plum (in their leaf, bark, and seeds); apple and pear (in their seeds); bamboo shoots and cherry laurel (in their leaves); cassava (topioca/manihot) and lima beans (in their fruit/bean and root). However, emulsin enzymes can hydrolyze these and release hydrocyanic acid. The burning of plastic furniture, silk, wool, and cigarettes (smoking) produces traces of cyanide.

Uses: HCN gas is used for fumigation of ships. It is often used in laboratories in various laboratory processes and in photography, electroplating, coating silver, case hardening of steel/iron, and tanning industries. Calcium cyanide is utilized as a fertilizer.

Absorption: Rapid absorption is possible through both skin and the mucous membrane of the respiratory tract and stomach. On ingestion of cyanide salts, they react with acids (eg, HCl) in the stomach and liberate HCN acid. Rhodanese enzymes present in the mitochondria of the liver and kidneys metabolize cyanides. They are excreted in the breath and sweat, producing a bitter almond odor.

Mode of action Cyanides are protoplasmic cytotoxic poisons. They act by inhibiting cytochrome oxidases for utilizing O_2 in a cell, leading to internal asphyxia (cellular asphyxia) and death (Fig. 8.1). Cyanides have mild action in other enzymes. They also act as a corrosive agent on mucosa. Death is mainly due to either respiratory paralysis or cytotoxicity.

Signs and symptoms

Acute Poisoning All symptoms reflect cellular hypoxia, and symptoms shift rapidly depending on the extent of cyanide exposure. Inhalation brings about death instantaneously by respiratory arrest.

Central Nervous System: Headache, giddiness, anxiety, agitation, confusion, convulsions, and coma are common. Eyes are glassy and prominent with unresponsive pupils. Violent convulsions, clenched jaw, loss of muscle power, loss of consciousness, and, ultimately, death can occur.

Cardiovascular System: Initially, symptoms include hypertension with reflex bradycardia and sinus arrhythmia, followed by tachycardia, hypotension ventricular dysarrhythmias, and cardiac collapse.

Gastrointestinal (GI): When taken orally, the victim may complain of a bitter, acidic, burning taste. Constriction and numbness of throat, salivation, nausea, and, rarely, vomiting occur. Frothing and corrosion of the mouth associated with the smell of bitter almonds occur around mouth and in the breath.

Respiratory System: The respiratory system shows initial tachypnea followed by dyspnea, bradypnea, severe respiratory depression, and cyanosis.

Skin: Skin and mucosa will be brick red in color and may be due to an increase in hemoglobin oxygen saturation in venous blood because of decreased utilization of oxygen by tissues. Skin will be cold and clammy; in late stages, it turns cyanotic.

Chronic Poisoning Chronic poisoning comprises exposure over a long period by inhalation of nonlethal doses of HCN acid vapors. Usual manifestations are headache, vertigo, nausea, vomiting, and visual defects such as scotoma and progressive loss of vision (tobacco amblyopia) in victims who are chronic smokers. Optic atrophy (Leber's hereditary optic atrophy) may be observed, which may be due to the sensitivity of the optic nerve to cyanide, a congenital defect of rhodanese deficiency seen only among men.

Tropical ataxic neuropathy is common. This is a condition with clinical manifestations of peripheral sensory neuropathy, optic atrophy, ataxia, deafness, glossitis, stomatitis, and scrotal dermatitis. It is common among the victims who eat large quantities of tuber topioca (Cassava/manihot), which contains cyanogens.

The fatal dose varies with the toxic substance used: pure acid, 60 mg; any pharmacological preparation, 30 drops; crude oil of bitter almond, 60 drops; and potassium cyanide, 200 mg.

Air pollution

1. 0.15 mg HCN/L: Death in 30–60 min
2. 0.3 mg HCN/L: Death instantaneously
3. 1:500 concentration: Death instantaneously

The fatal period in some cases may be immediate death. An average for HCN acid is 2–10 min, and for potassium cyanide it is 30 min. Prognosis of the survival of the victim at 4 h after poisoning is usually good and is followed by recovery.

Postmortem findings Postmortem appearances are mainly those of asphyxia.

Treatment Use of supportive therapy and antidotes are useful; for example, sodium nitrite is often used in conjunction with sodium thiosulphate to help form nontoxic compounds that can be excreted in the urine. Sodium nitrite converts hemoglobin to methemoglobin by the process of oxidation. Methemoglobin, in turn, reacts with the lethal cyanide ion of cyan-cytochrome oxidase to produce cyan-methemoglobin. This process reactivates the inactivated cytochrome oxidase enzyme. The cyan-methemoglobin in the presence of rhodanese enzymes takes sulfur from the donor sodium thiosulphate and forms sodium thiosulphate, which is nontoxic and eliminated through urine. Hemoglobin is released during this process. The mechanism of action of sodium nitrite in cyanide poisoning is shown in Fig. 22.1.

Decontamination can be performed by gastric lavage, preferably with 5% sodium thiosulphate solution, or activated charcoal followed by cathartics. In case of skin contamination, removal of clothes from the patient and washing the skin with soap and water are useful. Assisted ventilation using 100% oxygenation, cardiac monitoring treatment of metabolic acidosis, and vasopressors for hypotension help in stabilization of the victim of cyanide poisoning.

Administration of an antidote such as amyl nitrite therapy under the supervision of doctor is recommended. Other antidotes include: use of oral solution A and solution B, comprising ferrous sulfate dissolved in aqueous citric acid and aqueous sodium carbonate; dicobalt edetate (cobalt-EDTA 20 mL of 1.5%, maximum 300–600 mg) is given in a slow intravenous (IV) injection, followed by 20 mL of 50% glucose, which acts by chelating the cyanide and forming a

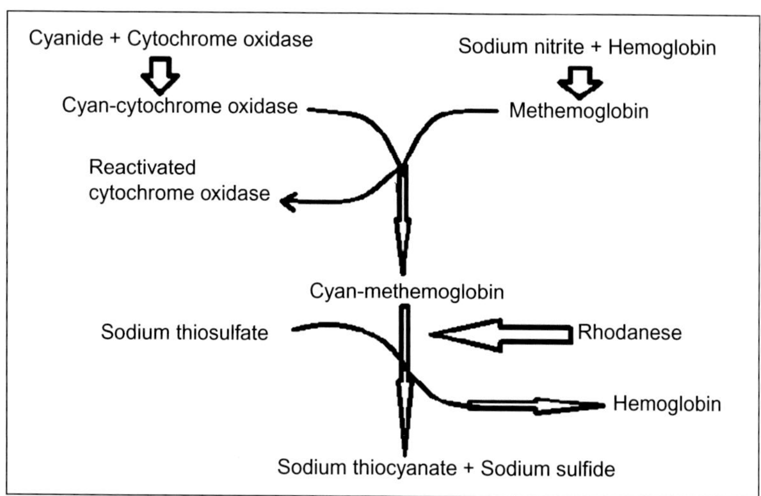

FIGURE 22.1

Proposed mechanism action of sodium nitrite in cyanide poisoning.

harmless product that is excreted in urine; and hydroxycobalamine (vitamin B_{12} precursor), which is available as a solution of 1000 mg/mL and given at a dosage of 50 mg/kg in a 3.5-L IV infusion and acts by the formation of cyanacobalmin (vitamin B_{12}), which is excreted in the urine.

Recently, PAPP (para-aminopropriophenone) has been recommended as an antidote to form methemoglobin. However, its action is somewhat slow.

22.6 AMMONIA (NH_3)

At room temperature, ammonia (NH_3) is a highly water-soluble, colorless, irritant gas with a unique pungent odor. Ammonia has a boiling point of $-33°C$ and an ignition temperature of 650°C. The farming industry uses anhydrous ammonia as a component of fertilizer and animal feed. Ammonia also is used in the production of explosives, pharmaceuticals, pesticides, textiles, leather, flame retardants, plastic, pulp and paper, rubber, petroleum products, and cyanide. Ammonia is also a major component of many common household cleaning and bleaching products (eg, glass cleaners, toilet bowel cleaners, metal polishes, floor strippers, wax removers, smelling salts). Ammonia is liberated during combustion of nylon, silk, wood, and melamine, thus rendering firefighters at risk for exposure to this irritant gas.

Cases of industrial accidental poisoning are more common with ammonia. Suicide with ammonia is also common. However, homicide is extremely rare due to its odor.

Permissible levels of exposure to toxic gases are defined by the time-weighted average (TWA), short-term exposure limit (STEL), and concentration at which toxic gasses are immediately dangerous to life or health (IDLH). Anhydrous ammonia has TWA of 25 ppm, STEL of 35 ppm, and IDLH of 500 ppm.

The fatal dose of the gaseous form is 0.5% in air. The fatal dose of the liquid form is 10–20 mL.

Mode of action The most common mechanism by which ammonia gas causes damage is when anhydrous ammonia (liquid or gas) reacts with tissue water to form the strongly alkaline solution ammonium hydroxide.

$$NH_3 + H_2O = NH_4OH$$

This reaction is exothermic and capable of causing significant thermal injury.

Although injury from ammonia is caused by inhalation, it may also result from ingestion or direct contact with eyes or skin. Because of its high water solubility, ammonia has a tendency to be absorbed by the water-rich mucosa of the upper respiratory tract. However, unlike most highly water-soluble irritant gases that tend to exclusively affect the upper respiratory tract, ammonia can damage proximally and distally.

Signs and symptoms *Inhalation*: Head, ears, eyes, nose, and throat (HEENT) symptoms include runny nose and increased salivation. Ammonia inhalation can produce tachypea, oxygen desaturation, stridor, drooling, cough, decreased air entry asthma, severe upper respiratory tract irritation, pneumonia, pulmonary edema, bronchitis, and obstructive lung disease. Death is usually due to bronchopneumonia.

Ingestion: HEENT symptoms include edema of the lips, oropharynx, and upper airway. Ammonia ingested can produce intense pain and dysphagia, followed by esophageal stenosis. Patients may experience epigastric tenderness; madiastinitis and peritoneal signs may be present with viscus perforation, which can occur as late as 24–72 h after ingestion.

Contact: Can result in skin burns (alkali burns) and cold injury. Facial and oral burns and ulceration may be seen. Alkali burns to the skin are yellow, soapy, and soft in texture. When burns are severe, the skin turns black and leathery.

Eye: Exposure results in watering of the eyes, corneal damage, conjunctivitis, and palpebral edema. Ammonia typically causes more corneal epithelium and lens damage than other alkalis. Intraocular pressure and pH of the anterior chamber increase, resulting in a syndrome similar to acute narrow-angle glaucoma. Other symptoms include iritis, corneal edema, semi-dilated fixed pupil, and eventual cataract formation. Blindness may be the serious consequence in severe cases.

Postmortem findings The postmortem changes indicate brownish staining, odor of ammonia, staining of affected skin, grayish sloughing of affected mucosa, congestion of GI walls (rarely perforations) and respiratory tract, and pulmonary edema.

Treatment Management of toxic exposure to ammonia is largely supportive, and medical therapy is directed toward the correction of hypoxia, bronchospasm, pulmonary edema, hypovolemia, and burns of the skin and eyes. Treatment includes:

1. Stomach wash and emetics use is not recommended.
2. Administering demulcents and dilute solution of vinegar are useful.
3. Tracheostomy, oxygen administration, and assisted ventilation may help to alleviate respiratory distress.

Antibiotics and corticosteroids are controversial therapies following ammonia inhalation and ingestion exposures. Corticosteroids are administered to decrease the incidence and severity of esophageal strictures that occur during healing from significant alkaline injuries. Antibiotics are administered because of increased risk of mediastinitis associated with full-thickness esophageal alkaline corrosive burns. If steroids are administered, then the recommended dose is 1–2 mg/kg per day of methyl prednisolone for 3 weeks, followed by gradual tapering. If antibiotics are administered, then a broad-spectrum antibiotic (second-generation cephalosporin) is appropriate. The decision to continue or stop corticosteroid and antibiotic therapy is based on endoscopic findings.

Lesions of the skin and eye need thorough washing with copious amount of water. Diluted vinegar may be applied to the skin after washing.

22.7 WAR GASES

War gases are chemicals that are used only as warfare agents. The term designates their applicability as agents befitted to carry destruction or damage, mostly in times of war or in dispersing unruly mobs. The characteristics of war gases along with examples are summarized in Table 22.2.

22.7.1 LACHRYMATORS (TEAR GASES)

Lachrymators need to be fired during an attack in artillery shells or pen guns to saturate the area of attack. Chloroacetophenone (CAP) is a solid or fine powder with a locust flower odor. It disintegrates rapidly. Bromobenzyl cyanide (BBC) is a heavy, oily, dark brown liquid with a fruity odor. The effect may persist for a maximum of 3 days. Ethyliodoacetate (KSK) is also a heavy, oily liquid; its effect persists for 10 days.

Mode of action War gases are harmless to life. They produce severe lacrimation due to intense irritation of the eyes with a copious flow of tears, spasm of the eyelids, and temporary blindness and irritation to respiratory passages. Long-term exposure can result in nausea, vomiting, blistering, and ulceration of the skin.

Treatment Treatment is supportive and symptom-based, such as moving the patient to fresh air, washing the eyes with normal saline or with boric acid solution, and application of a weak solution of sodium bicarbonate solution to the affected parts such as the skin, nose, and other sites.

22.7.2 LUNG IRRITANTS (ASPHYXIANTS, CHOKING GASES)

Lung irritants include chlorine (Cl_2) and phosgene ($COCl_2$) gases, but under pressure they are hot liquids. Chloropicrin and diphosgene are liquids. All of these war gases are used in shells. Phosgene is 10-times and chloropicrin is four-times more toxic than chlorine. Phosgene and diphosgene are called green cross.

Table 22.2 Types of War Gases and Examples

Lacrymators (tear gases)	Chloroacetophenone (CAP), bromobenzyl cyanide (BBC), ethyliodoacetate (KSK)
Lung irritants	Chlorine (Cl_2), phosgene ($COCl_2$)
Nasal irritants (sternutators)	Diphenyl chlorasine (DA), diphenylamine chlorasine (DM), dphenyl cyanasine (DC)
Nerve gases	Organophosphate (OP) compounds with acetylcholine-like actions
Paralysants	Carbon monoxide (CO), hydrocyanic acid (HCN), hydrogen sulfide (H_2S)
Vesicants	Mustard gas, lewisite
Miscellaneous	Yellow rain, methyl isocyanide

Mode of action These war gases can be fatal. They mainly act on the alveoli. Inhalation can cause dyspnea, tightness in the chest, cough, and irritation of conjunctivae, followed by restlessness, rapid and stertorous respiration (breathing with a heavy snoring sound), and cyanosis, followed by collapse and death within 1–2 days. The cause of death is acute pulmonary edema.

Postmortem findings Usually, findings are those of asphyxia. Other findings could be those of bizarre injuries due to bursting of shells containing the gas.

Treatment Treatment is supportive and symptom-based, such as the use of gas masks to prevent exposure, moving the patient to a clean atmosphere, providing oxygen and adrenaline, and washing of eyes/irrigation with normal saline/boric acid.

Symptom-based measures include use of codeine for cough and antibiotics for respiratory tract/lung infection.

22.7.3 NASAL IRRITANTS AND VOMITING GASES (STERNUTATORS)

These are solid compounds of arsenic that require firing in an artillery shell, such as diphenyl chlorarsine (DA) (or sickening gas), diphenylamine chlorarsine (DM), and diphenylcyanarsine (DC). Diphenyl chlorarsine is six-times heavier than air.

Mode of action Diphenyl chlorarsine can act on the vomiting center in the brain. Vapors can result in intense pain and irritation in the nose and sinuses, leading to sneezing, malaise, headache, and salivation, followed by nausea, vomiting, and chest pain. Additional symptoms similar to those of arsenic poisoning may also be observed.

Treatment Use of a gas mask, sodium bicarbonate for washing, and symptom-based treatment are recommended.

22.7.4 NERVE GASES

These are compounds related to organophosphate (OP) esters in action and toxicity. They are colorless and odorless volatile liquids. They are absorbed from the lungs, GI tract, skin, and conjunctiva. These nerve gases are chemicals with acetylcholine-like action by inactivating AChE, leading to accumulation of acetylcholine. Some of the known war gases are serin and tabun (for details, please refer to chapter: Toxic effects of pesticides (agrochemicals)).

22.7.5 VESICANTS (BLISTER GASES)

These gases mainly include mustard gas (dichloroethyl sulfide, yellow cross, etc.) and lewisite, which are in liquid form. Like the lachrymators, vesicants are also used during attacks with artillery shells to saturate the area of attack.

Mode of action Mustard gas can produce severe irritation of the eyes, nose, throat, and respiratory passages. It can also cause severe irritation of the skin, especially over the oily areas such as the face, axillae, pubis, and scrotum, resulting in redness, vesication/blister formation (of varying size), and ulceration, especially over the moist areas. It can even pass through clothes and produce intense itching of the skin.

These gases can cause inflammation of the stomach, leading to nausea, vomiting, pain in the abdomen, and diarrhea (mimics arsenic poisoning). Rarely, death can occur due to bronchopneumonia.

Treatment Use of a gas mask and special cloth covering (to protect skin), removal of contaminated clothing, washing of body with soap and water, and solution of sodium bicarbonate for the irrigation of the eyes (2%) and nose (5%) are recommended. BAL is a good antidote for lewisite.

22.7.6 PARALYSANTS (NERVE AND BLOOD POISONS)

Paralysants include hydrocyanic acid (HCN acid), CO, and hydrogen sulfide (H_2S). For details, please refer to the individual gas or agent in this book.

22.7.7 MISCELLANEOUS WAR GASES

These gases include yellow rain, red rain, and methyl isocyanate.

22.7.7.1 Yellow and red rain

Yellow rain and red rain are combinations of mustard gas, phosgene, chlorine, and nerve poison.

Signs and symptoms Victims feel as if their body is getting blown up. The patients have cough and hemoptysis, followed by painful breathing and burning in the throat that results in dysphagia. Eyes may turn yellow, with blurring of vision, nose tingling as if hot pepper has been inhaled, and necrosis of the gums with loosening of the teeth. The skin may necrotize with a red to blue coloration and there is an increase in body temperature.

The fatal period is usually 2 weeks.

Treatment Treatment is supportive and symptom-based.

22.7.7.2 Methyl isocyanate

Methyl isocyanate (MIC) has a pungent but sweet odor. It is a fairly stable liquid at room temperature (except in summer) and has a boiling point of 31°C. It reacts with water/moisture, alkaloids, and most other common solvents. Hence, it needs to be preserved under inert conditions. Poisoning is mostly accidental, for example, the Bhopal gas tragedy is a good example of poisoning due to MIC. MIC is a deadly substance used in pesticides and pharmaceutical industries that can kill in small doses. The chemical gets absorbed orally, through the respiratory tract, or through intact skin.

Signs and symptoms

Acute Poisoning In acute poisoning, MIC can locally produce irritation to the skin, eyes, and mucous membranes, resulting in a severe burning sensation in the throat and unbearable irritation of the eyes, followed by severe chest pain with labored breathing. Death is usually due to pulmonary edema in untreated cases.

Subacute Poisoning Subacute poisoning occurs when a person survives for more than 5–6 days after the exposure. The patient shows more of the neurological effects, such as motor weakness, paralysis, convulsions, coma, and cerebral edema, leading to death.

Delayed effects are observed in patients who survive for more than 1 week and show dyspnea, jaundice, and weakness of limbs, followed by exhaustion and death. In victims who are pregnant women, the delayed effects may include spontaneous abortion, congenital malformations, and stillbirth.

Treatment Treatment is supportive and symptom-based.

CHAPTER

Toxic effects of caustics (corrosives) 23

CHAPTER OUTLINE

23.1 INTRODUCTION

Corrosive poisons are those substances that corrode (or eat away) and destroy tissues through direct chemical action. They almost always act locally and have few systemic effects. The term caustic is often mistakenly presumed to denote an alkali; actually, it has a much broader meaning and refers to any substance that is corrosive and burning in nature. Obviously, this would also include the more important groups comprising acids. Table 23.1 summarizes the list of commonly used caustics/corrosive poisons.

23.2 CLASSIFICATION

1. Acids:
   a. Inorganic acids (mineral acids): Sulfuric, nitric, hydrochloric, and hydrofluoric acids.
   b. Organic acids: Carbolic, oxalic, and salicylic acids. These acids are weaker in action compared to inorganic acids and are usually absorbed into circulation, promoting local and remote action.
2. Alkalis: these include Alkalis include anhydrous ammonia, potassium hydroxide, sodium hydroxide, ammonium carbonate, potassium carbonate, and sodium carbonate.

Fundamentals of Toxicology. DOI: http://dx.doi.org/10.1016/B978-0-12-805426-0.00023-8

Table 23.1 Selective List of Commonly Used Caustics

Strong Acids	Strong Alkalis	Others
Inorganic acids (mineral acids): Sulfuric, nitric, hydrochloric, and hydrofluoric acids *Organic acids*: Carbolic, oxalic, and salicylic acids	Anhydrous ammonia, potassium hydroxide, sodium hydroxide, ammonium carbonate, potassium carbonate, sodium carbonate	Hydrogen peroxide, iodine, potassium permanganate, quaternary ammonium compounds

Table 23.2 Comparative Characteristics of Sulfuric, Nitric, and Hydrochloric Acids

	Sulfuric Acid	Nitric Acid	Hydrochloric Acid
Synonymous	Oil of vitriol	Aqua fortis, spirit of niter	Spirit of salts, muriatic acid
Physical properties	Heavy	Heavy	Heavy
	Colorless	Colorless	Colorless
	Viscid/oily	Not viscid/oily	Not viscid/oily
	Nonfuming	Fumes (yellow) in air	Fumes in air
	Gives heat with water	Not so	Not so
	Charring positive	Xanthroproteic reaction positive	Not so
	Burning acid taste	Choking odor	Not so
Fatal dose	5–10 mL	10–15 mL	15–20 mL
Fatal period	12–24 min	24–30 min	15–24 min
Commercial use	Textile, arts, and industry	Industries	Cleansing agent

23.3 ACIDS

23.3.1 INORGANIC ACIDS/MINERAL ACIDS

Sulfuric, nitric, and hydrochloric acid Acids are hydrogen-containing substances that, on dissociation in water, produce hydrogen ions. They are potent desiccants with the ability to produce coagulation necrosis of tissues on contact (except hydrofluoric acid, which produces liquefactive necrosis). When a strong acid is dissolved in a solvent, an exothermic reaction ensues, resulting in the emanation of heat, which is referred to as the heat of solution. Table 23.2 summarizes comparative characteristics of sulfuric, nitric, and hydrochloric acids.

Mode of action Strong acids act as corrosives, burning all tissues in the upper gastrointestinal (GI) tract when digested and sometimes resulting in esophageal or gastric perforation. They produce coagulation necrosis characterized by the formation of a coagulum (eschar) as a result of the desiccating action of the acid on proteins in superficial tissues. The coagulum formed limits the penetrating ability of acids. However, strong alkalis create injury to tissue by the mechanism of liquefaction necrosis. Alkalis, unlike acids, produce extensive penetrating damage. Squamous epithelium of the esophagus is more resistant to acids than is the columnar epithelium of the stomach. Therefore, esophageal strictures are more common in alkali poisoning, and pyloric and gastric strictures are more common in acid poisoning. Dilute acids and alkalis act as irritants, and corrosion is not really a prominent feature. The mode of action of acids is summarized in Fig. 23.1.

Signs and symptoms After oral consumption, corrosion of the GI and respiratory tracts is common but varies in intensity depending on the type and concentration of the acid. Fig. 23.1 shows the respiratory signs and symptoms after ingestion of all inorganic acid poisons, except hydrofluoric acid. The oral cavity shows chalky white teeth, swollen blackish tongue, and swollen lips. Acid burn (eschar) is

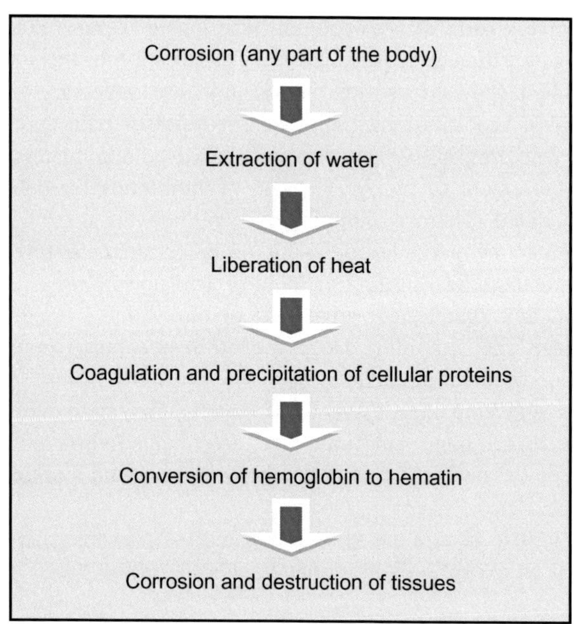

FIGURE 23.1

Schematic representation of the mechanism of coagulation necrosis.

commonly seen because vomited acid trickles down the angle of the mouth toward the neck and chest. The abdomen may be distended and tender.

Immediate death may be due to suffocation and asphyxia due to edema of the glottis; exhaustion and shock may be due to circulatory collapse or perforation of stomach; and delay in death may be due to starvation and dehydration because of stricture of the esophagus or pylorus. The victim may also die due to peritonitis or secondary infections. The mind remains sound until death.

Postmortem findings

External Corrosion of parts that come in contact with the acid, especially the lips, mouth, throat, chin, angle of mouth, and hands.

Internal The findings are restricted to the upper GI and respiratory tract and lead to corrosion.

Treatment The management of poisoning should be carefully undertaken. Certain general measures such as respiratory distress due to laryngeal edema should be treated with 100% oxygen.

Demulcents: Milk (canned condensed milk), egg white (beaten), vegetable oils, starch solution, barley water, and thin oatmeal should be administered.

Immediate dilution with milk or water within 30 min of ingestion is strongly recommended for oral ingestions. Do not attempt to neutralize the acid with weak bases/dilute alkalizers such as milk of magnesia or lime water (ie, calcium hydroxide in water), because an exothermic reaction may extend the corrosive injury. Do not give alkalis such as sodium bicarbonate because they can produce carbon dioxide gas, which increases the risk of perforation of the stomach.

Airway maintenance and artificial respiration are necessary if there is any respiratory distress. Use morphine/pethidine for relief of pain and IV fluids and electrolytes for dehydration. No oral feeding should be administered until endoscopy confirms the extent of injury. The use of antibiotics for controlling infections is recommended. There is controversy regarding the use of corticosteroids (although proven to be good for delaying or preventing stricture formation in experimental animal studies) in the treatment of acid poisoning.

Skin care for any skin lesions involves copious saline irrigation. Treat with nonadherent gauze and wrapping. Deep second-degree burns may benefit from topical application of silver sulfadiazine.

Eye care for any acid injuries requires copious irrigation with retraction of the eyelids for 20–30 min. Antibiotic eye drops can help combat infections. However, it may be necessary to refer the patient to an ophthalmologist for further treatment.

Emesis and gastric lavage are contraindicated (to prevent gastric perforation; however, there is an exception with organic acids).

23.3.1.1 Hydrofluoric acid

Hydrofluoric acid is a colorless gas that becomes a fuming liquid when dissolved in water. It is used for etching glass and clouding electric bulbs.

The fatal dose is approximately 15 mL. The fatal period varies from a few minutes to 2 h. However, there have been reports of deaths occurring within 7 h of poisoning.

Mode of action The mode of action of hydrofluoric acid exposure is quite different from that of other inorganic acids. The fluoride anion produces liquefaction necrosis by binding with calcium and magnesium in the tissues, thus resulting in hypocalcemia and rendering hydrofluoric acid poisoning more serious.

Signs and symptoms Following ingestion, the patient shows hematemesis, hypovolemic tonic convulsions, upper airway obstruction, severe hypocalcemia, acidosis, shock, and coma. Myocardial irritability and subsequent life-threatening cardiac arrhythmias may be due to binding of potassium, magnesium, and calcium ions. Skin exposure can result in severe and deep burns, which are extremely painful and slow to heal.

Postmortem findings The lips, tongue, and mouth may show white patches or may be charred. The esophagus may show shredded epithelium with ecchymosis, inflammation, ulceration, and blackening of the stomach. Liver and kidneys show fatty and parenchymatous degeneration.

Treatment The following treatment is recommended:

- Acid burn lesions need copious irrigation with water and application of calcium and gluconate gel. Debridement may also be needed.
- Intra-arterial infusion of 20% calcium gluconate or calcium chloride is effective.
- Oxygen inhalation after removal from fumes and tracheotomy, if needed, should be performed.

23.3.2 ORGANIC ACIDS

23.3.2.1 Carbolic acid (phenol)

Carbolic acid is a poison that can be identified by its smell, which is commonly referred to as a phenolic odor or hospital odor. Pure phenol has a colorless, short, prismatic, needle-shaped, crystalline form. On exposure to air, it turns pink and liquefies. It is fat-soluble; therefore, it can attack the nervous system. It is also soluble in glycerin, ether, and alcohol, and it is slightly soluble in water. It is known specifically for its antiseptic or disinfectant property.

Other members of phenol group: Phenol has several derivates, namely, cresol, creosote, lysol, and dettol. These are absorbed orally, through intact skin, by the GI tract, through inhalation by the respiratory tract, per rectum, and per vaginum. The toxicological actions of these compounds are similar to phenol but less severe.

- *Cresol* is a methyl phenol with meta, ortho, and para isomers. It is used as a disinfectant and antiseptic.
- *Creosote* is a mixture of phenols consisting mainly of cresol and guiacol. It is used as a household remedy for coughs and is found in many proprietary preparations.

- *Resorcinol* is a colorless crystalline substance used for the treatment of various skin diseases, including ringworm, psoriasis, and eczema.
- *Lysol* is a 50% solution of cresol (3-methyl phenol) in saponified vegetable oil.
- *Thymol* is an alkyl derivative of phenol obtained from volatile oils of *Thymus vulgaris*, *Monarda punctata*, or *Trachyspermum ammi*. It occurs in colorless crystals with a characteristic pungent odor and taste. Previously, it was used as an antihelminthic (for ankylostomiasis), antifungal, and antiseptic.

Mode of action Phenol is a protoplasmic poison. It enters into loose combination with proteins and penetrates deep into the tissue. When applied to the skin or mucosa, it causes necrosis and gangrene. The local nerve endings are first stimulated and then paralyzed, resulting in anesthesia. After absorption, it causes widespread capillary damage and clotting in superficial blood vessels. It also acts on the cells of the central nervous system, heart, and kidneys.

Phenol is mainly metabolized by the kidneys, wherein it gets converted into hydroquinone and pyrocatechol and then is excreted in urine. These products turn urine olive green or brown on standing, which is a phenomenon called carboluria. Complete elimination occurs in 36 h. Phenol is nephrotoxic (other nephrotoxics are heavy metals, methanol, oxalic acid, salicylates, phenacetin, EDTA, and penicillamine).

Signs and symptoms Poisoning by carbolic acid is known as carbolism. The usual signs and symptoms of carbolism include headache, giddiness, tinnitus, vomiting, diarrhea, abdominal pain, and a burning sensation. Inhalation of vapors leads to laryngeal edema and stertorous breathing with cyanosis. Pupils are dilated. If the patient survives for 48 h, then carboluria followed by anuria are seen. The victim will pass dark, smoky urine, which soon turns olive green on standing. Nervous symptoms are common. Methemoglobinemia is a characteristic feature in severe cases. Muscular spasms and convulsions, collapse/unconsciousness, and coma followed by death occur due to respiratory and circulatory failure.

Diagnosis: Corrosions on the face, around and inside the mouth (greyish white with phenol or brownish with lysol), phenolic odor (breath/vomit), carboluria, dilated pupils, and stertorous breathing.

The fatal dose is 5–15 g. The fatal period varies from 2 to 12 h (rapid death, if injected intrauterine).

Postmortem findings

External Greyish or brownish corrosions at the angle of the mouth and thin cracks in the body, arms, and hands (splashes), with characteristic phenolic odor.

Internal Corrosion of gastrointestinal mucosa and laryngeal and pulmonary edema have been observed in all orally ingested poisoning cases. However, there are certain specific findings, such as the stomach emitting a phenolic odor. Gastric mucosa will show marked corrosion and swelling of mucosal folds with coagulated greyish or brownish silvery mucus. Intervening normal mucosal folds appear dark red.

The kidneys will show hemorrhagic nephritis when the victim survives for some time after poisoning. Vomit and gastric lavage collection may show partially detached gastric mucosa.

Treatment Symptomatic treatment should include artificial respiration, tracheal aspiration of secretions, and glucose saline to induce diuresis.

In case of poisoning through skin absorption, use the following:

- Remove the contaminated garments.
- Cleanse the site by mopping with a wet cloth and wash with soap and water.
- Apply olive oil/methylated spirit/10% ethyl alcohol, which can prevent further absorption.
- Move the victim to fresh air.
- Give normal saline plus sodium bicarbonate (intravenous (IV) drip).

In case of poisoning through the oral route, perform the following:

- *Gastric lavage*: Although phenol corrodes the stomach wall, it also hardens it, unlike other corrosive poisons. Hence, gastric lavage is performed whenever possible with plenty of lukewarm water containing animal charcoal, olive oil, magnesium or sodium sulfate, or saccharated lime soap solution with 10% glycerin. When the lavage is completed, 30 g of magnesium sulfate or medicinal liquid paraffin should be left in the stomach.
- Give egg whites and Epsom salts/demulcents orally.

23.3.2.2 Oxalic acid (acid of sugar)

Oxalic acid is a colorless, prismatic, crystalline substance (similar to magnesium sulfate ($MgSO_4$) and zinc sulfate ($ZnSO_4$)). It acts locally as a corrosive on the skin and mucosa (more severe). After absorption, it affects blood electrolytes. It can remove tissue calcium, leading to hypocalcemia, followed by cardiovascular shock, tubular necrosis, uremia, and death.

The fatal dose is 15–20 mg. The fatal period ranges from 1 to 2 h.

Signs and symptom With large oral doses (15 g or more), it can lead to a sour and acidic taste, followed by a sensation of constriction around the throat and burning pain from the mouth to the epigastrium, which radiates all over the abdomen. There will be tenderness in the epigastrium, nausea followed by vomiting (coffee ground–colored vomit), severe thirst, diarrhea, electrolyte imbalance, and hypocalcemia, leading to muscle irritability, tenderness, tetany, convulsions, tingling of extremities, coma, collapse, and death. In case of slow poisoning, there is uremia. Urine is scanty, with traces of albumin. Microscopically, blood and calcium oxalate crystals are observed.

Postmortem findings

External There are no specific findings; however, sometimes, burns of the face and skin may be seen.

Internal Specific findings are that the mucosa of the mouth, tongue, pharynx, and esophagus may be bleached (whitened/scale/red) if a strong solution is consumed.

Stomach Changes The stomach mucosa is reddened and punctate due to erosions, giving a "velvety red" or blackish appearance. The wall of the stomach is softened, but there are no perforations. The stomach contents are gelatinous brown (due to acid hematin formation). All other viscera are congested. Kidneys are swollen and congested. On histopathology, tubules are filled with oxalate crystals.

Treatment General management should include gastric lavage with calcium lactate (two teaspoons per lavage), 10 mL calcium gluconate IV frequently, parathyroid extracts of 100 units IM, demulcent drinks, enema, and purgatives (castor oil). Symptom-based treatment should also be followed.

Antidotes such as lime water, calcium lactate, calcium gluconate, calcium chloride, and chalk suspension in water or milk may be administered orally. These form insoluble calcium oxalate and are excreted easily.

23.3.2.3 Formic acid (methanoic acid, formylic acid)

Formic acid is a colorless liquid with a pungent penetrating odor. It is completely soluble in water and is used as bath cleaner. Generally, airplane glue makers, cellulose format workers, and tanning salon workers are exposed to a 60% solution of formic acid.

Signs and symptoms Skin contact produces brownish discoloration, dermatitis, pustules, vesicles, and sometimes sloughing. Formic acid is unique for its ability, in many patients, to cause death after a prolonged (several weeks) course of classical acid-induced gastrointestinal damage. Certain other complications include severe metabolic acidosis, intravascular hemolysis, and disseminated intravascular coagulation. Accidental ingestion in children usually does not lead to fatalities because the pungent taste prevents ingestion of a lethal dose. Nevertheless, it is a problem when used deliberately for suicide. It causes acute trachea bronchitis, which is characterized by cough, sore throat, chest pain, and light-headedness. Formic acid skin burns may also result in systemic toxicity. When absorbed by the body, it causes systemic acidosis, hematuria, and renal damage. The metabolism of methanol can also produce toxic metabolites of formic acid.

Treatment Treatment is by correction of acidosis by infusion of sodium bicarbonate intravenously and hemodialysis for renal failure.

23.3.2.4 Salicylic acids

An important therapeutic preparation of this is acetyl salicylic acid (aspirin). Details are discussed in another chapter dealing with therapeutic agents.

23.4 ALKALIS

Like acids, alkalis also act as corrosive poisons when administered in the concentrated form, but they act as an irritant poison when diluted. Alkalis are present in a number of household products (eg, drain cleaners, oven cleaners, dishwasher products, some paint strippers, etc.) and are also used in industry. Alkalis commonly encountered in poisoning include ammonia (usually in the form of ammonium hydroxide) and carbonates of sodium and potassium. Hydroxides of sodium and calcium and sodium hydrochloride are also increasingly used in household cleaning agents such as detergent.

Mode of action Alkalis generally contain hydroxyl groups, which on dissociation in water produce hydroxide ions. Alkali agents injure the GI tract by saponification of fats and solubilization of proteins that allow deep penetration into tissue. Thus, unlike acids, they produce extensive penetrating damage. This pathogenesis of injury is rapidly progressive and may extend weeks after onset.

Alkalis have more severe corrosive effects on the esophagus (acids produce corrosive effects on the stomach). Severe esophageal damage can occur if the pH is lower than 11. However, with deliberate ingestion of large quantities, corrosive effects can be seen anywhere from the mouth to the small intestine.

Locally, alkalis produce liquefaction necrosis, which results in extensive penetrating damage because of saponification of fats and solubilization of proteins. Ulcers are common and may persist for several weeks.

Signs and symptoms The esophagus is often severely affected, resulting in dysphasia, vomiting, and hematemesis. Stridor is an important indicator of severe esophageal injury. Eye involvement can produce serious complications of ophthalmologic emergency.

The fatal dose is 10–15 g for most alkalis and 15 to 20 mL for ammonia.

Treatment Treatment involves removal from exposure and rest, and also symptom-based treatment. Corneal irrigation with water and topical use of antibiotics are recommended.

CHAPTER

Drug toxicity, dependence, and abuse 24

CHAPTER OUTLINE

24.1 INTRODUCTION

There are thousands of pharmaceutical substances (therapeutic drugs) that are potentially poisonous if taken in a large dosage and or for a long period. Although therapeutic use of chemicals is within the preview of pharmacology, essentially all therapeutic drugs can be toxic and produce deleterious effects at some dose. The three principal classes of cytotoxic agents used in the treatment of cancer, Melphalen (a nitrogen mustard), adriamycin (an antitumor antibiotic), and methotrexate (an antimetabolite), all contain carcinogens. Diethylstilbestrol, a drug formerly widely used, has been associated with cancer of the cervix and vagina.

Other toxic effects of drugs can be associated with almost every organ system. The stiffness of the joints accompanied by damage to the optic nerve (subacute myelo-optic neuropathy) that was common in Japan in the 1960s was apparently a toxic side effect of chloroquinol (Enterovioform), an antidiarrheal drug. Teratogensis can also be caused by drugs, with thalidomide being the most alarming example. Skin effects (dermatitis) are common side effects of drugs such as topically applied corticosteroids.

Fundamentals of Toxicology. DOI: http://dx.doi.org/10.1016/B978-0-12-805426-0.00024-X

A number of toxic effects on the blood have been documented, including agranulocytosis caused by chlorpromazine, hemolytic anemia caused by methyldopa, and megaloblastic anemia caused by methotrexate. Toxic effects on the eye have been noted and range from retinotoxicity caused by thioridazine to glaucoma caused by systemic corticosteroids.

Toxic and fatal consequences are largely accidental or suicidal. Some of the drugs that are commonly used are analgesics (aspirin, codeine, phenacetin, paracetamol, phenylbutazone, amidopyrine, etc.), antidepressants, sedatives, benzodiazepines, barbiturates, chloral, and insulin. Homicide by these compounds is very rare.

24.2 ASPIRIN AND OTHER SALICYLATES

Aspirin (acetyl salicylic acid) is a non-narcotic analgesic and antipyretic.

Signs and symptoms Most common symptoms of aspirin poisoning include vomiting, flushed face, facial edema, skin rash, tinnitus, deafness, hyperpnea, nausea, hematemesis, hypoprothrombinemia, acute renal failure, pulmonary edema, and respiratory arrest.

The fatal dose is 5–10 g. The fatal period is a few minutes to a few hours.

Treatment Treatment should include gastric lavage and correction of electrolyte volume. Alkaline dieresis can be used to increase urine flow. Patients are given a solution containing KCl and $NaHCO_3$; the K level should be maintained. Vitamin K, blood or platelet transfusion, and forced hemodialysis are useful.

24.3 PARACETAMOL

Paracetamol (acetaminophen) is a non-narcotic analgesic and antipyretic. It acts by inhibition of prostaglandin synthesis. It can produce severe liver damage due to the accumulation of a highly toxic intermediate metabolite, *N*-acetyl-para-benzoquinone imine.

Signs and symptoms Initially, within the first 24 h, the drug can produce anorexia, nausea, vomiting, and epigastric pain. This is followed by disappearance of all discomforts, thus giving a false sense of relief during the next 24 h (ie, total of 48 h). After 48–96 h, progressive hepatic encephalopathy can result, as is evidenced by vomiting, jaundice, hepatic pain, confusion, coma, coarse flapping tremors of the hands (asterixis), gastrointestinal (GI) hemorrhage, cerebral edema, and renal tubuler necrosis. There may be cardiac arrhythmias, hemorrhagic pancreatitis, and disseminated, intravascular coagulation; death often takes place during this stage. In cases where this does not happen, the patient goes into next stage, *recovery*, which begins in approximately 5–7 days. The patient gradually becomes completely normal in approximately 2–3 months.

The fatal dose is 10–25 g. The fatal period is up to 5 days.

Treatment Activated charcoal is given if acetaminophen is still in the GI tract. *N*-acetycysteine is an antidote for acetaminophen poisoning. The drug is most effective if administered within 8 h of acetaminophen poisoning.

In chronic poisoning, oral administration of *N*-acetylcysteine or intravenous (IV) therapy as a continuous infusion is useful. A loading dose of 150 mg/kg in 200 mL of 5% dextrose solution administered over 4 h is followed by 100 mg/kg in 100 mL of 5% dextrose administered over 16 h. Supportive treatment for hepatic failure is recommended.

Other general/supportive measures such as maintenance of electrolytes and rehydration, use of vitamin K for bleeding tendencies, and mannitol for cerebral edema should be provided.

24.4 DRUG DEPENDENCE AND ABUSE

24.4.1 DEFINITIONS AND TERMINOLOGY

World Health Organization Expert Committee in Addiction Producing Drugs has coined the terminology "drug dependence" in place of two older terminologies: (1) drug addiction and (2) drug habituation. The reason for this new terminology is due to the difficulty in demarcation between the two older terminologies.

However, although this newer terminology has been well accepted all over the world, the older terminology, especially "drug addiction," is still in use and is used to label a person who is addicted to some kind of addiction-forming drug as a "drug addict."

24.4.1.1 Drug dependence

Drug dependence is defined as a psychic and physical state of the person characterized by behavioral and other responses resulting in compulsions to use a drug on a continuous or periodic basis to experience its psychic effect and, at times, to avoid the discomfort of its absence.

Etiology of drug dependence:

1. Adults may take the drugs for the following reasons:

   Euphoria, improvements in the capacity to understand, improvements in creativity, better relaxation, improvements in the capacity to overcome the stress and strains of life, enhanced sexual capacity, experience of sexual pleasure without having actual sexual relations, and improvement in the power of meditation (religious).
2. Drug dependence is common among people with psychological disorders such as:

   Psychoneurosis, psychopathic state, frank psychoses, and unduly prolonged administration of drugs for therapeutic purposes (eg, analgesics, sedatives, etc.).

24.4.1.2 Drug addiction

Drug addiction is defined as a state of periodic or chronic intoxication harmful to the individual and to society resulting from repeated consumption of a drug, such as opium and its derivatives, pethidine, cannabis, heroine, alcohol, barbiturates, cocaine, lysergic acid diethylamide (LSD), amphetamine, and chloral hydrates.

Mode of drug addiction The mechanism of drug addiction is rather obscure. A diagrammatic representation of drug addiction is presented in Fig. 24.1.

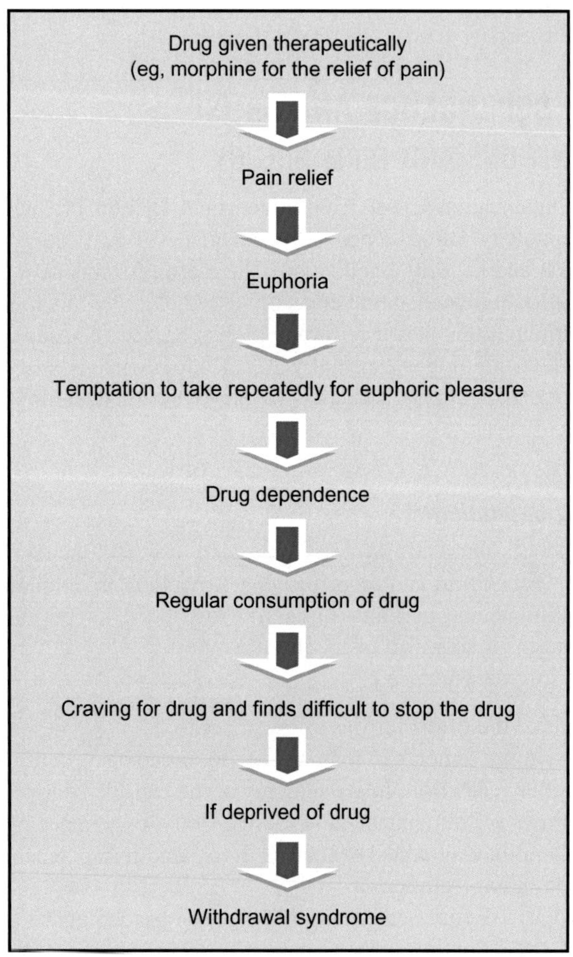

FIGURE 24.1

Steps that lead to drug addiction.

Signs and symptoms Signs and symptoms of drug addiction include the following:

- Irresistible desire to continue using the drug
- Development of tolerance
- A tendency to increase the dose
- Physical dependence on drug
- Desire to obtain drug by any means (even using criminal means)
- Withdrawal symptoms when the drug is stopped

24.4.1.3 Drug habituation

Drug habituation is defined as a condition resulting from repeated consumption of a drug that produces psychological or emotional dependency on the drug, such as caffeine and nicotine.

Mode of drug habituation Like drug addiction, the measures of drug habituation are obscure. However, the following facts are true:

- Common in people with an imitative curiosity
- Communicable from one person to another

Signs and symptoms A person habituated to a drug is called a drug habituate and presents with following:

1. A desire, but not irresistible, to continue to take the drugs
2. Little or no tolerance
3. Little or no tendency to increase the dose
4. Some degree of psychic, but no physical, dependence
5. A detrimental effect, if any, only on the person, but not on society
6. Absence of withdrawal symptoms

24.4.1.4 Drug abuse

Improper use of a therapeutic or nontherapeutic drug, which may or may not be harmful, even in the absence of addiction, constitutes drug abuse.

Hallucinogens, stimulants, and organic solvents are some of the important drugs of dependence and abuse (Table 24.1). In general, drugs of dependence and abuse either have no medicinal function or are taken at dose levels higher than would be required for therapy. Although some drugs of abuse may affect only higher nervous functions (change mood, reaction time, and coordination), many produce physical dependence and have serious physical effects, with fatal overdoses being a frequent occurrence. The drugs of abuse include central nervous system depressants, such as ethanol, methaqualone (Quaalude), and secobarbital, central nervous system stimulants, such as cocaine, methamphetamine (speed), caffeine, and nicotine, opioids, such as heroin and mependine (demerol), and hallucinogens, such as LSD, phencyclidine, and tetra-hydro-cannabinol, the most active principal of marijuana. A further complication of toxicological significance is that many drugs of abuse are synthesized in illegal and poorly equipped laboratories with little or no quality control.

Table 24.1 List of Substances of Dependence and Abuse

Alcohol	Hallucinogens: indole alkaloid derivatives (lysergic acid diethylamide, morning glory seeds; psilocine, psilocybine; ibogaine; harmine; DMT, DET, DPT; bufotenine); piperidine derivatives (datura, cocaine, phencyclidine, ketamine); phenylethylamine derivatives (mescaline, the psychotomimetic amphetamine); cannabinoids (delta tetrahydro cannabinol), mescaline, peyote, and nutmeg
Opium and its derivatives	Carbon tetrachloride
Chloral hydrate	Barbiturates
Cannabis	Caffeine
Cocaine	Nicotine

Therefore, the resultant products are often contaminated with compounds of unknown, but conceivably dangerous, toxicity. This chapter reviews only a few drugs, but others are discussed in different chapters in this book.

24.4.2 HALLUCINOGENS (PSYCHEDELICS)

The term hallucinogen is a misnomer because it is generally applied to certain group of drugs that produce visual illusions, sensory perceptual distortions, synesthesias, depersonalization, and derealization. This class of drugs is perhaps more appropriately termed illusionogenic, psychedelic, or mysticomimetic. These are drugs of both historical interest and immediate clinical concern (abused by many youngsters). The classic hallucinogens including LSD, morning glory seeds, the psychotomimetic amphetamine, psilocybin, dimethyl tryptamine, mescaline, peyote, and nutmeg are some of the hallucinogens of medicolegal importance (Table 24.1).

Numerous other hallucinogens, of both natural and synthetic origin, are frequently encountered. Clinicians should discard their assumption that all hallucination results from either drug abuse or psychiatric disorders because vast arrays of standard therapeutic agents have hallucinogenic potential in usual or moderate excessive doses, including drugs such as amantadine, anticholinergic drugs, carbamazepine, cephalexin, chlordiazepoxide, chloroquine, clonidine, dextramethorphan, dapsone, digoxin, diphenhydramine, disulfiram, ephedrine, griseofulvin, indomethacin, isoniazid, levodopa, lorazepam, methyldopa, methlprednisolone, minocycline, morphine, nalidixic acid, pentazocine, phenothiaznes, piperazine, procainamide, procaine penicillin G, propoxyphene, propranlol, streptokinase, and tricyclic antidepressants.

24.4.3 LYSERGIC ACID DIETHYLAMIDE

Synonyms: Lysergic acid diethylamide, LSD-25, d-LSD.

LSD is the most potent and widely abused hallucinogen. It was first prepared by Stoll and Hofmann in 1938 (at Sandoz Laboratories in Switzerland); its discovery was an outgrowth of their search for a pharmacologically active derivative of ergot. Ergot is a biologic product of the fungus *Claviceps purpurea*, a parasite of cereal grain (especially rye type).

Some of the common popular street names for LSD are acid, blotter acid, blue caps, blue dots, brown caps, crackers, deeda, green caps, orange wedges, paisley caps, pink dots, pink chief, the ghost, the hawk, white lightning, window panes, yellow caps, yellow dots, 25, and others.

LSD is synthesized from rye ergot. It is tasteless and odorless; it is the most potent hallucinogen, with effects occurring in minute doses. These doses can be supplied illicitly on sugar cubes, although it is available in the form of pills of varying colors, sizes, and shapes and also in ampoules.

Signs and symptoms

Acute Poisoning Physical symptoms including mydriasis, hippus, large pupils, nystagmus, vertigo, vomiting, diarrhea, sweating, piloerection, tachypnea, bronchiolar smooth muscle constriction (at high doses), muscle weakness, and cerebral artery spasm followed by coma may occur.

Psychologically, there may be euphoria, anxiety, behavioral changes, tremors, and in-coordination. There may be bizarre perpetual changes.

Chronic Poisoning Prolonged psychotic reactions, which are mainly schizophrenic in nature, severe depression, flashback phenomenon, a perceptual disorder (such as seeing images on floor or walls, floating faces hovering in space), and aeropsia (visualization of vibrating pinpoint dots) are the common features observed in chronic intoxication. The patient may enter the stage of bad trips.

Bad trips are defined as the adverse affects experienced by a person after consuming LSD. LSD mainly acts by interfering with the filtering mechanism of the mind. The victim's sense of perception alters uniquely, resulting in effects such as:

- Patient will hear noises with total disturbance of sense of time, space, and distance; patient will go into a dream-like state with loss of awareness of body boundaries
- He or she will experience fantasies and hallucinations of a varied nature and might present with a flight of ambivalent emotions such as depression and elation and happiness and sadness simultaneously.

Complication of bad trip Although these experiences cease after some time, they might result in a "flashback" of all the events of the dreamy state for several months to up to 2 years and require long-term therapy for total cure. There will be a hangover or after effects.

Although after effects with any hallucinogen is rare, there may be insomnia, headache, vertigo, and psychotic reactions.

Prolonged consumption of hallucinogens may lead to permanent damage of brain cells and chromosomal damage in peripheral blood smears (especially with LSD).

Because the dose required for desired effects of any of the hallucinogens is minimal, consumption of a lethal dose is rare. Therefore, death is exceptionally rare.
Treatment Management of poisoning needs special attention:

1. avoid gut contamination
2. do not use restrains for an agitated persons
3. elimination enhancement procedures are of little value because of the short half-life

Use of supportive care and administration of diazepam, neuroleptics such as haloperidol, and benzodiazepines such as clonazepam are recommended.

Sometimes prolonged treatment is essential because flashback effects last for a long time. Psychotherapy and use of tranquilizers can be the choice of treatment to minimize the flashback effects.

24.4.4 PEYOTE

Peyote is obtained from a variety of cactus plants (peyote). The toxic principle is present in its button-shaped growth. Peyote contains 1–6% mescaline. Each button contains approximately 45 mg of mescaline. They are just rolled into balls and kept in capsules. Synthetic mescaline is also available. Sometimes it may be served in hot tea. It is not as potent as LSD.
Signs and symptoms All hallucinogens are potentially hazardous to human psychology, resulting in disorders of the mind such as anxiety, panic, depressive and paranoid reactions, mood changes, confusion, inability to distinguish between reality and fantasy, and impairment of normal motivation do things in life such as studying, working, or other contributions to society.

Common symptoms of poisoning are unusual and bizarre behavior, hilarity, emotional swings, and suspiciousness. The patient may have nausea and vomiting (especially with peyote). There may be dilated pupils and tremors.
Treatment Treatment involves provision of a quiet environment and calm reassurance. Activated charcoal and diazepam are useful. Patients with suicidal intentions or psychotic behavior lasting longer than 12–24 h should be transferred to the care of psychiatrist.

24.4.5 AMPHETAMINES (CENTRAL NERVOUS SYSTEM STIMULANT, HALLUCINOGEN)

Signs and symptoms Intoxication with amphetamines leads to flushed face, sweating, excitement, restlessness, insomnia, tremors, ventricular tachycardia, hypertension, delirium, hallucinations, convulsions, and deep unconsciousness. Toxic psychosis is seen in chronic poisoning.

The fatal dose is 120–200 g. The fatal period is up to 5 days.

Treatment Use of charcoal, gastric lavage, and other symptomatic treatment should be given. In case of sedation, the use of chlorpromazine and benzodiazepines are helpful. Cardiorespiratory resuscitation and general measures should be undertaken. To combat central nervous system effects, slow IV administration of haloperidol 95–100 mg may be given.

24.4.6 CARBON TETRACHLORIDE

Carbon tetrachloride is both hepatotoxic and nephrotoxic.

Signs and symptoms Inhalation of carbon tetrachloride leads to irritation of eyes and throat, headache, nausea, vomiting, mental confusion, loss of consciousness, arrhythmia, slow respirations, and convulsions. When ingested, it can cause dizziness, headache, nausea, vomiting, colic, tremors, convulsions, and coma. The chemical is hepatotoxin as well as nephrotoxic.

The fatal dose is 2–4 mL (adult) or 1 mL (children). The fatal period is 1–2 days.

Treatment In case of inhalation, remove the patient from the source and administer oxygen, artificial respiration, gastric lavage, saline purgative, and treatment for hepatic and renal damage. *N*-acetylcysteine is administered in severe cases.

24.5 WITHDRAWAL SYMPTOMS (ABSTINENCE SYNDROME)

Withdrawal symptoms are self-explanatory. They develop in 6–48 h of withdrawal of drugs to which an individual has become an addict, and they are characterized by the restlessness, anxiety, vague pain in the abdomen and limbs, diarrhea, and increased libido. These symptoms last for variable periods depending on the drug used, dose consumed, and duration of the drug.

Treatment The following measures are effective:

- Institutional treatment is recommended
- Secret surveillance to prevent a further supply of drugs
- Gradual withdrawal of the drug in stages by using progressive tapering of dose
- Administration of small doses of sedatives (eg, barbiturates)
- Keep the victim engaged with physical and mental activities
- Psychotherapy in the form of encouragement
- Improve general health by consuming nutrient-rich food
- Symptom-based measures

CHAPTER

Toxic effects of domestic chemicals

25

CHAPTER OUTLINE

Poisoning from household products may be conveniently placed within three groups: (1) domestic or household poisons; (2) poisoning by medicine; and (3) food poisons. This chapter deals with some common domestic poisons.

25.1 DOMESTIC/HOUSEHOLD POISONS CLASSIFICATION

1. Hydrocarbons. These are a broad group of organic compounds that contain a carbon and hydrogen only. These may be:
   a. Aliphatic (straight chain).
   b. Aromatic (containing a benzene ring).
   c. Halogenated hydrocarbons.
2. Other than hydrocarbons: these include dishwashing powders and granules, dishwashing liquids and household detergents, disinfectants, metal polishes, and cosmetics.

25.2 HYDROCARBONS

25.2.1 ALIPHATIC HYDROCARBONS

These are petroleum distillates that are common constituents of several industrial and household products and are involved in accidental poisoning, especially among the children. It is reported that every year, nearly 28,000 children younger

Fundamentals of Toxicology. DOI: http://dx.doi.org/10.1016/B978-0-12-805426-0.00025-1

than age 5 years ingest petroleum distillates, accounting for 12–25% deaths due to all poisons in this age group. There are two types of aliphatic hydrocarbons low-molecular-weight hydrocarbons and high-molecular-weight hydrocarbons.

1. *Low molecular weight*: These include gaseous or nonliquid forms and liquid forms:

   Nonliquid forms (gaseous forms): These include methane (CH_4), ethane (CH_3CH_3), propane ($CH_3CH_3CH_3$), and butane ($CH_3(CH_2)_2CH_3$), all of which are flammable gases. Natural gas is primarily methane and ethane. Liquefied petroleum gas (bottled gas) contains propane and butane.

   Liquid forms (petroleum distillates): These are broken-down products that remain after processing crude oil. Some examples are fuels such as kerosene, diesel oil, gasoline (petrol), and furniture polish such as mineral seal oil and naphtha. Kerosene, diesel oil, and petrol are inebriant types of cerebral poison that are separated by distillation at various boiling points.
2. *High molecular weight*: These include hydrocarbons of petroleum distillate origin, such as petroleum jelly (Vaseline) and paraffin wax. They are petroleum distillates that are derived at boiling points of 300°C and higher. Toxicity decreases as the boiling point increases. Hence, these are relatively nontoxic.

   Hydrocarbons of nonpetroleum distillate origin do not necessarily have to be petroleum distillates. Turpentine and carbon tetrachloride are hydrocarbons, but they are not petroleum distillate products. Turpentine (paint thinner/paint remover) is a hydrocarbon made of pine oil and an aromatic hydrocarbon, but with the properties of an aliphatic hydrocarbon; therefore, it is dealt with under aliphatic hydrocarbons. Rectified turpentine has therapeutic uses as a counter-irritant.

Mode of action Low-molecular-weight hydrocarbons have very low viscosity, and toxicity is basically due to aspiration in the lungs. In the lungs, these liquid nongaseous hydrocarbons can spread rapidly throughout the pulmonary tree, resulting in fulminating pulmonary edema and bronchopneumonia. Aspiration can also occur during vomiting. The gaseous hydrocarbons can act directly as asphyxiants. Certain high-molecular-weight hydrocarbons also cause respiratory manifestations on aspiration. However, the resulting pneumonia is more localized and less inflammatory.

Toxic petroleum distillates are irritants that are absorbed orally as well as nasally. They dissolve in fat and, therefore, can act on nervous tissues. They can induce depression of the central nervous system (CNS) and also damage the liver, kidneys, and bone marrow. Thus, the presenting symptoms and signs are usually related to three main organ systems: pulmonary, central nervous, and gastrointestinal. The cardiovascular system, kidneys, liver, spleen, and blood also may be involved.

Signs and symptoms Vaseline and paraffin are nontoxic and used medicinally, whereas petrol, naphtha, and kerosene are highly toxic by ingestion or inhalation. Poisoning can be acute or chronic.

Acute Poisoning Oral ingestion of fatal doses can result in a characteristic odor specific to hydrocarbon ingestion. In general, the chronological order of symptoms is: intense excitement, hallucinations and convulsions, cyanosis, unconsciousness, profound coma, and death.

Pulmonary System: A peculiar odor is usually evident in the breath and vomit. Cyanosis can occur due to pulmonary complications such as bronchopneumonia. Aspiration can produce coughing, choking, gasping, bronchospasm, and hypoxia. Severe cases may present with hemoptysis. Hemorrhagic pulmonary edema can result in pink, frothy sputum and progress to shock and cardiac arrest.

CNS: Depression results in vertigo, giddiness, drowsiness, headache, tremors, and convulsions. Toluene sniffing may present with a drunken appearance. Pupils are usually constricted initially; later, when coma supervenes, they are dilated.

Gastrointestinal (GI) Tract: Ingestion of the poison results in pain, burning pain in throat, nausea, vomiting, colicky abdomen, and diarrhea.

Cardiovascular System (CVS): Cardiomyopathy, arrhythmias, and others.

Renal and Hepatic System: Less commonly involved.

Hemopoietic System: Blood may show aplastic anemia and agranulocytosis.

In Fatal Cases: Drowsiness merges into coma and death due to respiratory failure.

Chronic Poisoning Chronic poisoning usually occurs among those who inhale petroleum products while working in petroleum industries. This results in manifestations such as:

Skin: Chronic eczematoid dermatitis with redness, itching, and inflammation. Cutaneous exposure to gasoline and other hydrocarbons can cause second-degree burns.

General Symptoms: Dizziness, weakness, weight loss, anemia, nervousness, limb pain, peripheral numbness, and paraesthesias.

The fatal dose is 10–15 mL of kerosene. Even a few milliliters on aspiration can cause serious toxicity. The fatal period is a few hours to 1 day.

Postmortem findings The GI tract may show acute gastroenteritis; the stomach is congested and its contents produce a characteristic odor specific to the type of hydrocarbon ingested. Lungs smell of kerosene, with pulmonary edema and bronchopneumonia (ie, pneumonic consolidation and emphysematous changes). Liver and kidneys show degenerative changes and bone marrow will be hypoplastic. For chemical analysis, preserve the brain and other viscera.

Treatment

Acute Poisoning Wash the contaminated skin with copious amounts of water and soap and provide symptomatic treatment such as liquid paraffin orally at a dose of 250 mL. It dissolves kerosene and reduces its absorption. Activated charcoal in large doses is recommended, although petroleum distillers are not adsorbed. Saline purgatives may also be useful. Avoid gastric lavage because of the fear of aspiration. However, gastric lavage with warm water containing 5% sodium bicarbonate administered with extreme care to prevent entry into the respiratory tract is beneficial for large amount of kerosene consumption (more than 4 mL/kg weight). Avoid intravenous fluid overload because it may precipitate pulmonary edema.

Chronic Poisoning Prevention and symptom-based treatment. Avoidance of further exposure to prevent absorption of poison is recommended.

25.2.2 AROMATIC HYDROCARBONS

Most of the aromatic hydrocarbons are widely used in industry. Some examples are benzene, toluene, xylene, and styrene. Most of the aromatic hydrocarbons have characteristic odors and are absorbed through inhalation, ingestion, and direct skin contact. Both benzene and toluene are highly toxic, whereas xylene is relatively nontoxic. Domestic poisoning is not very common with these compounds. However, industrial exposure is common. Workers handling benzene need regular blood checks. Toluene is involved in glue sniffing.

Signs and symptoms The common signs of toxicity include:

CNS: Vertigo, lethargy, and convulsions, followed by coma

GI tract: Abdominal pain, vomiting, and diarrhea

Respiratory System: Pulmonary edema and pneumonia

CVS: Cardiac arrhythmias and blood dyscrasias

Renal and hepatic damage and metabolic acidosis are common in toluene poisoning. Chronic exposure, particularly to benzene, can result in anemia, leukemia, and CNS damage.

Treatment Treatment is symptom-based and supportive. The treatment line should be followed as in the case of aliphatic hydrocarbon toxicity.

25.2.3 HALOGENATED HYDROCARBONS

Halogenated hydrocarbons are not discussed in this chapter. For details, please refer to other chapters in this book.

25.3 OTHER THAN HYDROCARBONS

For details of individual chemicals, the readers may refer to other chapters covered in this book. However, a brief description of commonly used chemicals such as detergents and household substances (Table 25.1), medicines (Table 25.2), and household insecticides (Table 25.3) are summarized in tabular form.

Table 25.1 Domestic Use Chemicals (Other Than Hydrocarbons) With Slight Toxic Potential

Domestic Chemical	Nature of Chemical	Toxic Symptoms	Management
Dishwashing powders, granules	Irritant/ corrosive	Irritation of the mouth, throat, esophagus, and stomach is seen, especially in children	The stomach does not need to be emptied; give milk, water, or fruit juice; endoscopy is helpful in doubtful cases
Dishwashing liquids	Irritant/ caustic	Swallowing may lead to choking, retching, and coughing	Stomach wash, provide simple fluids to drink
Household detergents	Soaps	Vomiting when taken orally	Stomach wash, provide simple fluids to drink
Dettol and lysol (chlorinated phenols)	Chemicals/ or admixed with isopropyl alcohol	Usually low toxicity, but can act like ethanol when swallowed if admixed with isopropyl alcohol	Stomach wash and any sequelae should be treated as for ethanol overdose; avoid stomach wash
Metal polishes	May have petroleum hydrocarbon	Harmless when swallowed; however, bronchial aspiration can lead to major hazards	Low toxicity needs stomach wash; if large quantities are ingested, use palliative measures only
Cosmetics: Hair dyes, hair conditioners, shampoos, bath oils, soaps	Nontoxic	In practice, if these are nontoxic, then no special attention is required	Symptom-based

Table 25.2 Common Household Medicines Containing Toxic Substances

Preparations	Toxic Substances[a]
1. Antiseptics	Iodine, benzoin, phenol
2. Cough remedies	Codeine
3. Headache remedies	Asprin, phenacetin, analgin
4. Energy tablets	Benzedrine
5. Sleeping preparations	Barbiturates
6. Throat tablets	Potassium chlorate
7. Tonic syrup	Easton's syrup (strychnine)
8. Others	Antidepressants, tranquilizers, antibiotics, analgesics, etc.

[a]*For details of toxicity, please refer to individual chemicals in other chapters in this book.*

Table 25.3 Commonly Used Household Pesticides Containing Toxic Substances

Pesticides	Toxic Substances[a]
1. Fungicides	Lead arsenate, copper compounds, organic mercurials, lime, sulfur
2. Insecticides	Nicotine, tar oils, organochlorine and organophosphorus, carbamates, and pyrethroid insecticides
3. Weed killers (herbicides)	Sodium chlorate, arsenious oxide and arsenites, dinitrocresol, paraquat

[a]*For details of toxicity, please refer to individual chemicals in other chapters in this book.*

CHAPTER

Toxic effects of poisonous plants

26

CHAPTER OUTLINE

26.1 INTRODUCTION

Ingestion of poisonous plants may cause toxicity, and clinicians routinely have to deal with poisoning cases. The problem is made more intense by the fact that there is no accurate information available because very few cases are reported or published in literature. It is also well established that many of the experimental data are available regarding laboratory animals and reported in veterinary literature. The applicability of such studies in humans is an open challenge. It is also true that for many plant poisoning cases, the treatment is practically same (ie, symptom-based measures and supportive therapy). Rarely do these cases have an antidote therapy. There is chaos in the areas of plant identification and nomenclature. A few selective, important plants commonly involved in poisonings are discussed.

26.2 *ABRUS PRECATORIUS*

Abrus precatorius is a plant grown in many parts of the world.

Common name: Jequirity bean, rosary pea, Buddhist rosary bead, rosary bead, Indian bead, Indian liquorice, Seminole bead, prayer head, crab's eye, weather plant, lucky bean, gulagunchi, and rati.

Fundamentals of Toxicology. DOI: http://dx.doi.org/10.1016/B978-0-12-805426-0.00026-3

Family: Leguminoceae.

Plant characteristics: It is a slender vine and climber, with compound leaves and 10–15 pairs of narrow leaves, and small pinkish flowers with seedpods that split open when ripe, exposing 4–6 seeds within. These seeds are bright red (gray in print versions) in color with a black spot in one pole and weigh approximately 105 mg (Fig. 26.1).

Toxic part of the plant: The whole plant is poisonous. However, seeds are more often used.

Toxic principles: *N*-methyltryptophan, flycyrrhizin (lypolytic enzyme that is the active principle of liquorice), abrin (toxalbumin, also known as phytotoxin), abrine (amino acid), abralin (glucoside), and abric acid.

Signs and symptoms Signs and symptoms occur only if the seed is masticated and swallowed. It can act locally as well as systemically.

Local effects: The plant can lead to dermatitis, conjunctivitis, rhinitis, and asthma. Oral ingestion can produce severe gastroenteritis, hemorrhagic gastritis with severe pain, copious vomiting, diarrhea that may become bloody, severe thirst, and circulatory collapse. Death is reported to be due to persistent gastroenteritis.

Systemic effects: When implanted as "suis" or if the seed extract is injected parenterally, cardiac manifestations like a viperine snakebite can develop, with the site of injection turning edematous and hemorrhagic. The victim (animal/human) then becomes drowsy, unable to move, and goes into a coma; this is followed by convulsions and death. Abrin can lead to development of cardiac arrhythmias, convulsions, and cerebral edema.

The usual fatal dose is 60–120 mg of abrin (1–2 crushed seeds). The fatal period is 3–5 days. The toxicity rating is 5–6 (supertoxic).

Postmortem findings Postmortem inflammatory changes and congestion of the gastrointestinal (GI) tract are observed. At the site of injection, local signs of inflammation are seen.

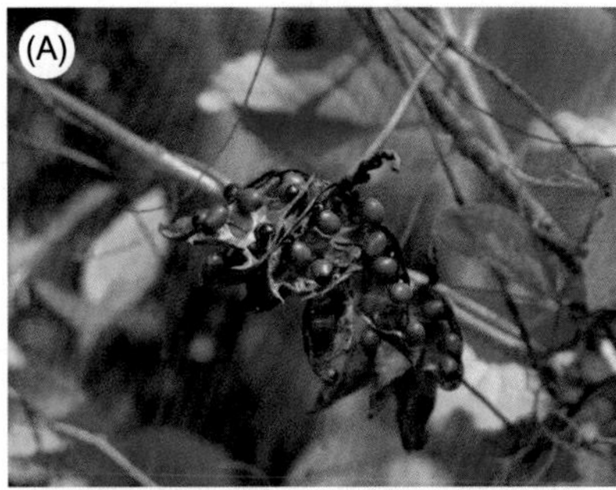

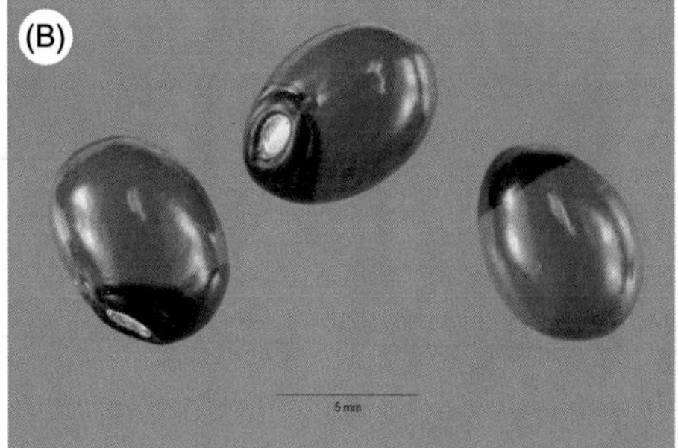

FIGURE 26.1

Abrus Precatorious plant leaves with seeds (A), and seeds (B).

Source: Wikimedia Commons. Available at: https://en.wikipedia.org/wiki/Abrus_precatorius.

Treatment All cases of ingestion should be given supportive therapy (lavage, charcoal, and cathartics). In the case of spontaneous diarrhea, cathartics should be avoided. In oral poisoning, an acid hydrochloric pepsin mixture and IV 10% sodium bicarbonate are recommended. In locally injected cases, dissect out the suis.

26.3 *RICINUS COMMUNIS* (CASTOR OIL PLANT)

Common names: Castor, arandi, mole bean.

Family: Euphorbiaceae.

Plant characteristics: It is a large shrub with greenish red leaves. Fruits are in clusters and are soft-spined greenish/brownish capsules with seeds. Seeds are oval or round in shape and are of two types: large and small. The large seeds are red with brown blotches (yielding 40% oil); the small seeds are gray with glossy, bright, polished, brown mottling (yielding 37% oil) (Fig. 26.2).

The toxic parts of the plant are the seeds and especially the seed oil (castor oil) extract, which is pale yellow and has a faint odor. Leftover oil cake after extraction is also highly toxic.

Active principle: The oil extract of the seeds has an acid called ricinoleic acid, and the leftover cake has a toxalbumin called ricin. Ricin is one of the most toxic parenteral substances in the plant kingdom. It contains two polypeptide chains held together by a single disulfide bond. Both these chains can bind with the cell surface, facilitating toxin entry into the cell and disrupting the protein synthesis. Because the cell binding and protein disruption need some time, its toxic effects are usually delayed but widespread. Ricin is more poisonous than cobra venom and is classified as a supertoxic poison.

(A)

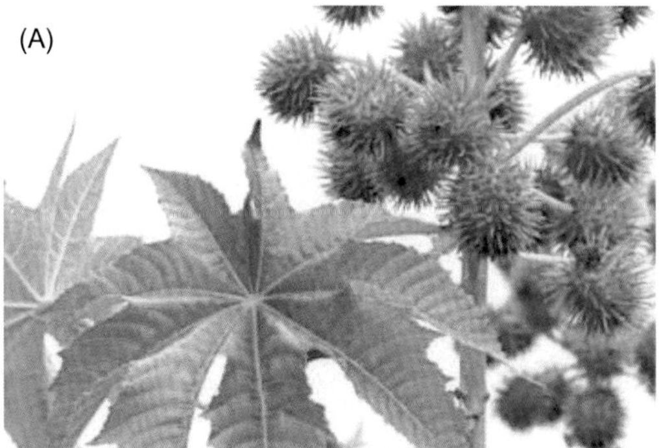

(B)

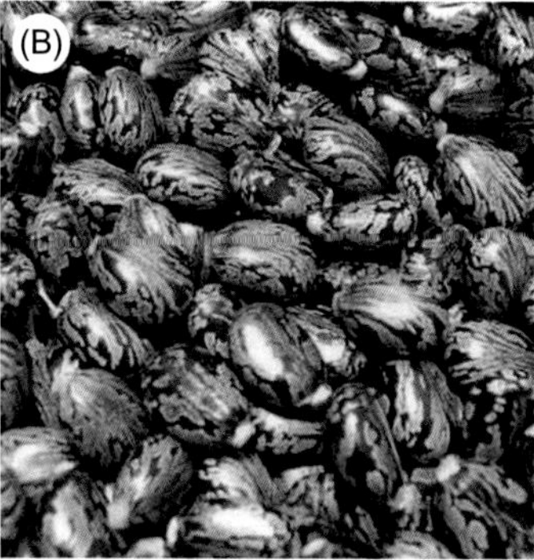

FIGURE 26.2

Castor plant leaves and pods (A), and seeds (B).

Source: (A) Horseback Riding worldwide. Available at: http://www.horsebackridingworldwide.com/the-castor-oil-plant-ricinus/wunderbaum-castor-oil-plant-11/; (B) Indo Exports. Available at: http://indoexports.tradeget.com/F38632/castor_bean_seeds.html.

Signs and symptoms *Local*: It can lead to dermatitis, conjunctivitis, rhinitis, and asthma. Castor bean dust is highly allergenic and may cause anaphylaxis.

Oral: Seeds, if masticated and swallowed, produce burning pain in the throat, followed by nausea, vomiting, colicky pain in the abdomen, and bloody purging. Both can ultimately lead to dehydration and muscular cramps.

Parenteral: Parenteral ingestion can produce the same manifestation as after oral ingestion, but the symptoms occur more rapidly than they do after being ingested via the oral route.

The fatal dose is 1 mg/kg body weight or 6 mg of ricin (approximately 8–10 seeds). The fatal period is several days.

Toxicity rating: Ricin has toxicity rating of 6 (super toxic); castor oil has a toxicity rating of 2 (slightly toxic).

Postmortem findings Inflammatory changes and congestion of the GI tract is common. The liver, kidneys, and pancreas are considered primary target organs. Postmortem findings may be inflammatory changes and congestion. Microscopic examination of the stomach contents reveals the prismatic appearance of the outer cells' coat of castor seeds (and also in croton, abrus, and jatropa seeds).

Treatment The patient should receive the supportive and general measures to prevent absorption (syrup ipecac, charcoal, cathartics). Recommended treatment for an asymptomatic patient who has chewed one or more seeds includes emergency treatment such as gastric decontamination, administration of activated charcoal, and observation for 4–6 h. However, all symptomatic patients need hospitalization for treatment with IV fluids, supportive care, and monitoring for hypovolemia. Most patients respond well to IV fluid therapy and recover without any permanent sequelae.

26.4 CROTON

Distribution: The croton plant grows all over, especially in wastelands. Grown in many varieties for their brightly colored foliage, it is widely cultivated as a houseplant.

Common names: Croton, jamalgota, and naepala.

Family: Euphorbiaceae.

Plant characteristics: It is an evergreen tree with smooth, ash-colored bark. The leaves of the tree are ovate-lanceolate (Fig. 26.3A). Flowers are small and oblong. Fruits are three-lobed and contain oval, dark brown seeds (Fig. 26.3B) and longitudinal striations. The seeds resemble castor seeds; the longitudinal striations mark their difference from castor seeds, which have mottling.

Toxic part: Seeds and oil extracted from the seeds are extremely toxic. Seed oil is known to have tumor-promoting properties.

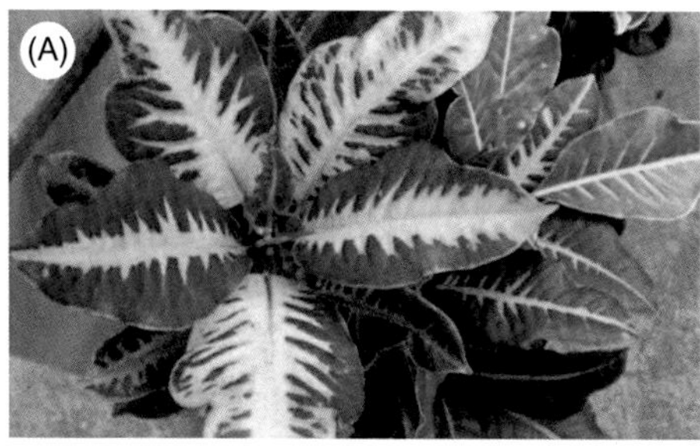

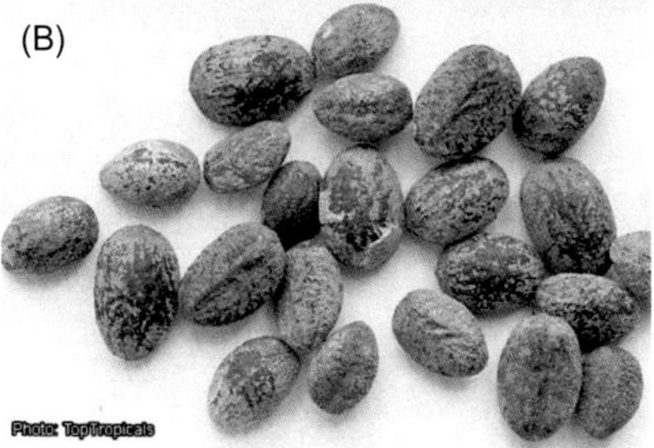

FIGURE 26.3

Croton plant leaves (A), and seeds (B).

Source: (A) Indian Nursery. Available at: http://indiannursery.in/indoor-plants/Codiaeum.html; (B) Prota 11(1): Medicinal plants/Plantes médicinales 1. Available at: http://database.prota.org/PROTAhtml/Croton%20sylvaticus_En.htm.

Active principles: There are two active principles: crotin (toxalbumin) and crotonoside (glycoside).

The fatal dose is 1–2 mL of oil or 4–6 crushed seeds. The fatal period is 4–6 h to 3–6 days.

The toxicity rating is 5 (croton oil).

Signs and symptoms Signs and symptoms resemble *Ricinus communis* (castor) poisoning.

Postmortem findings Inflammatory changes and congestion of the GI tract are common.

Treatment Same as for *Ricinus communis* (castor).

26.5 CALOTROPIS

Distribution: Grows all over, especially in wastelands and deserts.

Common name: Madar. It has two species:

1. *Calotropis gigantea*, which is a purple flowed plant
2. *Calotropis procera*, which is a white flowered plant

Family: Asclepiadaceae.

Plant characteristics: It is a tall shrub with yellowish white bark and oblong thick leaves and purplish (gray in print versions) or white flowers (Fig. 26.4). When stem, branches, and leaves are cut, crushed, or incised, it yields a milky white latex, which is an acrid juice called madar juice.

Toxic part: Stem, branches, leaves, and the milky white latex (madar juice).

Active principles: Uscharin, calotoxin, calotropin, and gigantin.

Signs and symptoms *Local*: It can give rise to lesions resembling bruises on the skin (called fabricated injuries), which at times can lead to the formation of

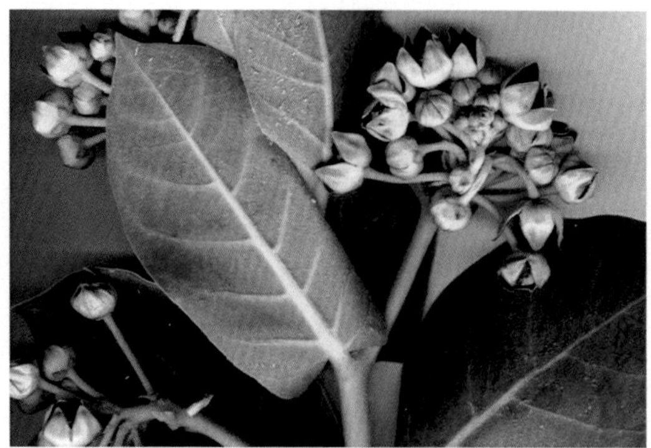

FIGURE 26.4

Calotropis leaves and flowers.

Source: Wikimedia Commons. Available at: https://en.wikipedia.org/wiki/Calotropis.

pustules and vesicles. When the juice comes in contact with the eyes, it can result in severe conjunctivitis.

Oral: Bitter in taste. Produces burning pain in the throat, salivation, nausea, and vomiting, followed by diarrhea, pain abdomen, mydriasis, tetanic convulsions, delirium, collapse, and death.

The fatal dose is uncertain. The fatal period is 12 h.

Postmortem findings Postmortem findings include froth at the nostrils, stomatitis, and inflammatory changes of the GI tract with ulceration; the stomach may show perforation. All viscera, including the brain, usually shows congestion.

Treatment Provide gastric lavage with warm water or potassium permanganate ($KMnO_4$), demulcent drinks, and washing with soap and water. Treat skin lesions. Cases of conjunctivitis can be managed by saline irrigations.

26.6 SEMECARPUS ANACARDIUM

Distribution: Grows all over, especially in wastelands and deserts.

Common names: Marking nut, bhilawan, bibva, bhela, and Oriental cashew.

Family: Anacardiaceae.

Plant characteristics: It is a small tree with flowers that are dull/greenish yellow (gray in print versions). The fruit is black and heart-shaped with a hard ring, within which is a thick, fleshy pericarp (Fig. 26.5) that yields brown oily resinous fluid. This turns black on exposure to air. This fluid is often used as “marking ink” on linen and cotton clothes by the washer men (Dhobis).

Active principles: Two active principles are isolated in the fluid extracted from the pericarp: semicarpol (monohydroxy phenol compound) and bhilawanol (alkaloid).

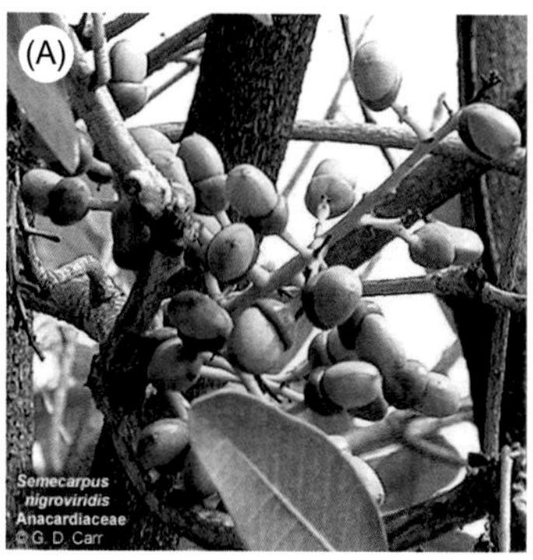

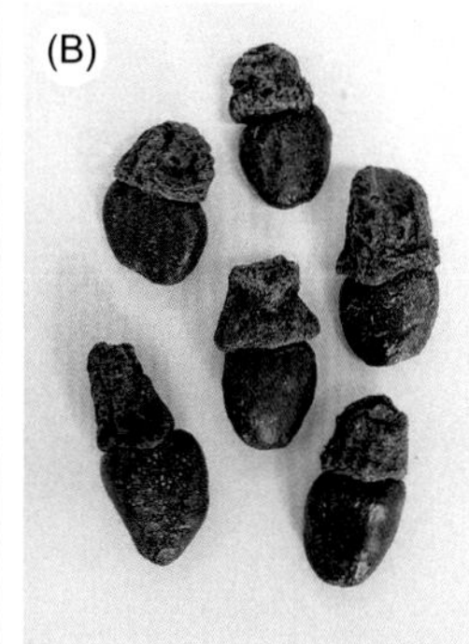

FIGURE 26.5

Semecarpus anacardium (A), and seeds (B).

Source: (A) Dr Gerlad Carr, University of Hawaii. Available at: http://www.botany.hawaii.edu/faculty/carr/images/sem_nig_2319.jpg; (B) Wikimedia Commons. Available at: https://commons.wikimedia.org/wiki/File:Semecarpus_anacardium_02.jpg.

Signs and symptoms *Local*: On skin, it produces bruise-like lesions that are actually raised blackish blisters or vesicular ecchymatous eruptions that are itchy. Scratching these can cause similar lesions on the tips of the fingers, on the nail beds, and below the nail tips. These can lead to pain, fever, and stranguria, with the excretion of brownish urine.

Oral: A large dose can produce blisters in the mouth and throat and gastroenteritis. It can also produce dyspnea, cyanosis, tachycardia, coma, and death.

The fatal dose is uncertain. The fatal period ranges from 12–24 h.

Postmortem findings There is inflammation of the GI tract and congestion of viscera and skin showing black vesicles with acrid serum.

Treatment For skin lesions, wash with water and apply liniments. For oral ingestion, perform gastric lavage and give demulcents, followed by other symptom-based measures as needed.

26.7 CAPSICUM ANNUUM

Common names: Chili peppers, Lal mirchi, red pepper, cayenne pepper.

Family: Solanaceae.

Plant characteristics: It is a small herb bearing somewhat long, tapering fruits that become red (dark gray in print versions) when ripe and posses a pungent odor and taste. The fruit (chili) contains a number of small, flat, yellowish (light gray in print versions) seeds that bear a superficial resemblance to datura seeds (Fig. 26.6).

Toxic part: Fruit and seeds.

Active principles: Capsicum (crystalline) and capsaicin are both acrid, volatile, and alkaloid substances.

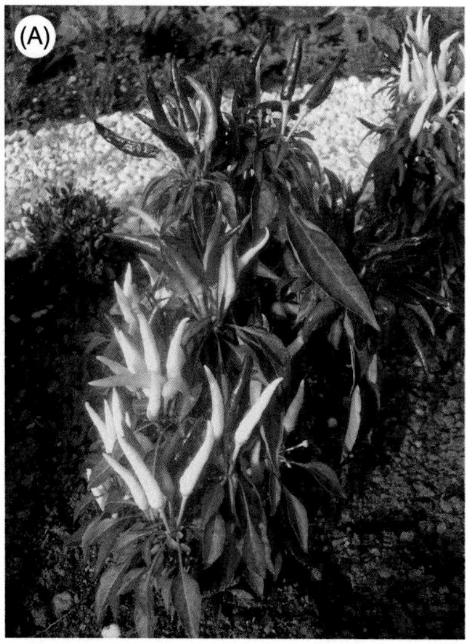
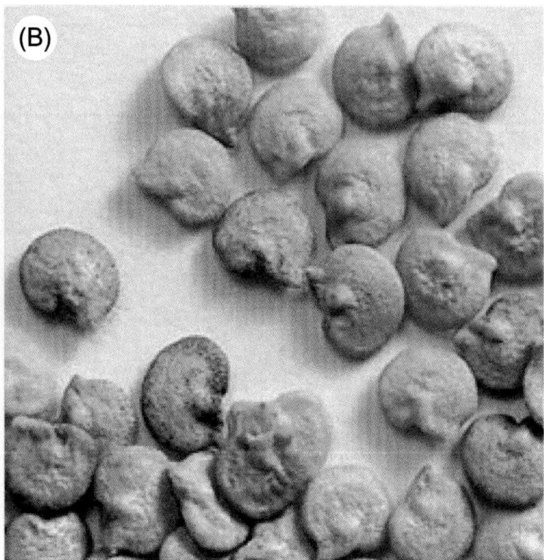

FIGURE 26.6

Capsicum annuum plant (A) and seeds (B).

Source: (A) Wikimedia Commons. Available at: https://en.wikipedia.org/wiki/Capsicum_annuum; (B) Indoor Gardening Club. Available at: http://indoorgardeningclub.com/product/giant-marconi-hybrid-sweet-pepper-seeds-capsicum-annuum-0-2-grams-approx-30-gardening-seeds-vegetable-garden-seed/.

Signs and symptom *Local*: It can produce irritation that results in burning and redness of skin and burning, redness, and lacrimation of eyes.

Oral: Large quantities can produce a burning and fiery hot sensation in the mouth, salivation, excessive perspiration, abdominal pain, vomiting, and diarrhea. Urine may also turn dark.

This can cause serious toxicity. The fatal period is unlikely.

Treatment In the case of oral ingestion, wash the stomach with warm water, followed by blunt scraping of the tongue, sucking on ice, and sipping ice-cold water.

In the case of local skin contamination, wash the area with copious amounts of water. Affected skin may be kept immersed in vinegar (5% acetic acid).

26.8 EUCALYPTUS GLOBULUS

Distribution: Grows in South India, especially in the hills of Nilgiris and Tamil Nadu.

Common names: Eucalyptus and bluc gum.

Plant characteristics: It is a tall tree with smooth bark, long curved leaves, and large flowers. Eucalyptus oil is obtained by steam distillation of the extract derived from the leaves.

Active principles: Eucalyptol (cineole).

Signs and symptoms Common symptoms include burning pain in the mouth, nausea, vomiting, diarrhea, abdominal pain, bronchospasm, tachypnea, chemical pneumonitis, respiratory depression, headache, vertigo, drowsiness, slurred speech, ataxia, convulsions, and coma. The breath and urine may smell of eucalyptus oil.

A dose of 5–10 mL can cause serious toxicity; however, death is unlikely.

Postmortem findings Nonspecific.

Treatment Symptomatic and supportive measures are needed.

26.9 COLCHICUM (*COLCHICUM AUTUMNALE*)

Common names: Autumn crocus, meadow saffron, and naked ladies.

Distribution: Eurasia and Africa.

Family: Liciaceae.

Plant description: Perennial herb (category: bulbs). Its height is 15–30 cm, with basal, slender leaves and long, tubular, flowers that are pink, violet/lavender, or white in color (Fig. 26.7).

Toxic part: All parts of the plant are highly poisonous and may be fatal if eaten.

Active principle: Alkaloid colchicines and demecolcin.

Signs and symptoms Usually, ingestion is by the oral route and the prominent symptoms are:

- Gastrointestinal system: Vomiting, diarrhea, abdominal pain, cramping, and hepatic dysfunction.
- Cardiovascular system: Increased blood pressure. Rarely, it can produce disseminated intravascular coagulation and bone marrow failure.
- Respiratory system: Rarely, it can produce respiratory failure.
- Urinary system: It may also cause signs and symptoms of renal dysfunction.
- Hair: It can produce alopecia.

This can cause serious toxicity; however, death is unlikely.

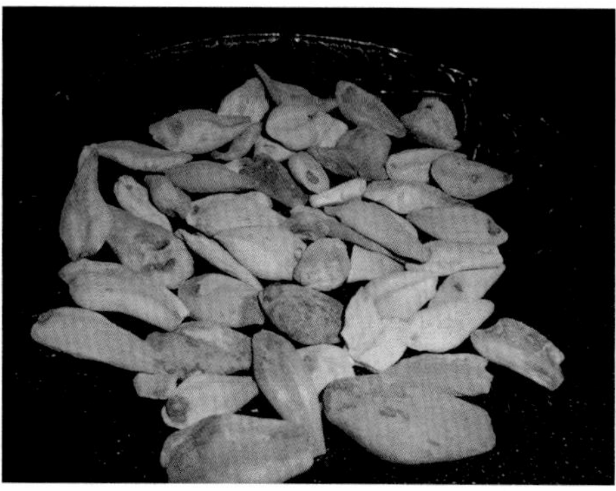

FIGURE 26.7

Colchicum plant seeds.

Source: Imran Usman Enterprises. Available at: http://iue.weebly.com/colchicum-bitter.html.

Treatment For oral poisoning, perform gastric lavage and use antihypertensives if blood pressure is increased. For renal failure, dialysis is recommended.

26.10 ERGOT

Common name: Mother of rye.

Characteristics: Ergot is an alkaloid. It is the sclerotium (mycelium) of a fungus *Claviceps purpurea*, which grows on many cereals like rye, barley, wheat, and oat fungus. It gradually replaces the whole grain to a dark purple (light gray in print versions)mass, which on drying yields ergo (Fig. 26.8).

Active principles: There are three active principles and all are ecbolics that can contract the gravid human uterus in late pregnancy. The active principles are ergotamine, ergotoxin, and ergometrine. They are known to contract arterioles, which can lead to gangrene of the part supplied.

Signs and symptoms

Acute Poisoning Acute poisoning is very rare. Some of the common symptoms include irritation of the throat, dryness, severe thirst, nausea, vomiting, diarrhea, pain in the abdomen, tingling in hands and feet, muscle cramps (all due to contraction of smooth muscles), dizziness, and a feeling of coldness. Sometimes symptoms of hypoglycemia, anuria, spontaneous abortion, and hemorrhages in a pregnant woman may be seen. Death is usually slow.

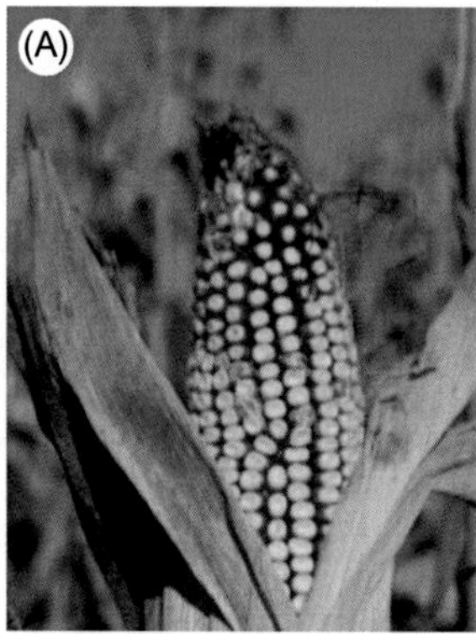

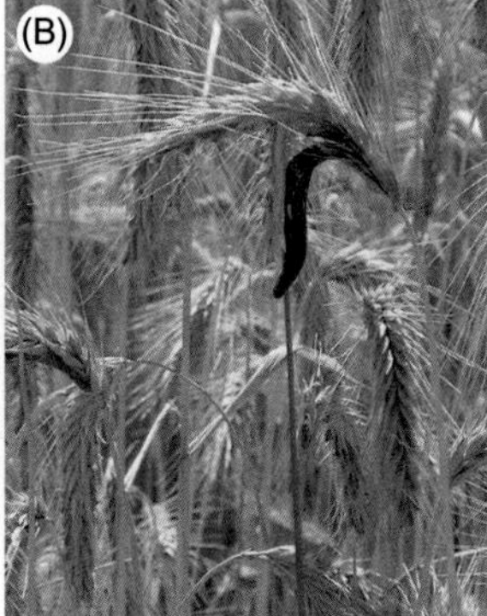

FIGURE 26.8

Fungus *Claviceps purpurea* on maize (A) and on rye (B).

Source: (A) Mycotoxins blog. Available at: http://mycotoxinsinfo.blogspot.in/2013_09_01_archive.html; (B) Wikimedia commons. Available at: https://en.wikipedia.org/wiki/Claviceps_purpurea#/media/File:Claviceps_purpurea.JPG.

Chronic Poisoning Chronic poisoning is called ergotism, and it is quite common. It occurs in two forms:

Convulsive form: Shows painful toxic contraction of voluntary muscles, followed by drowsiness, headache, giddiness, and madness. The victim may report feeling itchy/numb or the sensation of ants crawling under the skin.

Gangrenous form: Begins as pustules and swelling of limbs and feet, followed by intense hot feeling, severe pain, and numbness. This is followed by gangrenous changes (resembling Raynaud disease). Recovery is possible if ergot is withheld.

Fatal dose and period: Both are uncertain.

Toxicity rating: 4–5.

Treatment Symptom-based treatments such as washing of the stomach with tannic acid and magnesium sulfate are recommended. Other treatments include amyl nitrate inhalation, sodium nicotinate 140 mg IV, and withdrawal of ergot-contaminated substances in chronic cases.

CHAPTER

Poisonous foods and food poisoning 27

CHAPTER OUTLINE

27.1 INTRODUCTION

Food poisoning is a vague term. It includes illnesses resulting from ingestion of all foods containing nonbacterial or bacterial products. The nonbacterial products include poisons delivered from plants and animals and certain naturally occurring toxins. Foods containing such products are, by convention, known as poisonous foods (for animal poisons and plant poisons, please refer to other chapters).

27.2 MICROBIAL TOXINS

Bacterial products include bacteria and their toxins (microbial toxins). Poisoning resulting from microbial toxins is, by convention, known as bacterial food poisoning. The illness is characterized by: (1) simultaneous poisoning of many persons at the same time; (2) history of ingestion of common food by all sufferers; and (3) similarity of signs and symptoms in a majority of cases.

The term "microbial toxin" is usually reserved by microbiologists for toxic substances produced by microorganisms that are of high molecular weight and have antigenic properties; toxic compounds produced by bacteria that do not fit these criteria are referred to simply as poisons. Many of the former are proteins or mucoproteins and may have a variety of enzymatic properties. They include some of the most toxic substances, such as tetanus toxin, botulinus toxin, and diphtheria toxin. Bacterial toxins may be extremely toxic to mammals and may affect a variety of organ systems, including the nervous system and the cardiovascular system. A detailed account of their chemical nature and mode of action is

Fundamentals of Toxicology. DOI: http://dx.doi.org/10.1016/B978-0-12-805426-0.00027-5

beyond the scope of this volume. The range of poisonous chemicals produced by bacteria is also large. Again, such compounds may be used for beneficial purposes; for example, the insecticidal properties of *Bacillus thuringiensis*, due to a toxin, have been utilized in agriculture for some time.

27.3 FOOD POISONING

Microbial food poisoning is of three types:

1. infectious type
2. toxic type
3. botulism

Ptomaine poisoning due to advanced decomposition of food is not common. Ptomaine is proteolytic degradation of products formed in decomposing carcasses.

In the infectious type, food poisoning results from ingestion of viable microorganisms that multiply in the gastrointestinal tract, producing a true infection, for example, the *Salmonella* and *Shigella* groups of organisms. The organisms multiply in the gut and cause gastroenteritis. The common organisms responsible for the attack are the *Salmonella* group of organisms, such as *Salmonella typhimurium* (Aertrycke), *Salmonella enteritidis* (Gaertner), *Salmonella suipestifer* (cholera suis), *Salmonella thompson*, and *Salmonella newport*. Occasionally, the *Shigella* group of organisms, such as the *Shigella sonnei* and the *Shigella flexneri*, may be responsible.

The natural reservoirs of *Salmonella* organisms are certain birds, mammals, and reptiles; food may be contaminated with infected excreta of mice or rats, or infection may be transferred by flies or by human carriers employed in the handling of food. *Shigella* infection is the result of contamination of food or water supplies with the feces of the individuals who either have the disease or, less often, are asymptomatic carriers of the organism.

The types of foods that are particularly likely to be infected are twice-cooked meat dishes, fish dishes, soups, custards, milk, cream, ice cream, and canned foods. Canned foods, although initially sterile, may become infected if not immediately consumed after the can has been opened. Occasionally, but not usually, there may be visible change in the character of food. An outbreak of *Salmonella* food poisoning is likely to occur whenever large amounts of food are prepared and the unconsumed food is kept for future meals. Accordingly, such food poisoning is reported far more frequently from buffets, restaurants, hospitals, and institutions other than private houses.

In toxic type, the food poisoning results from poisonous substances produced by multiplying organisms that have gained access to the prepared food, such as enterotoxin produced by the *staphylococcus*. In botulism type, the food poisoning results from the ingestion of preformed Botulinum toxin in the preserved food. The toxin is produced by *Clostridium botulinum*.

Signs and Symptoms There is great variation in the susceptibility of individuals to *Salmonella* food poisoning. Hence, although some participants may remain free from symptoms, others may be severely affected.

The condition is not only toxemia but also gastroenteritis resulting from bacterial infection. The incubation period is longer than that for *staphylococcal* food poisoning. The organisms multiply in the intestine, and a delay of 12 h or more is usual before symptoms occur. The onset is sudden; sometimes chills may be the initial symptom, followed by headache, nausea, vomiting, severe abdominal cramps, and marked prostration.

Three characteristics that help to differentiate this poisoning with *staphylococcal* enterotoxin are muscular weakness, fever, and very foul-smelling and persistent diarrhea.

The diagnosis rests on the isolation of the causative organism from the patient and suspected articles of food.

Treatment The stomach should be washed by gastric lavage and the bowel should be emptied by a cathartic if diarrhea is not present. Most patients recover rapidly with bed rest and warmth. No food should be allowed until the acute symptoms are over. The rest of the treatment is symptom-based. The antibiotic of choice is chloramphenicol up to 2 g daily for an adult and for not more than 7 days.

27.4 MYCOTOXINS

The range of chemical structures and biologic activity among the broad class of fungal species is large and cannot be summarized briefly. Mycotoxins do not constitute a separate chemical category, and they lack common molecular features. Mycotoxins of most interest are those found in human food or in the feed of domestic animals. They include the ergot alkaloids produced by *Claviceps* sp., aflatoxins and related compounds produced by *Aspergillus* sp., and the trichothecenes produced by several genera of fungi imperfecti, primarily *Fusarium* sp.

The ergot alkaloids are known to affect the nervous system and cause vasoconstriction. Historically, they have been implicated in epidemics of both gangrenous and convulsive ergotism (St. Anthony's fire), although such epidemics no longer occur in humans due to increased knowledge of the cause and due to more varied modern diets. Outbreaks of ergotism in livestock still occur frequently, however. These compounds have also been used as abortifacients. The ergot alkaloids are derivatives of ergotine, with the most active being amides of lysergic acid (for details, the reader is referred to other chapters in the book).

Aflatoxins are products of species of the genus *Aspergillus*, particularly *Aspergillus flavus*, a common fungus found as a contaminant of grain, maize, peanuts, and other crops. First implicated in poultry diseases such as Turkey-X disease, they were subsequently shown to cause cancer in experimental animals and, according to epidemiological studies, in humans. Aflatoxin B_1, the most toxic of the aflatoxins, must be activated enzymatically to exert its carcinogenic effect.

Trichothecenes are produced by members of the genera *Fusarium* and *Trichoderma*. They are frequently acutely toxic, displaying bactericidal, fungicidal, and insecticidal activity, as well as causing various clinical symptoms in mammals, including diarrhea, anorexia, and ataxia. They have been implicated in natural intoxications in both humans and animals, such as Abakabi disease in Japan and Stachybotryotoxicosis in the former Union of Soviet Socialist Republics (USSR), and they are the center of a continuing controversy concerning their possible use as chemical warfare agents.

Mycotoxins may also be used for beneficial purposes. The mycotoxin avermectin is currently generating considerable interest both as an insecticide and for the control of nematode parasites of domestic animals.

27.5 ALGAL TOXINS

Algal toxins are broadly defined to represent the chemicals derived from many species of *cyanobacteria* (blue-green bacteria), *dinoflagellates*, and *diatoms*. The toxins produced by these freshwater and marine organisms often accumulate in fish and shellfish inhabiting the surrounding waters, causing both human and animal poisonings, as well as overt fish kills. Unlike many of the microbial toxins, algal toxins are generally heat-stable; therefore, they are not altered by cooking methods, which increases the likelihood of human exposures and toxicity. Many of the more common algal toxins responsible for human poisonings worldwide are summarized here.

Amnesic Shellfish Poisoning (ASP) was first identified in 1987 in Prince Edward Island, Canada, after four people died from eating contaminated mussels. It is caused by domoic acid, which is produced by several species of *Pseudonitzschia* diatoms. The main contamination problems include mussels, clams, and crabs of the Pacific Northwest of the United States and Canada.

Paralytic Shellfish Poisoning (PSP) was first determined to be a problem in 1942, after three people and many seabirds died from eating shellfish on the west coast of the United States, near the Columbia River. It is caused by the saxitoxin family (saxitoxin plus 18 related compounds) and produced by several species of *Alexandrium* dinoflagellates. The main contamination problems include mussels, clams, crabs, and fish of the Pacific Northwest and Northeast Atlantic.

Neurotoxic Shellfish Poisoning (NSP) is caused by a red-tide producer that was first identified in 1880 in Florida, with earlier historical references. It causes sickness in humans that lasts several days. NSP is not fatal to humans; however, it is known to kill fish, invertebrates, seabirds, and marine mammals (eg, manatees). It is caused by the brevetoxin family, including dinoflagellate, *Karenia brevis*, and *Gymnodinium breve*.

Diarrheic Shellfish Poisoning (DSP): Human poisonings were first identified in the 1960s. It causes sickness in humans lasting several days but is not fatal. It is caused by chemicals of the okadaic acid family (okadaic acid plus four related compounds) produced by several species of *Dinophysis* dinoflagellates. The main contamination problems include mussels, clams, and other bivalves of the cold and warm temperate areas of the Atlantic and Pacific Oceans, mainly in Japan and Europe. Only two cases of DSP have been documented in North America.

Ciguatera Fish Poisoning (CFP) was first identified in 1511. It is tropical-subtropical seafood poisoning that affects up to 50,000 people each year and is the most often reported food-borne disease of a chemical origin in the United States. Caused by consumption of reef fishes (eg, grouper, snapper), sickness in humans lasts several days to weeks, but the human fatality rate is low. It is caused by the ciguatoxin family (ciguatoxin plus three or more related compounds) and is produced by several species of dinoflagellates, including *Gambierdiscus*, *Prorocentrum*, and *Ostreopsis*. The main contamination problems include herbivorous tropical reef fish worldwide.

Cyanobacterial (Blue-Green Bacteria) Toxins: Cyanobacterial poisonings were first recognized in the late 1800s. Human poisonings are rare; however, it commonly kills livestock, other mammals, birds, fish, and aquatic invertebrates. It is caused by a variety of biotoxins and cytotoxins, including anatoxin, microcystin, and nodularin, produced by several species of cyanobacteria, including *Anabaena*, *Aphanizomenon*, *Nodularia*, *Oscillatoria*, and *Microcystis*. The main contamination problems include all eutrophic freshwater rivers, lakes, and streams.

Ambush Predator (Pfiesteria piscicida and Toxic Pfiesteria Complex) Toxins: Members belonging to this group of organisms were first identified in 1991 in estuaries in North Carolina. They were believed to produce a toxin that has been implicated in killing several large fish and is suspected of causing adverse human health effects. However, the toxin or toxins are not yet identified and toxicity tests are not universally conclusive. They are produced by several dinoflagellate species, including, *Pfiesteria piscicida*, *Pfiesteria shumwayae*, and perhaps several other unidentified and un-named dinoflagellates belonging to the potentially toxic *Pfiesteria* complex. The main problems include major killing of fish in North Carolina and Maryland and potential human health problems. The range may extend from the Gulf of Mexico to the Atlantic estuarine waters, including Florida, North Carolina, Maryland, and Delaware, and possibly outward to Europe.

CHAPTER

Poisons of animal origin

28

CHAPTER OUTLINE

28.1 INTRODUCTION

The action of natural toxins has long been recognized and understood throughout human history. It is important to understand the distinction between toxicant and toxin. A toxicant is any chemical, of natural or synthetic origin, capable of causing a deleterious effect on a living organism. A toxin is a toxicant that is produced by a living organism and is not used as a synonym for toxicant. All toxins are toxicants, but not all toxicants are toxins. Toxins, whether produced by animals, plants, insects, or microbes, are generally metabolic products that have evolved as defense mechanisms for the purpose of repelling or killing predators or pathogens. For example, ancient civilizations used natural toxins for both medicinal (therapeutic) and criminal purposes. Even today, we continue to discover and understand the toxicity of natural products, some for beneficial pharmaceutical or therapeutic purposes whose safety and efficacy are tested, and some for other less laudable

Fundamentals of Toxicology. DOI: http://dx.doi.org/10.1016/B978-0-12-805426-0.00028-7

purposes like biological or chemical warfare. Toxins may be classified in various ways depending on interest and need, such as by target organ toxicity or mode of action, but they are commonly classified according to source.

28.2 ANIMAL POISONS

The animal kingdom consists of more than 100,000 species spread through major phyla, including arthropods, mollusks, and chordates. At least 400 species of snakes are considered dangerous to humans. Myriad venomous and poisonous arthropods exist, and toxic marine animals are found in almost every sea and ocean. Envenomation can occur with these bites and stings, leading to toxic conditions that can be serious enough to cause death of the victim. There are a vast number of poisonous and venomous animals.

It is difficult to classify and characterize the vast numbers of poisonous and venomous animals; however, the poisonous and venomous animals have been defined as follows.

Venomous animal: A venomous animal can produce venom in specialized glands or cells and deliver it either by biting or by stinging, or in some cases by spitting.

Poisonous animal: A poisonous animal possesses a toxin (or toxins) within its tissues that can have deleterious effects when ingested.

The pharmacological and toxicological properties of most venom are incompletely understood because of their complexity, difficulties obtaining sufficient venom, and difficulties extracting individual components. For the sake of discussion, the properties of venoms produced by poisonous/venomous animals have several characteristics. Venoms are very complex, containing polypeptides, high-molecular-weight and low-molecular-weight proteins, amines, lipids, steroids, amino polysaccharides, quinones, glucosides, and free amino acids, as well as serotonin, histamine, and other substances. Some venom may consist of more than 100 proteins.

28.3 ARTHROPODS

There are more than 1 million species of arthropods, and they are generally divided into 25 orders, of which at least 12 are of importance to humans from an economic standpoint. However, medically, there are orders of venomous or poisonous animals that are of importance. These include:

1. Arachnids (scorpions, spiders, whip scorpions, solpugids, mites, and ticks)
2. Myriapods (centipedes and millipedes)
3. Insects: Heteroptera (true bugs), Hymenoptera (ants, bees, wasps, and hornets), Formicidae (ants), *Apidae* (bees), Vespidae (wasps), Lepidoptera (caterpillars, moths, butterflies, water bugs, assassin bugs, and wheel bugs)
4. Beetles (blister beetles)

28.3.1 ARACHNIDS

28.3.1.1 Scorpions

Of the more than 1000 species of scorpions, the stings of more than 75 can be considered of sufficient importance to warrant medical attention Scorpions spend the daylight hours under cover or in burrows. They emerge at night to ambush other arthropods or even small rodents, capture them with their pincers (Fig. 28.1), sting and paralyze them, tear them apart, and digest their body fluids. Because they are carnivorous, the larger ones often feed on the smaller ones. Many scorpion venoms contain low-molecular-weight proteins, peptides, amino acids, nucleotides, and salts, among other components. The neurotoxic fractions are generally classified on the basis of their molecular size, with the short-chain toxins composed of 20–40 amino acid residues with three or four disulfide bonds that appear to affect potassium or chloride channels; however, the long-chain toxins have 58–76 amino acid residues (6500–8500 Da) with four disulfide bonds and mainly affect the sodium channels. Scorpions are widely distributed all over the world.

In general, the scorpion is a poisonous insect with a crab-like body, eight legs, and a segmented tail with a bulbous expansion and a stinger in the last segment. The stinger has clear, colorless venom (toxalbumin) with two components, a hemolytic and a neurotoxic fraction. Fatality is rare because the dose in the stinger is not lethal.

Signs and symptoms The victim presents with nausea, vomiting, restlessness, and fever, followed by convulsions, paralysis, coma, and death (due to respiratory paralysis). Neurotoxic factors can mimic strychnine poisoning. Hemolytic factors can mimic viperine snakebite.

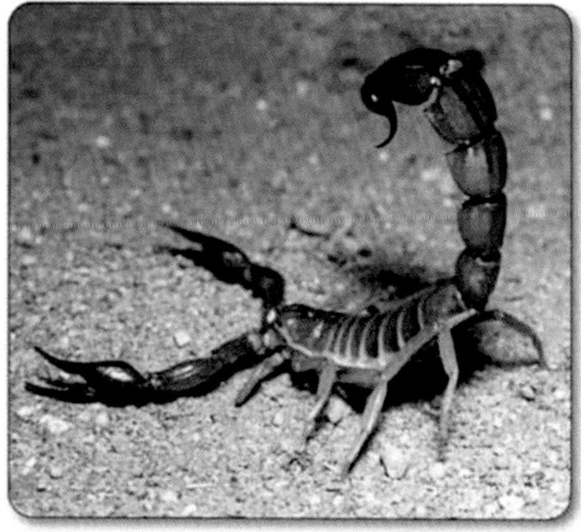

FIGURE 28.1

Poisonous insect: scorpion.

Source: Robert Frost Middle School. Available at: https://room42.wikispaces.com/Desert+Animals.

Diagnosis is by locating only one deep punctured wound (for snakebite wounds, there are always two fang marks) with a red surrounding area (inflammation), edema, and severe burning pain.

Treatment Attempts should be made to reduce the rate of absorption of the venom by:

- Tourniquet above the level of the sting
- Ice packing, incision, and suction (first aid)
- Washing with a solution of ammonia

Local anesthetics can also be helpful to reduce the pain and IV administration of calcium gluconate may reduce swelling. Use of a barbiturate can alleviate anxiety and atropine, and it may be given to reduce pulmonary edema (do not use morphine).

28.3.1.2 Spiders

Of the approximately 30,000 species, at least 200 have been implicated in significant bites to humans. Spiders are predaceous, polyphagous arachnids that generally feed on insects or other arthropods. All spiders except the Uloboridae family possess a venom apparatus that produces neurotoxins designed to paralyze or kill prey. Spider venoms are complex mixtures of low-molecular-weight components, including inorganic ions and salts, free acids, glucose-free amino acids, biogenic amines and neurotransmitters, and polypeptide toxins. Black widow spider venom contains various toxic proteins such as alpha-lactrotoxin, a labile neurotoxin that is the most important and potent toxin. The venom also contains several other lipoproteins and hyaluronidase. The venom of the black widow spider is one of the most potent biological toxins and is neurotoxic.

Treatment Most spiders are not very toxic to humans. Symptom-based and supportive treatment should be initiated. In the case of the black widow bite, antivenom is available.

28.3.1.3 Ticks

There are approximately 900 species of ticks that are associated with disease in humans and wild and domesticated animals Tick paralysis is caused by the saliva of certain ticks of the families Ixodidae, Argasidae, and Nuttalliellidae. Potentially 50 species of ticks are associated with clinical paralysis. Because tick bites are often not felt, the first evidence of envenomation may not appear until several days later, when small macules 3–4 mm in diameter develop that are surrounded by erythema and swelling, often displaying a hyperemic halo. Tick paralysis is rare, with ascending facial paralysis that occurs when toxin-secreting species of Ixodidae in the bite remain attached for several days. The patient often reports difficulty with gait, followed by paresis, and eventually locomotor paresis and paralysis. Problems in speech and respiration may ensue and lead to respiratory paralysis if the tick is not removed.

Treatment Treatment is symptomatic. After removal of ticks, apply an antiseptic. Sometimes the use of antibiotics is also recommended.

28.3.1.4 Mites

A number of biting mites have been reported to secrete toxin and cause a disease. Chiggers bite, feed in the skin, and then fall off. Common mite species that bite and burrow in the skin include *Sarcoptes scabiei*, which causes scabies; demodex mites cause a scabies-like dermatitis.

Treatment Treatment is symptom-based. Topical corticosteroids or oral antihistamines may be used.

28.3.2 MYRIAPODS (CENTIPEDES, CHILOPODA)

Found worldwide, these elongated, many-segmented (Fig. 28.2), brownish yellow (gray in print versions) arthropods have a pair of walking legs on most segments. They are fast-moving, secretive, and nocturnal. They feed on other arthropods and even small vertebrates and birds. Centipede venoms contain high-molecular-weight proteins, proteinases, esterases, 5-hydroxytryptamine, histamine, lipids, and polysaccharides. Such venom contains a heat-labile cardiotoxic protein of 60 kDa that produces, in humans, changes associated with acetylcholine release. Centipedes belong to the class Arthropods and are organic animal irritants. They have a long, segmented, dark to brownish black body with a pair of legs in each segment.

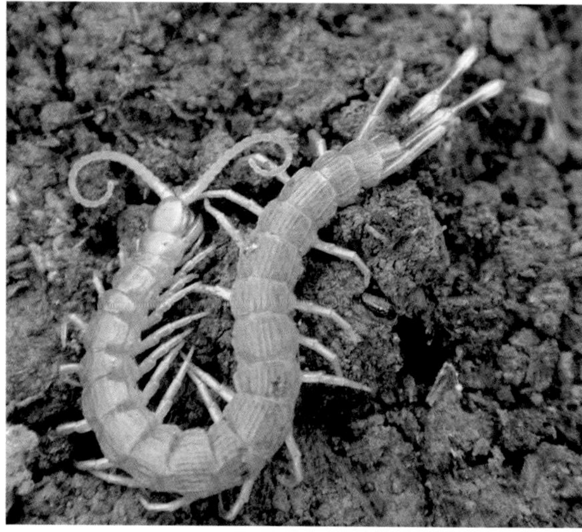

FIGURE 28.2

Poisonous insect: centipede in peat marshland.

Source: Wikimedia Commons. Available at: https://en.wikipedia.org/wiki/Centipede.

Signs and symptoms Usually, centipedes can inflict painful bites resulting in erythema, edema, and local lymphangitis.
Treatment Treatment consists of washing the bite site with soap and water and administration of analgesics.

28.3.3 INSECTS

Insects are a major group of arthropods with the greatest numbers of poisonous species. They are important from a toxicology point of view. A few of them include heteroptera (true bugs), hymenoptera (ants, bees, and hornets), vespidae (wasps; Fig. 28.3), and lepidoptera (caterpillars, moths, and butterflies).

The biting action of venoms of bees, wasps, hornets, and ants is usually local. It may be rarely fatal if the venom is a histamine (especially bites on the neck, face, etc.). However, the bite can result in laryngeal edema, leading to asphyxia and death when not treated immediately. Multiple stings can lead to severe systemic reactions, resulting in gastrointestinal disturbances, shock, unconsciousness, and death. A few species contain a complex mixture of biomedical compounds ranging from simple amines to complicated proteins or enzymes. Most ants have stingers, but those that lack them can spray a defensive secretion from the tip of the gaster, which is often placed in the wound of the bite. Ants of different species vary considerably in length, ranging from less than 1.5 mm to more than 35 mm. Clinically important stinging ants are the harvesting ants (*Pagonomyrmex*), fire ants (*Solenopsis*), and little fire ants (*Ochetomyrmex*). The harvester ants are large, red, dark brown, or black and range in size from 6 to 10 mm. They have fringes of long hairs on the posterior of their heads. The venoms of the ants vary considerably. The venoms of the *Ponerinae*, *Ecitoninae*, and *Pseudomyrmex* are proteinaceous in character.

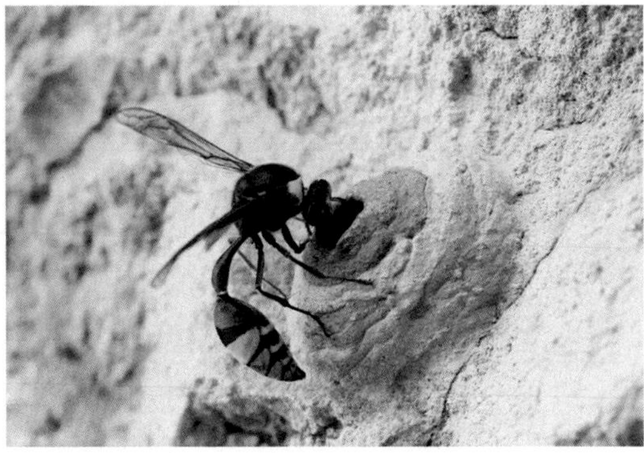

FIGURE 28.3

Poisonous insect: wasp building mud nest.

Source: Wikimedia Commons. Available at: https://en.wikipedia.org/wiki/Wasp.

The *Myrmecinae* venoms are a mixture of amines, enzymes, and proteinaceous materials, histamine, hyaluronidase, phospholipase A, and hemolysins, which hemolyze erythrocytes and mast cells. Other peptides named waspkinins cause immediate pain, vasodilation, and increased vascular permeability, leading to edema. These venoms also contain phospholipases and hyaluronidases, which contribute to the breakdown of membranes and connective tissue to facilitate diffusion of the venom. These proteins also contribute to the allergenicity of the venoms.

Treatment Treatment of ant stings is dependent on their number, whether an allergic reaction is involved, and whether there are possible complications. The following measures should be taken to reduce the rate of absorption of venom:

Use a tourniquet above the level of stinging or incision and suction.

Use drugs such as adrenaline, apply tincture iodine/antihistaminic (to reduce inflammation), administer IV adrenocorticotrophic hormone 25 mg in 1000 mL normal saline, and administer IV calcium gluconate.

28.3.4 CANTHARIDES (SPANISH FLY BLISTER BEETLE, LYTTA)

Beetles are winged insects that have a body of length 2 cm and a width 0.6 cm. They are greenish black with shiny wings of the same color. The insect, or the powder of its dried body, has a toxic (active) principle called cantharidin. The route of absorption is through the skin and all other mucosa.

Signs and symptoms Within 2 to 3 h of coming in contact with the skin, the poison produces burning pain, redness, and vesication. If taken orally, symptoms manifest within 30 min to 2 h.

The fatal dose is 15–30 mg of cantharidin or 1.5 g of powdered cantharides.

Postmortem findings The mouth, stomach, and intestines may show inflammation and vesication; particles of insect may be found in the stomach contents. The heart, lungs, and kidneys are inflamed and hemorrhagic.

Treatment: Stomach wash, demulcents, symptomatic.

28.4 MOLLUSKS

28.4.1 CONE SNAILS

Human interest in this group of mollusks has been due to the beautiful patterns on their shells. Cone snails were known to Roman scholars and natural history collectors, because the shells were often made into jewelry. The genus *Conus* is a group of approximately 500 species of carnivorous predators found in marine habitats that use venom as a weapon for prey capture. Cone snails (Fig. 28.4) may be divided into three groups depending on preferred prey. The largest group contains worm-hunting species that feed on polychaetes (segmented marine worms in the phylum Annelida).

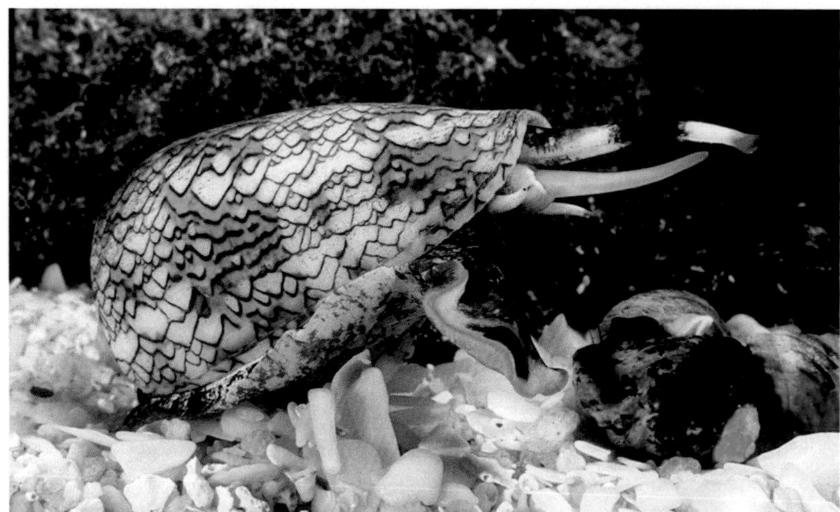

FIGURE 28.4

Australian cone snail.

Source: David Paul, Melbourne University, AAP Image. Available at: http://www.australiangeographic.com.au/news/2014/03/cone-snail-pain-drug-is-non-addictive.

The second group is molluscivorous and hunts other gastropods. The final group is piscivorous and has venoms that rapidly immobilize fish. There are probably more than 100 different venom components per species. Components have become known as conotoxins, which may be rich in disulfide bonds and conopeptides. Some components have enzymatic activity. Conopeptides also target ligand-gated ion channels that mediate fast synaptic transmission, resulting in poisoning.

28.5 REPTILES

28.5.1 LIZARDS

Gila monsters (*Heloderma suspectum*) and beaded lizards (*Heloderma horridum*) are divided into five subspecies. These large, relatively slow-moving, and largely nocturnal reptiles have few enemies other than humans. They are far less dangerous than is generally believed. Their venom is transferred from venom glands in the lower jaw through ducts that discharge their contents near the base of the larger teeth of the lower jaw. The venom is then drawn up along grooves in the teeth by capillary action. The venom of this lizard has serotonin and several enzymes with fibrinogen coagulase activities. The bite can lead to pain, edema, hypotension, nausea, vomiting, weakness, and diaphoresis.

No antivenin is commercially available. Treatment is supportive.

28.5.2 VENOMOUS SNAKES

Snakes are ectothermic (cold-blooded), limbless vertebrates of the class Reptilia. Snakes have a three-chambered heart and rely almost exclusively on an enlarged right lung (that spans approximately half of their body length) for respiration. Of the approximately 2700 known species of snakes, approximately 20% are considered to be venomous, which means that most of them are nonvenomous. Venomous snakes primarily belong to the following families:

1. *Viperida*e (vipers)
2. *Elapidae*
3. *Atractaspidae*
4. *Colubridae*

There are several poisonous species of snakes in the world, and they belong to three families:

- Elapidae, which includes common cobra, king cobra, and krait
- Viperidae, which includes Russell's viper, pit viper, and saw-scaled viper
- Hydrophiidae (the sea snakes)

However, among these, the majority of bites and consequent mortality are attributable to only five species: king cobra (Ophiophagus hannah), common cobra (Naja Naja), Russell's viper (Daboia rusellii), krait (Bungarus coeruleus), and saw-scaled viper (Echis carinatae). Venomous snakes have certain common features and some other features that are unique to each of them. Cobra venom is also a potential source of medicines, including anticancer drugs and painkillers.

Snake venoms These venoms are complex mixtures of proteins and peptides, consisting of both enzymatic and nonenzymatic compounds and comprising more than 90% of the dry weight of the venom. Snake venoms also contain inorganic cations such as sodium, calcium, potassium, and magnesium, and small amounts of zinc, iron, cobalt, manganese, and nickel. The metals in snake venoms are likely catalysts for metal-based enzymatic reactions.

Snake venoms are of three types: neurotoxic, hemotoxic, and myotoxic. Different types of toxic principles in the snake venom are summarized in Table 28.1.

Mode of action Actions of snake venoms have a broad range and can be grouped as neurotoxins, coagulants, hemorrhagins, hemolytics, myotoxins, cytotoxins, and nephrotoxins. Neurotoxins produce neuromuscular paralysis, dizziness, ptosis, phthalmoplegia, flaccid facial muscle paralysis, inability to swallow, paralysis of larger muscle groups, and, finally, paralysis of respiratory muscles and death by asphyxiation. Coagulants may have initial procoagulant action that uses clotting factors, leading to bleeding. Coagulants may directly inhibit normal clotting in the clotting cascade or via inhibition of platelet aggregation. In addition, some venom components may damage the endothelial lining of blood vessels, leading to hemorrhage.

Table 28.1 Types of Toxic Principles in Snake Venom

Toxins	Enzymes	Toxalbumins
Low-molecular-weight peptides and proteins	Cholinesterase	Cardiotoxin
	Anticholinesterase	Neurotoxin
	Hyaluronidase	Cytolysin
	Lecithinase	Hemorrhagin
	Phosphatidases	Hemolysin
	Phospholipase A	Fibrinolysin
	Proteases	Proteolysin
	Proteinases	Thromboplastin
	Ribonuclease	

Signs and symptoms In general, the venoms of rattle snakes and crotalids produce alterations in the resistance and often in the integrity of blood vessels, changes in blood cells and blood coagulation mechanisms, and direct or indirect changes in cardiac and pulmonary dynamics (Fig. 28.5). In addition, crotalids like *Crotalus durissus terrificus* and *Crotalus scutulatus* can cause serious alterations in the nervous system and changes in respiration. In humans, the course of the poisoning is determined by the kind and amount of venom injected, the site where it is deposited, and the general health, size, and age of the patient. Death in humans may occur within less than 1 h or after several days, with most deaths occurring between 18 and 32 h. Hypotension or shock is the major cause of death after North American crotalid bites. Table 28.2 summarizes the fatal dose of venom, amount of venom injected with a bite site, and fatal period due to snake venoms.

1. **Neurotoxic venomous snake**

   The neurotoxic symptoms are common in Elapidae snakes (eg, krait, cobra, etc.; Figs. 28.6 and 28.7). The toxins act like curare, affecting mainly the motor nerve cells and resulting in muscular paralysis. The muscles are affected in the following order: muscles of mouth, muscles of the throat, and, finally, muscles of respiration.

   Local action: Local manifestations of neurotoxic venoms that may be observed are severe burning at the bite site, rapid edema, and inflammatory changes, followed by oozing of serum.

   Systemic action: Within 15–30 min to 2 h of biting, convulsions may be seen with cobra venom, whereas krait venom produces only paralysis. Recovery is complete if the patient survives.

   The flow chart presents the neurotoxic effects of venom produced by neurotoxic venomous snakes (Fig. 28.8). The patient shows giddiness, weakness, lethargy, and muscle weakness, followed by paralysis and death.

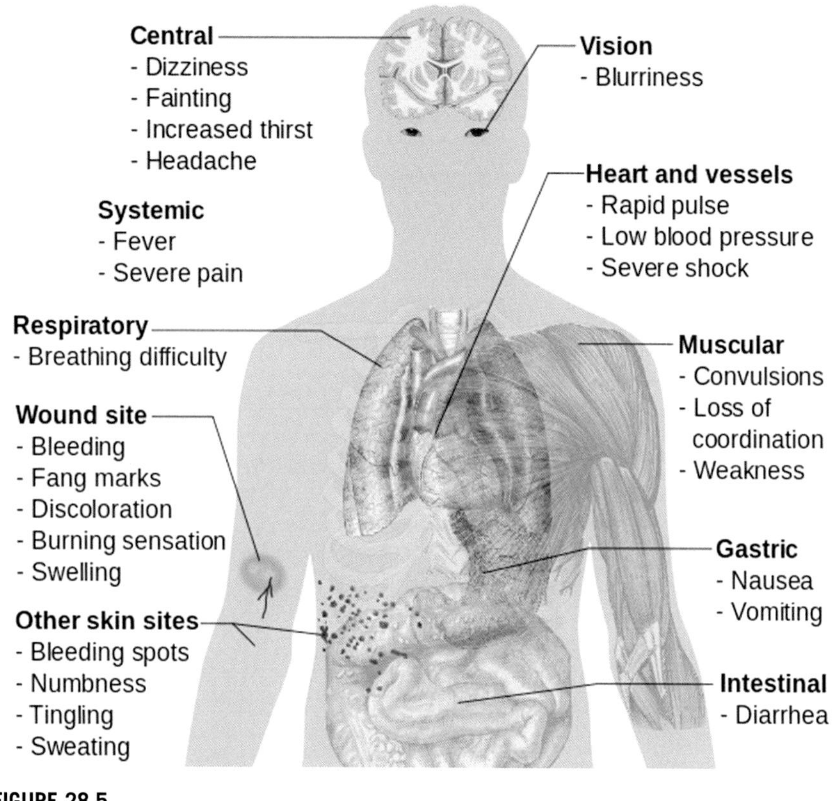

FIGURE 28.5

General symptoms observed after the bite of a venomous snake.

Source: Wikimedia Commons. Available at: https://upload.wikimedia.org/wikipedia/commons/a/a4/Snake_bite_symptoms.svg.

Table 28.2 Fatal Doses, Amount of Venom Injected with a Bite Site, and Fatal Period after Snake Bites

Venoms	Fatal Doses (Dried Form) (mg)	Amounts of Venom Injected With a Bite Site (Dried Form) (mg)
Cobra[a]	15	200–350
Viper[b]	40	150–200
Krait	6	22
Echis carinata	8	4.5

[a] *A few minutes to hours.*
[b] *A few hours to days.*

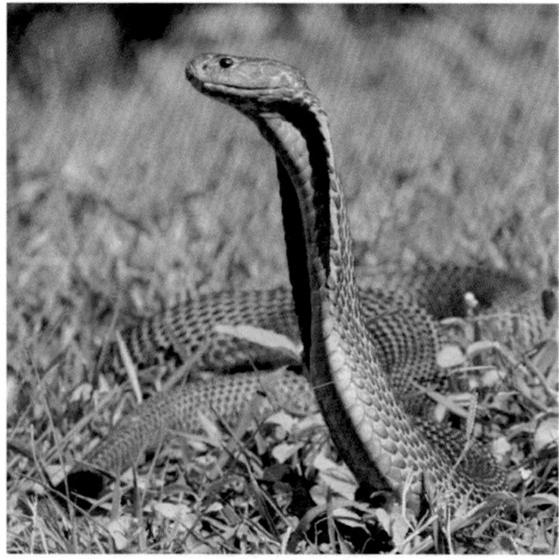

FIGURE 28.6

Naja philippinensis in defensive posture.

Source: Wikimedia Commons. Available at: https://en.wikipedia.org/wiki/Philippine_cobra.

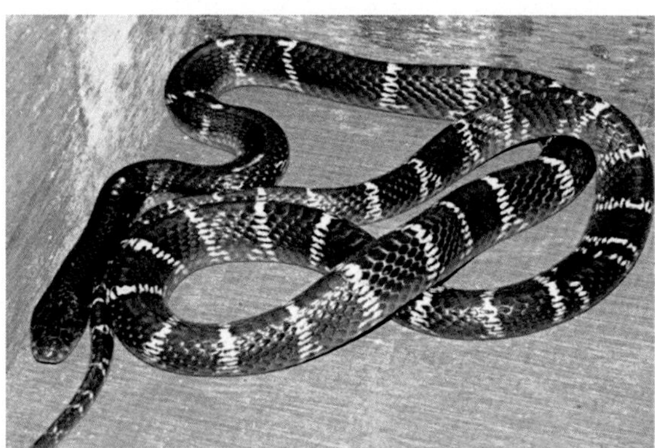

FIGURE 28.7

Venomous snake: krait.

Source: Wikimedia Commons. Available at: https://en.wikipedia.org/wiki/Common_krait.

2. Hemotoxic venomous snake

Hemotoxic symptoms are common in Viperidae snakes (Fig. 28.9), such as the pit viper (Crotalidae), pit-less viper (Russell's viper, saw-scaled viper/Phoorsa/Echis/Echis Carinata), and bamboo snake (common green (light gray in print versions) pit viper).

Local action: Severe pain at the bite site followed by swelling, ecchymosis, cellulitis, and severe hemorrhage are common.

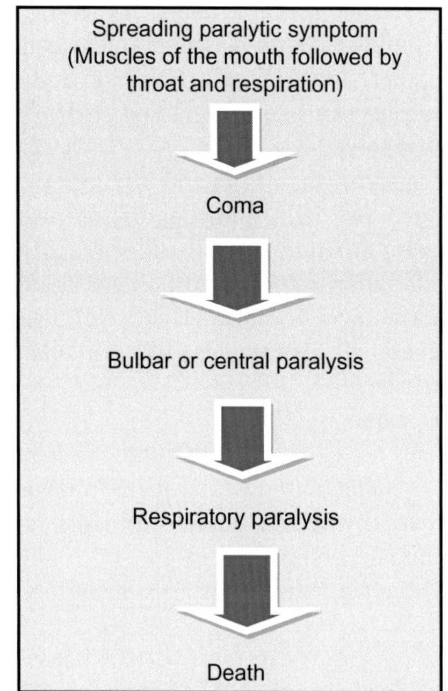

FIGURE 28.8

Schematic representation of symptoms produced by neurotoxic venom.

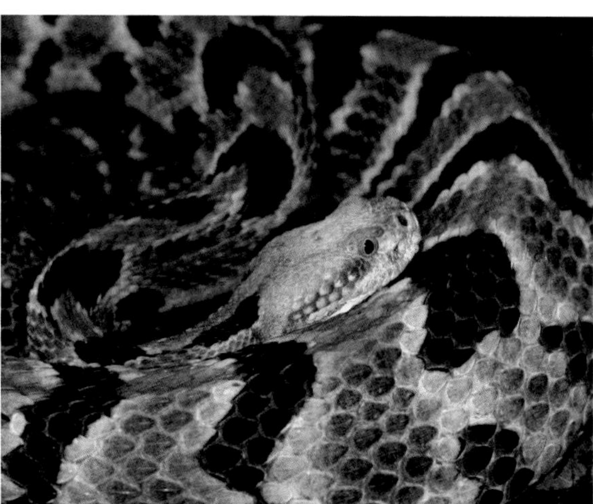

FIGURE 28.9

Hemotoxic venomous snake: *Crotalus horridus*

Source: Wikimedia Commons. Available at: https://commons.wikimedia.org/wiki/File:Crotalus_horridus_(1).jpg.

Systemic action: Systemic action is due to hemolytic effects on the heart and blood vessels, resulting in cardiovascular collapse and death. If the patient survives suppuration, then sloughing with infection at the site of bite, hemorrhage from the mucosa of the rectum and other natural orifices, and gangrene of the parts involved can occur.

The venom acts by cytolysis of the endothelium of blood vessels, lysis of red cells and other tissue cells, and coagulation disorders. This can lead to severe swelling, with oozing of blood and spreading cellulitis at the bite site. Blood from such patients fails to clot, even on adding thrombin, because of the very low level of fibrin. This is followed by necrosis of renal tubules and functional disturbances like convulsions due to intracerebral hemorrhage.

3. Myotoxic venomous snake

Myotoxic symptoms are common with hydrophiidae or sea snakes. The venom produces generalized muscular pain, followed by myoglobinuria within 3–5 h. Death usually occurs due to respiratory failure.

Local action: Minimal swelling and pain.

Systemic action: Myalgia, muscle stiffness, myoglobinuria, and renal tubular necrosis.

Postmortem findings At the site, there are two bite marks (1 cm deep for colubrine bite and 2.5 cm deep for viperine bite). In the case of a bite from a viperine snake, there may be some edema, cellulitis, and bleeding.

- In case of death due to a colubrine bite, changes seen will be that of asphyxia.
- In case of death due to a viperine bite, there will be hemorrhaging in the lungs, pleura, and pericardium. Kidneys will show renal tubular necrosis, desquamation, and cloudy swelling.

Treatment The treatment of bites by venomous snakes is highly specialized, and almost every envenomation requires specific recommendations. However, three general principles for every bite should be kept in mind: (1) snake venom poisoning is a medical emergency requiring immediate attention and exercise of considerable judgment; (2) the venom is a complex mixture of substances, of which the proteins contribute the major deleterious properties, and the only adequate antidote is the use of specific or polyspecific antivenom; and (3) not every bite by a venomous snake ends in an envenomation. Sometimes venom may not be injected by the snake. In almost 1000 cases of crotalid bites, 24% did not end in poisoning. In addition to a specific antidote, treatment should include a general approach such as supportive therapy and the specific therapy.

28.5.3 NONVENOMOUS SNAKES

- They have no poison apparatus
- They have four longitudinal rows of teeth in the upper jaw and two rows in lower jaw

- Tail is not compressed
- Ventral shields are small/moderately large
- Head scales are usually larger and without any special features
- Fangs are short and solid
- They are not nocturnal
- The bite marks show more than two teeth markings

28.5.4 OTHER REPTILE BITES

Among the other reptiles that are of significance are venomous lizards, alligators and crocodiles, and iguanas. Venomous lizards include the gila monster (*Heloderma suspectum*) and the beaded lizard (*Heloderma horridum*). This species is found in the southwestern United States and Mexico. Their complex venom contains serotonin, arginine, esterase, hyaluronidase, phospholipase A_2, and one or more salivary kallikreins, but it lacks neurotoxic components or coagulopathic enzymes. Bites are rarely fatal.

Signs and symptoms Signs and symptoms may include intense pain, swelling, edema, ecchymosis, lymphangitis, and lymphadenopathy.

Treatment Treatment is symptom-based and supportive. No antivenom is available. The wound should be probed with a small needle for broken or shed teeth and then cleaned.

28.5.5 ALLIGATORS AND CROCODILE

Bites are venomous and need preventive treatment with clindamycin and trimethoprim-sulfamethoxazole or tetracycline.

28.5.6 IGUANA

Iguana bites are claw injuries and treatment is local.

CHAPTER

Chemical food poisoning 29

CHAPTER OUTLINE

29.1 INTRODUCTION

Chemical food poisoning is caused by eating plants or animals that contain a naturally occurring toxin containing chemicals such as acetylcholine, alkaloids, serotonin, histamines, sulfur, lipids, phenols, and glycocides. Chemical food poisoning often involves mushrooms, poisonous plants, or marine animals. The toxicity of some of plants has already been discussed in other chapters in this book. The reader may refer to chapters dealing with toxic agents.

29.2 MUSHROOMS

Mushrooms are fungi with umbrella-shaped tops and stems. *Stropheria semeglobata*, *Hypholoma froomasciculare*, and *Lactarius vellereus* are among the poisonous varieties of mushrooms.

Symptoms of poisoning All toxic mushrooms cause vomiting and abdominal pain; other manifestations vary significantly depending on the type of mushroom ingested. Mushroom poisoning causes nausea, vomiting, diarrhea, bloody vomit and stools, enlarged tender liver and jaundice, oliguria, pulmonary edema, mental confusion, convulsions, and coma.

Generally, mushrooms that cause early symptoms (within 2 h) are less dangerous than those that cause later symptoms (usually after 6 h). Certain mushrooms act by parasympathomimetic action or may be due to hypersensitivity. The little brown mushrooms that grow in lawns cause gastroenteritis, sometimes with headache or myalgias. Diarrhea is occasionally bloody. Usually, symptoms vary with the type of mushroom ingested. Some mushrooms contain psilocybin, which may

Fundamentals of Toxicology. DOI: http://dx.doi.org/10.1016/B978-0-12-805426-0.00029-9

cause hallucinations, tachycardia, and hypertension. Some mushrooms cause muscrinic symptoms such as miosis, diarrhea, and bradycardia. Members of Amanita genera cause hypoglycemia and hepatic and renal failure.

Treatment Supportive and symptom-based treatment such as gastric lavage, atropine, exchange transfusion in children, charcoal, and hemoperfusion in adults are used. In the case of central nervous system toxicity resulting in neurological symptoms, pyridoxine 25 mg/kg (maximum daily dose, 25 g) is recommended.

29.3 POISONOUS PLANT TOXINS

The many toxic chemicals produced by plants, usually referred to as secondary plant compounds, often have chemicals that are used as defense mechanisms against herbivorous animals, particularly insects and mammals. This chapter focuses only on the human toxicity of some of the more well-known plants. These compounds may be repellent but not particularly toxic, or they may be acutely toxic to a wide range of organisms. They include sulfur compounds, lipids, phenols, alkaloids, glycosides, and many other types of chemicals. Many of the common drugs of abuse such as cocaine, caffeine, nicotine, morphine, and the cannabinoids are plant toxins (for details, see the other chapters). Many chemicals that have been shown to be toxic are constituents of plants that form part of the human diet. For example, the carcinogen safrole and related compounds are found in black pepper. Solanine and chaconine, which are cholinesterase inhibitors and possible teratogens, are found in potatoes, and quinines and phenols are widespread in food. Livestock poisoning by plants is still an important veterinary problem in some areas.

Some plants are known to cause damage to various organs of the body. For example, there are a several plants that affect the skin and make contact painful. This occurs either through an allergic antibody-mediated response or through direct action by chemicals. For an allergic type of response, it is not the first contact that produces the reaction, but rather the next contact. For example, poison ivy produces a class of chemicals called urushiol, which causes a widely variable allergic response in approximately 70% of people exposed. Similarly, pollen of ragweed, mugwort, or grasses causes an allergic response in many people. Dieffenbachia or dumb cane, a common houseplant, produces a juice that is released when a stem is broken or chewed and causes painful, rapid swelling and inflammation of the tongue and mouth. The symptoms can take several days to resolve and are caused by oxalate crystals coated with an irritating protein. Stinging nettle (Urtica) releases histamine, acetylcholine, and serotonin from fine tubes with bulbs at the end that break off onto the skin, causing an intense burning or stinging sensation.

Some plants cause direct irritation of the stomach lining. For example, the chemical colchicine stops cell division (an antimitotic), producing severe nausea, vomiting, and dehydration, which can lead to delirium, neuropathy, and kidney failure. However, colchicine is used in the treatment of gout and as an anticancer agent because it stops cell division. Most toxic of all plants are the ones that produce lectins, and the most toxic of these is the chemical ricin, which is produced by castor beans. Only five to six seeds are necessary to kill a small child. Ricin is extremely toxic and 0.1 μg/kg of body weight can be fatal. Another example is the medically important drug digitalis, which is derived from foxglove (*Digitalis purpurea*). Digitalis slows and stabilizes the heart rate, but at high dose it produces an irregular heart rate and decreased blood pressure. Likewise, there are several other poisons such as "mad honey poisoning," which is caused by bees. The cardiovascular effects are caused by grayanotoxin, which is produced in the leaves and nectar of rhododendrons and are concentrated in the honey by the bees.

Hepatitis and cirrhosis of the liver from contaminated grain caused by ragwort or pyrrolizidine alkaloids are well known. Children are often the most susceptible to many of the naturally occurring toxins, just as they are to other toxicants. The caffeine from a can of cola will have a much larger effect on a small child than it will on an adult. Health status and age, both young and old, also influence the response. Aflatoxin from contaminated nuts has a greater likelihood of causing cancer in some with a liver disease such as hepatitis. It is important to develop a knowledge of which plants and animals can be dangerous and to learn how to avoid dangerous contact with them.

29.4 POISONOUS MARINE BITES AND STINGS

Some marine bites and stings are toxic, and all create wounds at risk for infection with marine organisms. Shark bites result in jagged lacerations with near-total or total amputations and should be treated as traumas.

29.4.1 POISONOUS FISHES

There are several species of venomous fish that are capable of producing poisoning. Fish poisoning may occur due to attacks and bites (eg, sharks and barracudas), by injecting toxic venom through their venomous spines or tentacles (eg, stingrays), and through eating fish whose flesh is toxic. There are three common types of fish whose flesh is toxic and cause poisoning. They are described here.

Ciguatera poisoning may result from eating any of the more than 400 species of fish in which a dinoflagellate produces a toxin that accumulates in the flesh of the body. Symptoms may begin 2–8 h after eating; intravenous (IV) mannitol has been suggested as a treatment.

Scombroid poisoning is caused by high histamine levels in fish flesh due to bacterial decomposition after the fish is caught. Commonly affected species include tuna, mackerel, bonito, skipjack, and mahi mahi. Symptoms include facial flushing, nausea, vomiting, and urticaria. Treatment may include administration of antihistamines.

Tetrodotoxin poisoning is most common due to eating puffer fish, but more than 100 fresh water and salt water species contain tetrodotoxin. Symptoms are similar to ciguatera and may produce fatal respiratory paralysis.

Tetrodotoxin is found in all organs of the fish but is highest in the liver, skin, and intestine. The origins of the toxin are not clear, but one possibility is that the fish has come in contact with bacteria that produce tetrodotoxin. Puffer fish may also have elevated levels of saxitoxin, a neurotoxin responsible for paralytic shellfish poisoning. Saxitoxin is produced by dinoflagellates (algae) and most often contaminates mussels, clams, and scallops. Both saxitoxin and tetrodotoxin are heat-stable, so cooking does not reduce toxicity.

Mode of action Tetrodotoxin causes paralysis by affecting the sodium ion transport in both the central and peripheral nervous systems. A low dose of tetrodotoxin produces tingling sensations and numbness around the mouth, fingers, and toes. Higher doses produce nausea, vomiting, respiratory failure, difficulty walking, extensive paralysis, and death. As little as 1–4 mg of the toxin can kill an adult. Saxitoxin has a very different chemical structure than tetrodotoxin, but it has similar effects on transport of cellular sodium and produces similar neurological effects. Saxitoxin is less toxic than tetrodotoxin. Some people, particularly in Asia, consider the puffer fish a fine delicacy if it is carefully prepared by experienced chefs. The trick is to get just a small dose to feel mild tingling effects, but not the more serious symptoms of tetrodotoxin poisoning. In the United States tetrodotoxin poisoning is rare, but a recent US report indicated several cases of people catching and consuming puffer fish containing elevated levels of these toxins and suffering the ill effects.

Treatment Treatment is supportive and symptom-based. Activated charcoal may be helpful.

29.4.2 SHELLFISH

Shellfish such as mussels, clams, oysters, and scallops are not naturally toxic, but they can become so after feeding on plankton contaminated with a toxin. When visible, the blooming of the plankton (dinoflagellate) is called red tide and can cause significant death among marine animals. There are several types of toxins, mostly affecting the nervous system. The newest, domoic acid, first appeared in 1987 off Prince Edward Island in Canada. This neurotoxin caused confusion and memory loss, particularly in the elderly. Several elderly people died after seizures and coma. Domoic acid is heat-stable, so cooking does not affect the toxin. Government agencies now monitor for contaminants of shellfish and move quickly to restrict harvesting. The puffer fish is probably the best known neurotoxic fish. Several related species of fish as well as other marine life, such as some frogs, starfish, octopus, and others, contain tetrodotoxin. Many people consider these fish a delicacy despite the occasional reported death from poor preparation. Tetrodotoxin is heat-stable but water-soluble, so careful preparation is necessary to limit neurological effects. Symptoms of poisoning include rapid onset of numbness in the lips and mouth that then extends to the fingers and toes, followed by general weakness, dizziness, respiratory failure, and death. The mechanism of action is similar to that of saxitoxin and affects sodium channel permeability.

It should also be remembered that fish high in the food chain such as tuna, swordfish, and shark accumulate toxic substances like mercury or PCBs. Mercury affects the nervous system and is a proven reproductive hazard.

Treatment Supportive and symptom-based treatment such as gastric lavage, IV mannitol, atropine, exchange transfusion in children, charcoal, and hemoperfusion in adults are administered. In some cases, treatment may include H1 and H2 blockers.

CHAPTER

Health effects of radioactive materials

30

CHAPTER OUTLINE

30.1 INTRODUCTION

All life is dependent on small doses of electromagnetic radiation. Radiation is produced by disintegration of unstable naturally occurring or human-made elements. Radiation has been utilized for many beneficial effects, but direct or indirect exposure to ionizing radiations produce several deleterious effects on the health of humans and animals. Ionizing radiation can cause different types of damage in mammalian systems, including effects on both proliferative and nonproliferative tissues. At the same time we are surrounded by and depend on radiation-emitting devices, including the sun, our cell phones, radios, medical X-rays, and the electricity that powers our homes. Radiation-emitting devices have many benefits, but we are still learning about some of the health effects.

30.1.1 HISTORICAL BACKGROUND

The cave dwellers were probably the first to manage radiation when they learned to control and use fire. The control and use of electricity was another huge step forward. However, the turn of the twentieth century really marked the beginning of rapid progress in the understanding and harnessing of the power of radiation. This period also ushered in a growing understanding of the potential adverse effects of radiation exposure. In 1895, Wilhem Conrad Roentgen discovered

Fundamentals of Toxicology. DOI: http://dx.doi.org/10.1016/B978-0-12-805426-0.00030-5

X-rays, and in 1901 he was awarded the first Nobel Prize for physics. These discoveries led to significant advances in medicine.

In 1903, Marie Curie and Pierre Curie, along with Henri Becquerel, were awarded the Nobel Prize in physics for their contributions to understanding radioactivity, including the properties of uranium. To this day, the "curie" and the "becquerel" are used as units of measure in radiation studies. Subsequently, this knowledge was used to develop the atomic bombs that were dropped on Japan in an effort to end World War II. Much of our understanding of the effects of nuclear radiation exposure has come from the victims in Japan as well as the many workers in uranium mines.

A great deal was learned from the atomic bomb survivors. The US military dropped the first atomic bomb on Hiroshima, Japan, on August 6, 1945, and then a second on Nagasaki, Japan, 3 days later. The bombs used two different types of radioactive material, 235 U in the first bomb and 239 Pu in the second. It is estimated that 64,000 people died from the initial blasts and radiation exposure. Approximately 100,000 survivors were enrolled in follow-up studies, which confirmed an increased incidence of cancer.

X-rays were also used to treat disease. From 1905 to 1960, X-rays were used to treat ringworm in children. Subsequently, during the 1950s X-rays were used to treat a degenerative bone disease called ankylosing spondylitis. It was learned from these incidences that the greater the dose, the greater the likelihood of developing cancer. In addition, there could be a very long delay in the onset of the cancer, from 10 to 40 years. It is estimated that 1 in 100 cancers results from this background exposure.

30.1.2 REGULATORY ASPECTS OF RADIATION

The first organized effort to protect people from radiation exposure began in 1915, when the British Roentgen Society adopted a resolution to protect people from X-rays. In 1922, the United States adopted the British protection rules and various government and nongovernmental groups were formed to protect people from radiation. In 1959, the Federal Radiation Council was formed to advise the President and recommend standards. In 1970, the US Environmental Protection Agency was formed and took over these responsibilities. Now, several government agencies are responsible for protecting people from radiation-emitting devices.

30.1.3 STANDARDS FOR RADIATION EXPOSURE

Recommended exposure limits are set by the US National Council on Radiation Protection (NCRP) and worldwide by the International Council on Radiation Protection (ICRP). The occupational exposure guidelines are 100 mSv in 5 years (average, 20 mSv/year), with a limit of 50 mSv in any single year. For the general public, the standard is 1 mSv/year. This must be put in the context of natural

Table 30.1 Comparison of Older Units of Measure With Standard International Unit System of Radiation Energy

Item	Previous Unit	SI Unit	Ratios
Activity (ie, quantity of rays or particles)	Curie (Ci)	Becquerel (Bq)	(Ci) 1 Ci = 3.7×10^{10} Bq 1 mCi = 37 MBq 1 μCi = 37 KBq *U78*
Exposure	Roentgen (R)	X (Coul/kg)	1 R = 2.58×10^{-4} Coul/kg
Absorbed dose	Rad	Gray (Gy) Gy = 1 J/kg	1 Gy = 100 rad 1 rad = 10 mGy
Gray (Gy)	Gray (Gy) Rem Sievert (Sv)	1 Sv = 100 rem	1 rem = 10 mSv

m, *milli (one one-thousandth);* SI, *International system of units (Systeme Internationale).*

background radiation, which is approximately 3 mSv/year depending on location (such as elevation) as well as other variables.

In the United States, the Food and Drug Administration (FDA) and the Federal Communications Commission (FCC) share regulatory responsibilities related to mobile devices and set a SAR limit of 1.6 W/kg.

30.1.4 UNITS OF RADIATION

The units that are used to describe the exposure and dose of ionizing radiation have changed to an international system (SI), which stands for Systeme Internationale. Table 30.1 compares the previous unit, the older system, and the SI system. Recommended limits on radiation exposure are expressed in Sv.

30.2 TYPES OF RADIATION

Electromagnetic radiation has two types, nonionizing and ionizing. The range of the electromagnetic spectrum is summarized in Fig. 30.1.

Nonionizing Radiation: Nonionizing radiation includes ultraviolet, visible, infrared, radio, television, and power transmission. We depend on the sun's radiation for photosynthesis and heat.

Ionizing Radiation: Ionizing radiation includes high-energy radiation such as cosmic rays, X-rays, or gamma rays generated by nuclear decay. Ionizing radiation also includes several types of subatomic particles such as beta radiation (high-energy electrons) and alpha radiation (helium ions). Medical X-rays are an example of a common beneficial exposure to ionizing radiation. Nuclear radiation is used to generate electricity and cure disease, but it is also an important element in military weapons. Uses of nuclear radiation pose serious problems of human exposure and environmental contamination.

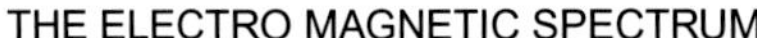

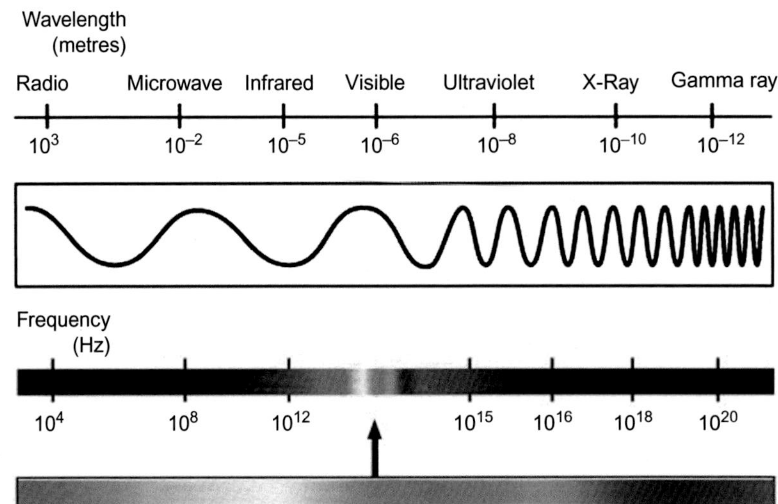

FIGURE 30.1

Electromagnetic spectrum.

Source: Shapley, P, 2012. Light and the Electromagnetic Spectrum. University of Illinois, IL. Available at: http://butane.chem.uiuc.edu/pshapley/GenChem2/A3/3.html.

30.2.1 NONIONIZING RADIATION

Uses: Power transmission, television, radio, and satellite transmissions, radar, light bulbs, heating, cooking, microwave ovens, lasers, photosynthesis (sunlight), mobile phones, and WiFi networks.

Source: Ultraviolet light, visible light, infrared radiation, microwaves, radio, television, mobile phones, and power transmission.

Recommended Daily Intake: Different depending on the source (ie, sunlight can damage skin).

Absorption: Depends on source.

Sensitive Individuals: Variable (eg, fair-skinned children sunburn more easily).

Biological effects Nonionizing radiation has no serious ill effects. The visible light from the sun, in-house light bulbs, radio and television transmissions, and electric appliances all contribute to our background exposure to nonionizing radiation. Most evidence indicates that this radiation is harmless, although some studies have found possible effects. However, at higher levels and longer durations of exposure, nonionizing radiation can be harmful. The classic example is sunlight or solar radiation. Ultraviolet radiation from the sun, part of the electromagnetic spectrum with wavelengths less than 400 nm, can damage the skin. Sunburn (erythema) is the result of excessive exposure of our skin to UV radiation when we lack the protection of UV-absorbing melanin. Acute cellular damage causes an inflammatory type of response and increases vascular circulation (vasodilation) close to the skin. The increased circulation causes redness and a hot feeling on the skin. Lightly pressing on the skin pushes the blood away and the spot appears white. People with darker skin have an ongoing production of melanin, which protects them to some extent from UV radiation. In people with lighter skin, UV radiation stimulates the production of melanin, producing a tan and protection against UV radiation. Extreme exposure can result in blistering and severe skin damage. UV radiation can also damage cellular DNA, and repeated damage can overwhelm the DNA repair mechanism, resulting in skin cancer. Skin cancer accounts for approximately one-third of all cancers diagnosed each year. Thinning of the atmospheric ozone layer, which filters UV radiation, is suspected of being one cause of the increased incidence of skin cancer.

30.2.2 IONIZING RADIATION

Description: Higher-energy radiation, with enough energy to remove an electron from an atom and damage biological material.

Uses: Nuclear power, medical X-rays, medical diagnostics, scientific research, cancer treatment, and cathode ray tube displays.

Source: Radon, X-rays, radioactive material producing alpha, beta, and gamma radiation, and cosmic rays from the sun and space.

Recommended Daily Intake: None (not essential).

Absorption: Interaction with tissue atoms.

Sensitive Individuals: Children and developing organisms.

Mechanism of action Ionizing radiation has sufficient energy to produce ion pairs as it passes through matter, freeing electrons and leaving the rest of the atoms positively charged. In other words, there is enough energy to remove an electron from an atom. The energy released is also enough to break bonds in DNA, which can lead to significant cellular damage and cancer. The health effects and dose/response relationship for radiation exposure are well established from human exposure to radiation and from other research. The four main types of ionizing radiation are:

1. alpha particles
2. beta particles (electrons)
3. gamma rays
4. X-rays

Alpha particles are heavyweight and relatively low-energy emissions from the nucleus of radioactive material. The transfer of energy occurs over a very short distance of approximately 10 cm in air. A piece of paper or layer of skin will stop an alpha particle. The primary hazard occurs in the case of internal exposure to an alpha-emitting material: cells close to the particle-emitting material will be damaged. Typical sites of accumulation include bone, kidney, liver, lung, and spleen. Radium is an alpha-particle emitter that accumulates in the bone following ingestion, causing bone sarcoma. Airplane travel increases our exposure to cosmic and solar radiation that is normally blocked by the atmosphere. Radiation intensity is greater across the poles and at higher altitudes; therefore, individual exposure varies depending on the route of travel. Storms on the sun can produce solar flares that release larger amounts of radiation than normal. For the occasional traveler, this radiation exposure is well below recommended limits established by regulatory authorities.

Biological effects Ionizing radiation is more harmful than nonionizing radiation because it has enough energy to remove an electron from an atom and thereby directly damage biological material. The energy is enough to damage DNA, which can result in cell death or cancer. The study of ionizing radiation is a large area of classical toxicology, which has produced a tremendous understanding of the dose/response relationship of exposure. The primary effect of ionizing radiation is cancer. It can also affect the developing fetus of mothers exposed during pregnancy. Radiation exposure has a direct dose/response relationship: the more radiation one receives, the greater is the chance of developing cancer.

Radon is a radioactive gas that is present in uranium mines and can also be found in high concentrations in soil in some places. Radon exposure results in lung and esophagus cancer. The actual carcinogens are daughter products of radon that adhere to the internal tissue and emit alpha particles.

Diagnosis Diagnosis may be made from a history of exposure to radiation or radioactive materials, clinical signs, and postmortem changes. Absolute lymphocyte count is considered the most useful screening measurement of total dose and prognosis. In humans, a lymphocyte count of 1000 cells/mL^3 at 24 h or 500 cells/mL^3 at 48 h indicates severe exposure to radiation.

Postmortem findings Lesions may be present on the specific organ or system depending on their exposure to the radiation. There may be gastroenteritis, ulceration, petechiae hemorrhages, hematomas, and degenerative lesions. All soft tissues, organs, and bones of the body show the presence of radioactive material.

Treatment and management There is no specific treatment. The treatment and management should be aimed at reducing the exposure by:

- Limiting the amount of time of exposure to the source of radiation. One of the easiest examples is to avoid getting sunburned by limiting the amount of time in bright sunlight. This same principle applies to ionizing radiation, such as emitted by radioactive material.
- Increasing the distance from the source of radiation. Emissions from the source of radiation decrease in intensity rapidly.
- Using shield. The effectiveness of shielding depends on the type of radiation and the shielding material itself, but placing absorbent shielding material between you and the radiation source reduces exposure. This can be as simple as wearing a hat to protect your face from the sun or using a lead apron in the dentist's chair to shield other parts of your body from the dental X-rays.

Supportive and symptomatic treatment Supportive and symptomatic treatment such as antibiotics, corticosteroids, and antihistamines should be administered. Transfusion of fresh bone marrow cells may be performed. Parathyroid extracts and low-calcium diets are recommended to increase the rate of excretion of radioactive material from the body.

UNIT

V

CHAPTER

Basic concepts of forensic toxicology 31

CHAPTER OUTLINE

31.1 INTRODUCTION

Forensic toxicology refers to the use of toxicology for the purposes of law. Therefore, it can be defined as the science that deals with medical and legal aspects of the harmful effects of the chemicals on the human body. It is considered a hybrid of analytical chemistry and fundamental toxicology. The efforts and activities are diverse, including detection of drugs in urine, regulatory toxicology, occupational disease, identification of agents causing death or injury in humans and animals, and courtroom testimony and consultation concerning toxicoses to provide support for diagnosis, identification of poison and management/treatment, and prognosis of poisoned individuals.

31.2 HISTORY AND BACKGROUND

The knowledge of poisons is perhaps as old as the history of humankind. Until the 1700s, convictions associated with homicidal poisoning were based only on circumstantial evidence rather than the identification of the actual toxicant within the victim. In 1781, Joseph Plenic stated methods for the detection and identification of the poison in the organs of the deceased. Several years later, in 1813, Mathieiv Orfila (considered the father of toxicology) published the first complete work on the subject of poisons and legal medicine. By 1836, James M. Marsh developed a test for the

Fundamentals of Toxicology. DOI: http://dx.doi.org/10.1016/B978-0-12-805426-0.00031-7

presence of arsenic in tissues. Subsequently, in 1839, Orfila successfully used Marsh's test to identify arsenic extracted from human tissues. Fifty years later, Ernst Wilhelm Heinrich Gutzeit developed a method (Gutzeit test) to quantitate arsenic in tissues. By 1918, the Medical Examiner's Office and Toxicology Laboratory was established in New York. The chief forensic toxicologist was Alexander O. Gettler, who headed the laboratory and is considered the father of American forensic toxicology. Since then, the science of forensic toxicology has expanded and several new techniques to identify chemicals in tissues have been developed.

The purpose of this chapter is to introduce some fundamental concepts of forensic toxicology. Analytical and clinical toxicology are discussed in subsequent chapters.

31.3 COURTROOM TESTIMONY

The reports provided by forensic toxicology personnel and expert consultants are ultimately produced as evidence in a court of law. These reporting individuals may be asked to interpret and substantiate their findings and any associated opinions. It is therefore necessary for the forensic toxicologist to be thoroughly knowledgeable or familiar with legal practices and to be professionally comfortable in a courtroom environment.

31.4 INVESTIGATION

There are basic phases when conducting an investigation of a suspected toxicant-induced/related death. When conducting an investigation, there are primary questions that must be answered. These include:

1. What was the route of administration?
2. What was the administered dose?
3. Is the concentration enough to have caused death or injury or to have altered the victim's behavior enough to cause death or injury?

31.4.1 COLLECTION OF INFORMATION

As much information as possible concerning the facts of the case must be collected. Due to the limited material available for analysis, it is essential to obtain as much historical information as possible. In addition to any witness accounts of events, one must accurately record information such as the age, sex, and weight of the victim, medical history, identification of any medications or other drugs/substances used before death, and the time interval that elapsed between the intake of these substances and death.

31.4.2 COLLECTION OF SPECIMENS

When collecting the specimens, many different body fluids and organs should be collected because xenobiotics have different affinities for body tissues; therefore, multiple extractions (for specific analyses) may be needed. Specimens should be collected before embalming because embalming may destroy or dilute the xenobiotic. It is possible to obtain useful specimens from burned or burial remains (such as bone marrow, skeletal muscle, vitreous humor, hair, and maggots). For example, using hair samples, it is possible to detect the presence of antibiotics, antipsychotics, and drugs of abuse. However, the information is primarily qualitative in nature. Using maggots, barbiturates, benzodiazepines, phenothiazines, morphine, and malathion can be detected.

It is often necessary to add preservatives to specimens to protect against postmortem changes. For example, the addition of sodium fluoride to a tissue specimen can prevent the production of bacterial growth, whereas use of ethanol can yield a false-positive result for the presence of ingested ethanol.

31.4.3 TOXICOLOGICAL ANALYSIS

The decision concerning which analytical methods are to be used depends greatly on a number of factors. One can imagine that a given method may need more sample volume or weight than another method. Therefore, the amount of specimen available is a critical determinant of methods to be selected for proper toxicological analysis. It is necessary to know the nature of the toxicant to be tested. In a particular case, is it relevant to detect the parent compound, its metabolites, or all of these? Furthermore, toxicant biotransformation must be taken into account when performing the analyses and making interpretations. A low concentration of a toxic parent compound may reflect biotransformation as opposed to a low level of exposure. Conversely, a low-level presence of a nontoxic parent compound may be associated with a sufficient concentration of a biotransformation product that was high enough to cause the insult. Furthermore, both forms (parent and metabolites) may have contributed to the diverse outcome. For details of analytical toxicology, the reader is referred to subsequent chapters dealing with analytical toxicology.

31.4.4 DOCUMENTATION AND DATA INTERPRETATION

The record of documents including labeling and the name of the victim (if known) must be recorded, along with the name of the medical examiner. The condition of the body and the time and date of death should be recorded. Additionally, the date of the toxicological analyses request should also be stated on the report. Each collected specimen should be identified, as should the tests that are to be performed. In the results section, it is necessary for the analyst of each test to sign the form identifying the actual results for the tissue tested and the date when the results were obtained.

CHAPTER

Applications in toxicology 32

CHAPTER OUTLINE

32.1 INTRODUCTION

Until the 19th century, doctors and scientists believed that if a dead body was black, blue, or spotted in places, or if it "smelled bad," then the cause of death was a poison. This is because the first Dutch physician Hermann Boerhoave pointed out that various poisons in hot vaporous conditions yield typical odors. He placed substances suspected of being poisons on hot coals and tested their smells. In 1936, Marsh developed the test for arsenic poisoning in body tissues. Now, several analytical techniques are available for all kinds of poisons.

32.2 OBJECTIVES OF ANALYTICAL TOXICOLOGY

Analytical toxicology is aimed at providing support for the following:

1. Diagnosis (D)
2. Identification of poisons (I)
3. Management and treatment of poisoning (M)
4. Prognosis (P)
5. Law enforcement (L)
6. Education and research (E)

These six indications can be remembered by using the mnemonic DIMPLE. The toxicology laboratory has the following important functions:

1. *Prognosis*: to assess the outcome of a case of poisoning
2. *Research*: to study toxicokinetics and mechanism of action

Fundamentals of Toxicology. DOI: http://dx.doi.org/10.1016/B978-0-12-805426-0.00032-9

3. *Order*: to follow the order from the court of law/law enforcement office
4. *Monitoring*: to monitor the treatment and its efficacy
5. *Identification*: of the nature of poison
6. *Severity*: to assess the seriousness of the case
7. *Exclusion*: confirmation of toxic response

These seven indications can be remembered by using the mnemonic PROMISE.

In developed countries, analytical services are provided by a specialized laboratory attached to a clinical toxicology unit with a well established biochemistry laboratory, an analytical pharmacy unit, and a university department of forensic medicine. In many developing countries, such services are not available on a regular basis; where they are available, the physician is generally dependent on a national or regional health laboratory established for other purposes that operates only part of the time. In these countries, the government forensic science laboratory mostly caters to the needs of the required services, and there are very few laboratories in the private sector. Most government laboratories use very simple analytical techniques that do not require any sophisticated equipment, expensive reagents, or even a continuous supply of electricity.

32.3 ANALYTICAL SCHEMES FOR TOXICANT DETECTION

The circumstances surrounding the case will usually determine the types of analytical toxicological tests that are required. There are different screens specific for the type of substance to be assayed. A given laboratory will follow an algorithm to perform the analysis. The list of drugs included in most toxicological screens is summarized in Table 32.1. The volatile screen is frequently used for the detection of ethanol. A drugs of abuse screen is commonly used for amphetamines, cocaine, marijuana, and others. When the cause of death is unclear, a general drug screen is used. An acidic/neutral screen is primarily used to detect barbiturates, muscle relaxants, and others. Basic drug screens are more specific for the detection of drugs such as cocaine and antidepressants. It is recommended that the presence of a drug or toxicant should be verified in more than one specimen. However, if only one specimen is available, then replicate analyses on different occasions should be performed with adequate concurrent positive and negative controls.

32.4 LABORATORY ANALYSES

The nonspecific initial tests in a series are valuable for determining the presence or absence of a particular class of compounds. The steps to be undertaken in an analytical procedure are given in Table 32.2. For example, colorimetric tests to detect the presence of phenothiazines provide initial information about a drug

Table 32.1 Common Drugs Included on Most Toxicology Screens

Alcohol	Ethanol, methanol, isopropanol, acetone
Barbiturates/ sedatives	Amobarbital, secobarbital, pentobarbital, butalbital, butabarbital, phenobarbital, glutethimide, ethchlorvynol, methaqualone
Antiepileptics	Phenytoin, carbamazepine, primadone, phenobarbital
Benzodiazepines	Chlordiazepoxide, diazepam, alprazolam, temazepam
Antihistamines	Diphenhydramine, chlorpheniramine, brompheniramine, tripelennamine, trihexiphenidyl, doxylamine, pyrilamine
Antidepressants	Amitriptyline, nortriptyline, doxepin, imipramine, desipramine, trazedone, amoxapine, maprotiline
Antipsychotics	Trifluoperazine, perphenazine, prochlorperazine, chlorpromazine
Stimulants	Amphetamine, methamphetamine, phenylpropanolamine, ephedrine, MDA, MDMA (other phenylethylamines), cocaine, phencyclicline
Narcotic analgesics	Heroin, morphine, codeine, oxycodone, hydrocodone, hydromorphone, meperidine, pentazocine, propoxyphene, methadone
Other analgesics	Salicylates, acetaminophen
Cardiovascular drugs	Lidocaine, propranolol, metoprolol, quinidine, procainamide, verapamil
Others	Theophylline, caffeine, nicotine, oral hypoglycemics, strychnine

Table 32.2 Steps to be Followed in an Analytical Toxicological Investigation

Phases and Steps
Step 1
Based on circumstantial evidence: biochemical and blood investigation
Step 2
Based on medical history: decide priorities for the analysis
Step 3
Analytical phase
Step 4
Interpretation of the results
Step 5
Perform additional analysis of the original samples/of further samples from the patient, if necessary

class present. This is followed by more specific tests to identify the actual compound as well as to provide quantitative data. Another example of a type of initial test would be an immunoassay that determines the presence of barbiturates. Confirmatory tests are mandatory to identify the particular drug within the class detected. The analytical aspects of toxicology testing and the procedures used are discussed in the chapter dealing with analytical toxicology.

32.4.1 GENERAL PRECAUTIONS

- Strong acids or alkalis should always be added to water and not vice versa
- Strong acids and alkalis should never be preserved together
- Organic solvents should not be heated over a naked flame, but rather in a water bath
- Use fume cupboards/hoods when organic solvents are heated

32.5 WET CHEMISTRY

Traditional wet chemistry refers to the wet chemical methods of analysis. This comprises painstaking testing and retesting of unknown materials using different reagents until the composite behavior patterns provide a clue to the identity of the material/poison. Wet chemistry also refers to the analytical techniques in which various chemical reagents, such as acids, bases, and salts, are applied to a sample and identified on the basis of its reactions with the reagents. These tests are of two types: qualitative analytical tests and quantitative analytical methods.

32.5.1 QUALITATIVE ANALYTICAL TESTS

Toxicology laboratories use several methods to screen for poisons/drugs because there is no single, accurate, inexpensive method for this purpose. Each method differs in cost, accuracy, complexity, speed, and specificity. Certain color tests (bedside tests) are used in routine practice and cover a number of important drugs and other poisons for detection. Table 32.3 summarizes 13 qualitative analytical tests commonly performed. These are performed to detect poisonous substances in the blood, urine, feces, saliva, cerebrospinal fluid, gastric lavage, vomit, and available residue.

32.5.1.1 Thin-layer chromatography

Thin-layer chromatography (TLC) is also a qualitative technique that involves the movement via capillary action of a liquid phase (usually an organic solvent) through a thin, uniform layer of a stationary phase (usually silica gel) held on a rigid support (usually a glass, aluminum, or plastic sheet). Compounds are separated by a partition between the mobile and stationary phases. A TLC tank is filled with a suitable developing solvent to a depth of approximately 1 cm from the bottom. The properly spotted plate is then dipped into the solvent, the lid is firmly closed, and the atmosphere is allowed to saturate with vapor. When the solvent front just touches the horizontal mark at 10 cm, quickly remove the plate and spray with appropriate reagents to bring out the characteristic color spot. The characteristic fluorescence or absorbance is examined under UV light. the

Table 32.3 Recommended Qualitative Color Tests (Bedside Tests)

1. Trinder's test (salicylic acid, including acetyl salicylic acid (aspirin), salicylamide, or methyl salicylic acid): Add 100 mL of Trinder's reagent, which is a mixture of 40 g of mercuric chloride in 850 mL of water and 120 mL of aqueous hydrochloric acid (1 mol) and 40 g of hydrated ferric nitrate diluted to 1 L with warm water, to 2 mL of urine and mix for 5 s. A violet color indicates the presence of salicylate. If only stomach contents or scene residues are available, then first hydrolyze the same by heating with 0.5 mol/L hydrochloric acid on a boiling water bath for 2 min and neutralize with 0.5 mol/L sodium hydroxide before performing the test. If a positive result is obtained, then perform a qualitative assay on plasma/serum.
2. Ferric chloride test: Add 1 mL of 5% ferric chloride solution to 2 mL urine. A persistent purple color indicates the presence of phenol, phenothiazine, phenylbutazone, oxyphenobutazone, or salicylates.
3. FPN test (phenothiazines): Add 1 mL of FPN reagent, which is a mixture of 5 mL of aqueous ferric chloride solution (50 g/L), 45 mL of aqueous perchloric acid (200 g/kg), and 50 mL of aqueous nitric acid (500 mL/L), to 1 mL of urine or stomach contents and mix for 5 s. Colors ranging from pink to red, orange, violet, or blue suggest the presence of phenothiazines (tricyclics give a green or blue color). Thin-layer chromatography (TLC) should confirm positive results.
4. Forrest test (imipramine and related compounds): Add 1 mL Forrest reagent, which is a mixture of 25 mL of aqueous potassium dichlorate (2 g/L), 25 mL of aqueous sulfuric acid (300 mL/L), 25 mL of aqueous perchloric acid (200 g/kg), and 25 mL of aqueous nitric acid (500 mL/L), to 0.5 mL of sample and mix for 5 s. A yellow–green color deepening to dark green to blue indicates the presence of imipramine or related compounds. TLC should confirm positive results.
5. Fujuwara test (trichloro compounds, including chloral hydrate, chloroform, dichloral phenazone, and trichloroethylene): Use three 10-mL tubes. Label those three 10-mL tubes as A, B, and C. Add, respectively, 1 mL of the sample, purified water (blank test essential), and aqueous trichloroacetic acid (10 mg/L). Add 1 mL of sodium hydroxide solution (5 mol) and 1 mL of pyridine to each test tube. Mix carefully and heat in a boiling water bath for 2 min. An intense red/purple color at the top (pyridine) layer of tube A as in tube C indicates the presence of trichloro compounds. Tube B (blank test) should show no coloration.
6. O-cresol/ammonia test (paracetamol, phenacetin): Add 0.5 mL of concentrated hydrochloric acid to 0.5 mL of the sample, heat in a boiling water bath for 10 min, and cool. Add 1 mL of the aqueous O-cresol solution (10 g/L) to 0.2 mL of hydrolysate; add 2 mL of ammonium hydroxide solution (4 mol/L) and mix for 5 s. A strong blue to blue–black color, which forms immediately, indicates the presence of paracetamol or phenacetin. If a positive test result is obtained, then a quantitative assay may be performed.
7. Dithionite test (paraquat, diquat): Add 0.5 mL of aqueous ammonium (hydroxide 2 mol/L) to 1 mL of test solution, mix for 5 s, and add approximately 20 mg of solid sodium dithionite. A strong blue to blue–black color indicates paraquat; diquat gives a yellow–green color, but this is insignificant in the presence of paraquat. If the color fades on continued agitation in the air and is restored by adding further sodium dithionite, then paraquat or diquat is confirmed.

(Continued)

Table 32.3 Recommended Qualitative Color Tests (Bedside Tests) *Continued*

8. Dichromate test (ethanol and other volatile reducing agents): Apply 50 mL of potassium dichromate (25 g/L in aqueous sulfuric acid 500 mL/L) to a strip of glass fiber filter paper in the neck of test tube containing 1 mL urine. Lightly place the stopper on the tube and place in a boiling water bath for 3 min. A change in color from orange to green indicates the presence of a volatile substance. If positive, then perform a quantitative assay.
9. Diphenylamine test[a] (chlorates and other oxidizing agents): Carefully add 0.5 mL of diphenylamine (10 g/L in concentrated sulfuric acid) to 0.5 mL of filtered stomach contents or scene residue. A strong blue color, which develops rapidly, indicates the presence of oxidizing agents.
10. Ferricyanide/ferrocyanide test[a] (ferrous and ferric iron): To 50 mL of filtered stomach contents or scene residue, add 100 mL of aqueous hydrochloric acid (2 mol/L) and 50 mL of aqueous potassium ferricyanide solution (10 g/L). A deep blue precipitate with potassium ferricyanide or ferrocyanide indicates the presence of ferrous or ferric iron. If a positive result is obtained, then perform a quantitative assay for iron.
11. Meixner test (poisonous mushroom): This test is performed with a stool sample. To a stool sample, add methanol, centrifuge it, and filter it. Place one or two drops of this on a piece of filter paper and then add a few drops of hydrochloric acid. A bluish coloration indicates the presence of amatoxins, which are present in most poisonous mushrooms.
12. Reinsch test (arsenic, antimony, bismuth, and mercury): Applicable to urine, stomach contents, and scene residues. Take a copper foil mesh (5 × 10) or wire (2–3 cm) and clean it in nitric acid until the copper acquires a bright surface. Rinse the same with purified water. Add 10 mL of concentrated hydrochloric acid and 20 mL of the test solution in a 100-mL conical flask along with a strip of copper. Heat on a boiling water bath in a fume cupboard for 1 h. Maintain the volume of the solution by adding dilute hydrochloric acid as necessary. Color staining on the copper can be interpreted as follows:
    - Purple black: antimony
    - Dull black: bismuth
    - Shiny black: bismuth
    - Silvery: mercury
13. Marquis reagent test (morphine and other opium): Applicable to scene residue (fragments of suspected residue) and stomach contents. Place a drop of Marquis reagent (prepared by adding 3 mL of concentrated sulfuric acid and 3 drops of formalin) on the suspected scene residue or add a few drops to the stomach contents. A purple coloration that gradually turns to violet and finally to blue indicates the presence of opium and its derivatives.

[a]*Tests for stomach contents or residues only.*

Rf value is calculated (the distance traveled by the compound divided by the distance traveled by the solvent). This value and the color reactions are used as qualitative results.

$$\text{Rf is the ratio} = \frac{\text{Solute front}}{\text{Solvent front}} \times 100$$

Approximate quantitation can be performed to compare standards of materials similarly prepared on the same plate, and then the Rf value is calculated.

32.5.2 QUANTITATIVE ANALYTICAL METHODS

This comprises methods wherein the tests are performed not only to exactly identify the poison but also to estimate the concentration of the poison in the body of the poisoned victim; for example, a quantitative analysis is performed using whole blood or plasma to confirm the poisoning. However, these tests may not be possible in laboratories where facilities are limited. Some of the quantitative analytical assays are described here. The following tests are performed by using some simple instruments and sophisticated equipment such as:

- Chromatography
- Ultraviolet spectrophotometry
- Mass spectrometry
- Enzymatic immunoassay

32.5.2.1 Colorimetric screening tests

These tests require little sample preparation and are usually performed directly on the specimen. This is a rapid procedure, but it requires confirmation.

32.5.2.2 Thermal desorption

In addition to the analysis of arson crime scene evidence, thermal desorption has been used for the analysis of residual volatile agents in street drugs and for the analysis of stains on forensic evidence. Samples are heated to volatilize water and organic compounds. The organic analytes may then be separated by gas chromatography (GC).

32.5.2.3 Thin-layer chromatography

As explained, this is a qualitative test, but to some extent the quantities can be estimated by eluting the spots with appropriate solvents. Estimation is performed using UV spectrophotometry.

32.5.2.4 Gas chromatography

The basic principle of GC involves vaporization of the sample and injection into the head space of the chromatographic column. The sample is transported through the column by the flow of an inert gas (mobile phase). The column itself contains a liquid stationary phase that is adsorbed onto the surface of an inert solid. Retention time with the detection technique (spectrophotometer, mass spectrometry, fluorescence) identifies the compound.

32.5.2.5 High-performance liquid chromatography

The mobile phase is a solvent that is pumped at high pressure through a packed column. As described for GC, retention time with various detection techniques identifies the compound.

32.5.2.6 Enzymatic immunoassay

An enzyme-linked drug derivative is added to the specimen to be tested. This competes with the drug in question for the antibody. The more of the drug that binds to the antibody, the less that is bound to the enzyme-linked drug. Enzyme activity is proportional to the amount of the drug that was already in the specimen.

Detailed procedures and the use of other test procedures are beyond the scope of this book.

CHAPTER

Clinical toxicology

33

CHAPTER OUTLINE

33.1 INTRODUCTION

Analytical toxicology approaches play important roles in the clinical setting. The methods and instrumentation used in a clinical toxicology laboratory are similar to those used in forensic toxicology laboratories. The approaches discussed previously have the following benefits in clinical toxicology:

1. Aid the diagnosis and treatment of toxicoses
2. Allow the monitoring of treatment effectiveness
3. Identification of the nature of exposure
4. Quantification of toxicant

33.2 HISTORICAL BACKGROUND

The first documentation of use of a specific antidote may be found in Homer's *Odyssey* (600 BC), in which it is suggested to Ulysses that he should use moli to protect himself from poisoning. Moli may actually be *Galanthus nivalis*, a plant-derived

Fundamentals of Toxicology. DOI: http://dx.doi.org/10.1016/B978-0-12-805426-0.00033-0

cholinesterase inhibitor that might counteract the effects of the anticholinergic plant *Datura stramonium.* Galen (AD 129–200) wrote three books that described the development of a universal antidote. The use of these ancient antidotes included treatment of acute poisoning and prophylactic treatment to make one "poison-proof." One of the earliest writings on the prevention of the gastrointestinal absorption of poisons was by Nicander. In this ancient writing, the induction of emesis by ingestion of an emetic agent or mechanical stimulation of the hypopharynx was described as a method to prevent poison absorption. Subsequently, in the 1600s, the use of ipecacuanha for induction of emesis was recommended by William Piso. The use of oral charcoal, now a mainstay in the treatment of human poisoning, can be dated to early Greek and Roman civilizations when wood charcoal was used for the treatment of maladies such as anthrax and epilepsy. By the 1960s, the use of activated charcoal was routinely recommended for the treatment of patients poisoned with substances thought to be adsorbed by charcoal.

33.3 INTRODUCTION OF THE POISON CONTROL CENTER

Because of the growing concern over the burgeoning incidence of poisoning worldwide, coupled with a lack of public awareness about its seriousness, Poison Information Services made their first appearance in the Netherlands in 1949, in England in 1961, and in the United States in 1963. Since then, all around the world, similar centers have emerged that perform the invaluable functions of generating public awareness of poisoning and impart much needed toxicological diagnostic and therapeutic assistance to doctors. Today, there are approximately 80 such certified centers in the United States alone, providing almost any information within a matter of seconds through the use of an intricate, computerized information resource system (POISINDEX) regarding more than 800,000 poisonous products.

In other countries such as Ireland, Spain, India, and the Netherlands, the poison centers are integrated with diagnostic laboratories, unlike those in the United States, which function independently. In England, France, and Germany, the centers work in conjunction with acute poisoning treatment units as well as diagnostic laboratories. Some other countries also have poison centers, but many developing countries are still making efforts to establish them.

Poison centers provide immediate, around-the-clock toxicity assessments and treatment recommendations over the telephone for all kinds of poisoning situations affecting people of all ages, including: ingestion of household products; overdose of therapeutic medications or illegal, foreign, or veterinary drugs; chemical exposures on the job or elsewhere; hazardous material spills; bites from snakes, spiders, and other venomous creatures; and plant and mushroom poisoning. Nearly 75% of poisoning incidents reported to poison centers are managed entirely by telephone consultations without further necessity of additional costs for the health care system.

33.4 ACUTE POISONING DEATHS

Acute poisoning may be intentional, accidental, or occupational. Although there are no reliable estimates of how many people suffer every year from acute chemical poisoning (drugs, pesticides, and other chemicals), it is clear that pesticide poisoning accounts for significant morbidity and mortality worldwide, particularly in developing countries Since 1992, organophosphorus, carbamate, and aluminum phosphide (fumigant, redenticide) pesticides have become the most common agents used in suicide poisoning in developing countries (65–70% of the total poisoning incidents), but estimates of the total number of events show a high degree of variability depending on the author and time reported. This varies from country to country depending on the kind of poisons encountered, the extent of awareness about poisoning, the availability of treatment facilities, and the presence of qualified personnel. In developed countries the rate of mortality from poisoning may be as low as 1%; however, it may vary from a shocking 15–35%.

Children younger than age 15 years account for most cases of accidental poisoning; fortunately, these are associated with relatively low mortality. In developing countries, most suicidal exposures are seen in individuals older than age 15 years, but these are associated with high mortality.

33.5 CAUSES OF POISONING

Poisoning is most commonly caused by ingestion but can result from injection, inhalation, or the exposure of body surfaces (eg, skin, eye, mucous membrane). Most commonly ingested food substances are generally nontoxic; however, any substance can be toxic if ingested in excessive amounts.

Accidental poisoning is common among young children who are curious and ingest items indiscriminately despite the noxious taste and odor. Usually, only a single substance is involved. Poisoning is also common among adolescents and adults attempting suicide, and among those who consume multiple drugs, including alcohol, acetaminophen, and other over-the-counter drugs. Accidental deaths may occur in the elderly because of confusion, poor eyesight, mental impairment, or multiple prescriptions of the same drug by different physicians.

Occasionally, people are poisoned by someone who intends to kill or disable them (eg, for the purpose of rape). Drugs used to disable (eg, scopolamine, benzodiazepines) tend to have sedative or anesthetic properties, or both.

Most poisons are metabolized, pass through the gastrointestinal (GI) tract, or are excreted. Occasionally, some of them remain for a longer time and continue to be absorbed, thus leading to toxicity.

33.6 PRINCIPLES OF DIAGNOSIS

Most poisoning incidents are dose-related; poisoning or toxicity may vary from exposure to excess amounts of normally nontoxic substances. Some poisoning incidents occur from exposure to substances that are poisonous at all doses. Poisoning should be distinguished from hypersensitivity and idiosyncratic reactions, which are undesirable and not dose-related, and distinguished from intolerance, which is a toxic reaction to an unusually nontoxic dose of a substance.

Diagnosis is the evaluation of signs and symptoms of a disease or dysfunction to arrive at a cause. Diagnosis of poisoning is a difficult task and cannot be based on a single observation. Diagnosis often rests on appropriate findings and should take into account several points. The majority of poisoned patients presenting to the casualty (emergency) department are victims of acute exposure. Most of them are usually coherent enough to tell the doctor what the problem is and what they have taken or have been exposed to; however, in an unconscious or uncooperative patient, the diagnosis will have to be made on the basis of circumstantial or third-party evidence. Generally, clinical examination gives some valuable clues that can help to narrow the differential diagnosis. A seasoned clinician usually takes into account the following points to arrive at any conclusion.

33.6.1 CLINICAL HISTORY

Performing a thorough general history of the patient aids in the effective treatment of intoxication. Often, it may not be possible to communicate directly with the patient. Sometimes this is due to a lack of consciousness or altered mental state leading to inaccurate information, or deliberate submission of misleading information, which may lead to complications in diagnosis. Generally, the type of information that is essential and helpful include:

1. Identification of what was taken and when, how much, and by what route
2. Presence of preexisting conditions or allergies
3. Whether the patient is currently using any medications or substances of any kind
4. Whether the patient is pregnant

Historical information can include information obtained from family, friends, law enforcement, medical personnel, and any observers.

33.6.2 PHYSICAL EXAMINATION

A thorough examination of the patient is required to assess the patient's condition. If the patient's mental status is altered, then determine possible additional explanations for the abnormal mental status, such as trauma or central nervous

Table 33.1 Characteristic Odors Associated With Poisoning

Odor	Potential Poison
Bitter	Almonds, cyanide
Rotten eggs	Hydrogen sulfide, mercaptans
Garlic	Organophosphates DMSO, thallium
Mothballs	Naphthalene, camphor
Vinyl	Ethchlorvynol
Winter green	Methylsalicylate
Phenolic	Phenol and phenolic disinfectants
Stale tobacco	Nicotine
Shoe polish	Nitrobenzene
Sweet	Chloroform and other halogenated hydrocarbons

system infection. One very helpful tool for the clinical toxicologist is to categorize the patient in broad classes such as narcotic, cholinergic, sympathomimetic, and anticholinergic. Categorization of the patient's presentation into toxic syndromes allows for the initiation of rationale treatment based on the most likely category of toxin responsible. For example, if a patient presents in a coma and with miosis (pinpoint pupils), hypotension, bradycardia, markedly reduced respiratory rate, and slight hypothermia with an otherwise nonlocalizing neurological examination, then the clinical toxicologist can characterize the patient's presentation as consistent with narcotic toxic syndrome. The presence of needle tracks on the skin would support this categorization. The treatment would then be directed at support of respiration and pharmacological reversal with a mu-receptor opioid antagonist such as naloxone. In this example, life-saving treatment can be administered in a timely manner, even in the absence of definitive identification of the ingested poison. Critical examination of other clinical signs may help determine the proper diagnosis.

1. *Odor*: Occasionally, a characteristic odor can be detected on the poisoned patient's breath or clothing that may point toward exposure or poisoning by a specific agent. Table 33.1 lists some of the better recognized odors and the substance associated with the odor. Several toxins have a characteristic odor and may help detect the poison consumed. However, the odor may be subtle and the ability to smell the odor may vary (eg, only approximately 50% of the population can smell the "bitter almond" odor of cyanide).
2. *Record of vital organs*: This includes recording of pulse, respiratory rate, blood pressure, body temperature, and papillary manifestations. For example, several drugs/poisons affect the pupil of the eye, producing either miosis or mydriasis; a few produce nystsagmus (Table 33.2).
3. *Color of urine*: Observation of the urine passed may also give some clue about the type of poison ingested by the patient (Table 33.3).

Table 33.2 Examples of Some Poisonous Drugs Showing Pupillary Manifestations

Miosis (Papillary Constriction)	Mydriasis (Papillary Dilatation)	Nystagmus
Barbiturates	Alcohol (constricted in coma)	Alcohol
Caffeine	Amphetamines	Barbiturates
Carbamate	Antihistamines	Carbamazepine
Carbolic acid (phenol)	Carbon monoxide	Phencyclidine
Clonidine	Cocaine	Phenytoin
Methyl dopa	Cyanide	
Nicotine	Datura	
Opiates	Ephedrine	
Organophosphates		
Parasympathomimetics		

Table 33.3 Color of Urine Versus Toxins

Urine Color	Toxin/Substance
Green or blue	Methylene blue
Gray–black	Phenols or cresols
Opaque appearance that settles on standing	Primidone cresols
Orange or orange–red	Rifampicin, iron (especially after administering desferrioxamine)

Skin Marks: Some poisons have characteristic dermal manifestations in acute toxicity, whereas others demonstrate skin signs on chronic exposure such as irritant dermatitis or dermal lesions/allergy, as seen in some drug poisoning incidents. In some cases, examination of mouth can give some clue about the type of poison.

33.6.3 ANALYTICAL EVIDENCE

The common proof of poisoning lies in the detection of a significant amount of toxic material in the body tissues. Confirmation of poisons responsible for the poisoning will help in the proper management and treatment of the patient. For further details, the reader is referred to previous chapters in this book.

33.7 GENERAL MANAGEMENT OF POISONING

The following concepts are central to approaching a toxicosis patient:

1. Ensure airway is clear so that breathing and circulation are adequate
2. Remove unabsorbed material
3. Limit the further absorption of toxicant
4. Hasten toxicant elimination

The initial survey should always be directed at the assessment of and correction of the life-threatening problems, if present; attention must be given to the airways, breathing, circulation, and disability (ABCD).

33.7.1 INITIAL STABILIZATION

Treatment of any systemic poisoning begins with airways, breathing, and circulatory stabilization. If patients have apnea or compromised airways (eg, foreign material in the oropharynx, decreased gag reflex), then an endotracheal tube should be inserted. If patients have respiratory depression or hypoxia, then supplemental O_2 or mechanical ventilation should be provided as needed.

In patients with apnea, intravenous (IV) naloxone (2 mg in adults; 0.1 mg/kg in children) should be tried while airways support is maintained in opioid addicts; naloxone may precipitate withdrawal, but withdrawal is preferable to apnea. If respiratory depression persists despite the use of naloxone, then endotracheal intubation and continuous mechanical ventilation are required. If naloxone relieves respiratory depression, then patients are monitored. If respiratory depression reoccurs, then patients can be treated with another bolus of IV naloxone or mechanical ventilation. Using continuous naloxone infusion to maintain the respiratory drive is controversial.

If patients have altered consciousness, then plasma glucose or IV dextrose (50 mL of a 50% solution for adults; 2–4 mL/kg of a 25% solution for children) should be given. For adults with suspected thiamin deficiency (eg, alcoholics, malnourished patients), thiamin 100 mg IV is given with or before glucose.

Hypotension is treated with IV fluids. If fluids are ineffective, then invasive hemodynamic monitoring may be necessary to guide fluid and vasopressor therapy. The first-choice vasopressor for most poison-induced hypotension is norepinephrine 0.5–1 ug/min IV infusion, but treatment should not be delayed if another vasopressor is more immediately available.

33.7.2 SPECIFIC MEASURES

Specific measures are in relation to removal of the poison from the body. They depends on whether the poison is ingested, inhaled, injected, or a contact poison. The methods of removal of poisons from the body are summarized in Table 33.4.

Table 33.4 Methods of Removal of Poisons From the Body

Poisoning	Suggested Methods of Removal
Ingested	Gut decontamination
Inhaled	Provide fresh air, artificial respiration
Injected	Give first aid, followed by specific antidote, diuretics, dialysis, etc.
Contact	Wash with water, neutralize with antidotes etc.

Toxicologists recommend the following principal lines of treatment: decontamination, emesis, and a symptom-based line of treatment. Each of these is discussed in detail.

33.7.3 DECONTAMINATION

The majority of patients who present after an overdose require only meticulous supportive care. It is important for patients to be observed closely for signs of deterioration. Overall, the mortality from acute poisoning is less than 1%. It occurs in patients who have taken significant overdoses and in whom further measures such as decontamination may be required.

Decontamination refers to skin/eye decontamination, gut evacuation, and administration of activated charcoal. However, removal of poison from the GT tract demands maximum attention in managing an overdose. This comprises various gut decontamination procedures such as gastric lavage, emesis, administration of activated charcoal, catharsis, and whole-bowel irrigation. These procedures should only be used in patients who, left untreated, would risk serious poisoning, because they can be associated with complications.

Activated Charcoal: Charcoal is usually administered, particularly when multiple or unknown substances have been ingested. Use of charcoal adds little risk unless patients are at risk for vomiting and aspiration; however, its use may not substantially reduce overall morbidity or mortality. When used, charcoal is administered as soon as possible. Activated charcoal adsorbs most toxins because of its molecular configuration and large surface area. Multiple doses of activated charcoal may be effective for substances that undergo enterohepatic recirculation (eg, phenobarbital, theophylline) and for sustained-release preparations. Charcoal may be administered at 4- to 6-h intervals for serious poisoning with such substances unless bowel sounds are hypoactive. Charcoal is ineffective for caustics, alcohols, and simple ions (eg, cyanide, iron, other metals, lithium). The recommended dose is 5- to 100-times that of the suspected toxin ingested. The amount of toxin ingested usually is unknown; therefore, the usual dose should be 1–2 g/kg, which is almost 10–25 g for children younger than age 5 years and 50–100 g for older children and adults. Charcoal is administered as a slurry in water or soft drinks. It may be unpalatable and results in vomiting in 30% of patients; administration via a gastric tube should be considered. Activated charcoal should probably be used without sorbitol or other cathartics, which have no clear benefit and can cause dehydration and electrolyte abnormalities.

Gastric Emptying: Catharsis is known to reduce the transit time of drugs in the GT tract. Two types of cathartics are routinely tried in poisoning victims to induce catharsis: ionic/saline cathartics and saccharide cathartics.

Ionic/Saline Cathartics: These cathartics alter the physicochemical forces within the intestinal luman, leading to osmotic retention of fluid, which activates mortality reflexes and enhances expulsion. However, excessive doses of magnesium-based cathartics can result in hypermagnesemia, which is a serious complication. The doses of ionic/saline cathartics are as follows: magnesium citrate 4 mg/kg; magnesium sulfate 30 g (250 mg/kg in children); or sodium sulfate 30 g (250 mg/kg in children).

Saccharides Cathartics: This comprises administering sorbitol (D-glucitol), which is the cathartic of choice for adults because of its better efficacy than saline cathartics. However, this is not indicated in small children because it can result in fluid and electrolyte imbalance (hypernatremia). The recommended dose for catharsis by sorbitol for an adult is 50 mL of a 70% solution.

Whole-Bowel Irrigation: This procedure is used to flush the GI tract for pills and tablets. Irrigation is indicated for some serious poisoning incidents due to sustained-release preparations or substances that are not adsorbed by charcoal such as heavy metals or drug packets (latex-coated packets of heroin cocaine ingested by body packers). A commercially prepared solution of polypropylene glycol (which is nonabsorbable) and electrolytes is given at a rate of 1–2 L/h for adults or at 25–40 mL/kg/h for children until the rectal effluent is clear. This process may require many hours or even days. The solution is usually given via a gastric tube, although some motivated patients can drink these large volumes.

Elimination of Toxins: In a limited number of poisoning incidents, it may be necessary to consider the use of one of the following methods available to increase elimination of poisons:

1. Urinary alkalization
2. Multiple doses of activated charcoal
3. Extracorporeal techniques
4. Diaphoresis

Urinary Alkalization: This is also known as alkaline dieresis. It is used for chlorpropamide, mecoprop, phenoxyacetate herbicides, and salicylates, including aspirin.

Prior to the procedure, check the patient's plasma potassium concentration and renal function tests. Give IV bicarbonate 1 L of 1.26% (for an adult) over the course of 3 h. Check plasma potassium because it is very difficult to produce alkaline urine if the patient is hypokalemic. Once adequate levels of urinary alkalization commences, potassium will decrease precipitously. It is wise to add 20–40 mmol potassium to each liter of IV fluid given.

However, never force dieresis because pulmonary edema will ensue. Also, never give acetazolamide diuretic to induce alkaline urine because it produces a systemic acidosis that enhances the toxicity of certain drugs, such as salicylates.

Multiple-Dose Activated Charcoal: Clinical studies have shown that multiple-dose activated charcoal increases the elimination of certain drugs. The dose given is 50 g (1 g/kg in children) of activated charcoal every 4 h. Indications for multiple-dose activated charcoal include life-threatening overdose of carbanazepine, dapsone, phenobarbitone, quinidine, or theophyline.

Extracorporeal Techniques: Hemodialysis, charcoal hemoprofusion, and hemofiltration are some extracorporeal techniques. There are a limited number of poisoning incidents in which one of these procedures may be indicated.

Diaphoresis: Diaphoresis means inducing excessive perspiration so that the poison is excreted through sweat. In addition to physical methods, perfuse perspiration can be induced by giving a subcutaneous injection of 5 mg of pilocarpine nitrate. Administering alcohol, salicylates, or antipyretic is also used.

33.8 DIALYSIS

Common toxins that may require dialysis or hemoperfusion include ethylene glycol, lithium, methanol, salicylates, and theophyline. These therapies are less useful if the poison is a large or charged (polar) molecule, has a large volume of distribution (ie, stored in tissues), or is extensively bound to tissue proteins (as with digoxin, phencyclidine, phenothiazines, or tricyclic antidepressants).

33.9 NURSING AND PSYCHIATRIC CARE

General nursing care is especially important for comatose patients and for those who have been incapacitated by the poison. Because some cases of poisoning leave behind persisting sequelae, adequate follow-up for a period of time may be necessary. Psychiatric intervention is frequently essential in the case of suicidal doses.

CHAPTER

Treatment of poisoning

34

CHAPTER OUTLINE

34.1 INTRODUCTION

Poisoning occurs infrequently, but it is often life-threatening. Therefore, treatment and management of poisoning are very important to save the lives of poisoned patients. The treatment should be started as soon as possible because any delay may cause irreparable damage to the patient. Treatment of poisoning differs from other diseases because all cases are emergency cases. The first priority in poisoning is to establish and maintain the vital functions. Specific antidotes like receptor antagonists or chelating agents are available for a few drugs and poisons; however, for the majority of drugs and chemicals, there is no specific treatment. Symptom-based therapy that supports vital functions is the only approach. This chapter deals with the specific management of poisoning to provide relief from poisonous symptoms, such as atropine sulfate for colicky pain, morphine or pethidine for severe pain, and oral or intravenous fluids for dehydration.

34.2 SPECIFIC TREATMENT (ADMINISTRATION OF ANTIDOTES)

An antidote to poisons may be chemical, pharmacological, or physiological in nature. These countcract or neutralize the effect of a poison. Despite popular misconceptions, antidotes are available for only a small number of poisons. Actions of antidotes can be classified according to the mode of action. Different mechanisms of antidotal action with their specific antidotes are summarized in Table 34.1.

Inert Complex Formation: Some antidotes interact with the poison to form an inert complex, which is then excreted form the body, such as chelating agents for heavy metals (Table 34.2), Prussian blue for thallium, specific antibody fragments for digoxin, and dicobalt edentate for cyanide.

Accelerated Detoxification: Some antidotes accelerate the detoxification of a poison. For example, thiosulphate accelerates the conversion of cyanide to

Fundamentals of Toxicology. DOI: http://dx.doi.org/10.1016/B978-0-12-805426-0.00034-2

Table 34.1 Common Antidotes Based on the Mode/Mechanism of Action

Toxin	Antidote
Acetaminophen	*N*-acetycystein
Benzodiazepines	Flumazenil[a]
Blockers	Glucagon
Ca channel blockers	Ca, intravenous (IV) insulin at high doses with IV glucose
Organophosphates and (cholinesterase inhibitors)	Pralidoxine, physostigmine[a]
Carbamates	Atropine and protopam
Heparin	Protamine
Ethylene glycol	Ethanol fomepizole
Tricyclic antidepressants	$NaHCO_3$
Isoniazide	Pyridoxine (vitamin B_6)
Digitalis glycosides (digoxin, digitoxin, oleander, fox glove)	Steroid-binding resins, potassium salts, beta adrenergic blocking agents, procaine amide
Formaldehyde	Ammonia (by mouth)
Cyanide	Methehemoglobin (formed by nitrite administration), thiocyanide
Botulinum	Botulinus antitoxin, guanidine
Merthyl alcohol	Ethanol
Selenocystthionine	Cystine
Fluoroacetate	Acetate, monoacetin
Bromide	Chloride
Strontium, radium	Calcium salts
Neuromuscular blocking agents (eg, curare)	Neostigmine, edrophonium
Morphine and other related narcotics (opioids)	Naloxone and others
Coumarin anticoagulants	Vitamin K
Thallium	Potassium salts
Amino acid analogs	Amino acids
Carbon monoxide	Oxygen
Cyclopropane	Alpha adrenergic blocking agents (ie, haloalkylamine), antihistamines
Histamine	Antihistamines
Agents that produce methemoglobinemia (eg, aniline dyes, some local anesthetics, nitrites, nitrates, pheacetin, sulfonamides)	Methylene blue
Antitumor agents such as methotrexate and other folic acid antagonists	Glycine
5-Fluorouracil	Thymidine
6-Mercaptopurine	Purines

[a]*Use is controversial.*

Table 34.2 Metals That Make Complexes (Inert Complex Formation) With Poison: Guidelines for Therapy

Metal	Chelating Drug[a]	Dosage[b]
Antimony, arsenic, bismuth, chromates,[c] chromic acid,[c] chromium trioxide,[c] copper salts, gold, nickel, tungsten, zinc salts	Dimercaprol 10% in oil	3–4 mg/kg via deep intramuscular (IM) injection every 4 h on day 1, 2 mg/kg every 4 h on day 2, 3 mg/kg IM every 6 h on day 3, then 3 mg/kg every 12 h for 7–10 days until recovery
Cadmium, lead, zinc, zinc salts	Edentate (Ca disodium edathamil), diluted to 5%	25–35 mg/kg intravenous slowly (1 h) every 12 h for 5–7 days, followed by 7 days without the drug, then repeated
Arsenic, copper salts, gold, lead, mercury,[c] nickel, zinc salts	Penicillamine	20–30 mg/kg/day in 3–4 divided doses (usual starting dose is 250 mg qid) to a maximum adult dose of 2 g/day
Arsenic, occupational exposure to bismuth; lead if children have blood levels >45 μg/dL (>2.15 μmol/L); lead occupational exposure in adults; mercury, occupational exposure in adults	Succimer	10 mg/kg oral every 8 h for 5 days, then 10 mg/kg oral every 12 h for 14 days

[a]*Iron and thallium salts are not chelated effectively.*
[b]*Dosages depend on type and severity of poisoning.*
[c]*Chelating drug of choice.*

nontoxic thiocyanate and acetylcysteine acts as a glutathione substitute that combines with hepatotoxic paracetamol metabolites and detoxifies them.

Reduced Toxic Conversion: The best example of this mode of action is provided by ethanol, which inhibits the metabolism of methanol to toxic metabolites by competing for the same enzyme (alcohol dehydrogenase).

Receptor Site Competition: Some antidotes displace the poison from specific receptor sites, thereby antagonizing the effects completely. The best example is provided by naloxone, which antagonizes the effects of opiates at stereospecific opioid receptor sites.

Receptor Site Blockade: This mode of action is best exemplified by atropine, which blocks the effects of anti-ChE agents, such as organophosphorus compounds at muscrinic sites.

Toxic Effect Bypass: An example of this type of antidotal action is provided by the use of 100% oxygen in cyanide poisoning.

Further Reading

CHAPTER 1

Gallo, M.A., 2013. History and scope of toxicology. In: Klaassen, C.D. (Ed.), Casarett and Doull's Toxicology: The Basic Science of Poisons, eighth ed. McGraw-Hill, New York, pp. 1–10.

Gupta, P.K., 1988. Veterinary Toxicology. Cosmo Publications, New Delhi, India (Chapter 1).

Gupta, P.K., 2010. Introduction and brief history. In: Gupta, P.K. (Ed.), Modern Toxicology: Basis of Organ and Reproduction Toxicity, vol. 1. second reprint, PharmaMed Press, Hyderabad, India, pp. 1–26.

Gupta, P.K., 2016. Essential Concepts in Toxicology. BSP Pvt Ltd., Hyderabad, India (Chapter 1).

Hodgson, E.A., 2010. Introduction to toxicology. In: Hodgson, E.A. (Ed.), A Textbook of Modern Toxicology, fourth ed. John Wiley, New Jersey, pp. 3–12.

Oehme, F.W., 2012. Veterinary toxicology: a historical perspective. In: Gupta, R.C. (Ed.), Veterinary Toxicology: Basic and Clinical Principles, second ed. Academic Press/ Elsevier, Amsterdam, pp. 3–7.

CHAPTER 2

Bert Hakkinen, P.J., Kennedy, G., Stoss, F.W., 2000. Information Resources in Toxicology, third ed. Academic Press.

Gupta, P.K., 1988. Veterinary Toxicology. Cosmo Publications, New Delhi, India (Chapter 2).

Gupta, P.K., 2010. Epidemiology of anticholinesterase pesticides: India. In: Satoh, T., Gupta, R.C. (Eds.), Anticholinesterase Pesticides: Metabolism, Neurotoxicity, and Epidemiology. John Wiley & Sons, USA, pp. 417–431.

Gupta, P.K., 2010. Introduction and brief history. In: Gupta, P.K. (Ed.), Modern Toxicology: Basis of Organ and Reproduction Toxicity, vol. 1. second reprint, PharmaMed Press, Hyderabad, India, pp. 1–26.

Hodgson, E.A., 2010. Introduction to toxicology. In: Hodgson, E.A. (Ed.), A Textbook of Modern Toxicology, fourth ed. John Wiley, New Jersey, pp. 3–12.

Rao, G.N., 2010. Textbook of Forensic Medicine & Toxicology. Jaypee Brothes Medical Publishers, New Delhi, India (Chapter 31).

Thorne, P.S., 2013. Occupational toxicology. In: Klaassen, C.D. (Ed.), Casarett and Doull's Toxicology: The Basic Science of Poisons, eighth ed. McGraw-Hill, New York, pp. 1274–1292.

van der Merwe, D., Pickrell, J.A., 2012. Toxicity of nanomaterials. In: Gupta, R.C. (Ed.), Veterinary Toxicology: Basic and Clinical Principles, second ed. Academic Press/ Elsevier, Amsterdam, pp. 1383–1390.

CHAPTER 3

Cope, W.G., Leidy, R.B., Hodgson, E., 2010. Classes of toxicants: use classes. In: Hodgson, E.A. (Ed.), A Textbook of Modern Toxicology, fourth ed. John Wiley, New Jersey, pp. 49–73.

Hodgson, E.A., 2010. Introduction to toxicology. In: Hodgson, E.A. (Ed.), A Textbook of Modern Toxicology, fourth ed. John Wiley, New Jersey, pp. 3–12.

Rao, G.N., 2010. Textbook of Forensic Medicine & Toxicology. Jaypee Brothes Medical Publishers, New Delhi, India (Chapter 32).

CHAPTER 4

Gupta, P.K., 2010. Natural laws concerning toxicology. In: Gupta, P.K. (Ed.), Modern Toxicology: Basis of Organ and Reproduction Toxicity, vol. 1. second reprint, PharmaMed Press, Hyderabad, India, pp. 17–70.

Nebbia, C., 2012. Factors affecting chemical toxicity. In: Gupta, R.C. (Ed.), Veterinary Toxicology: Basic and Clinical Principles, second ed. Academic Press/Elsevier, Amsterdam, pp. 48–61.

Rao, G.N., 2010. Textbook of Forensic Medicine & Toxicology. Jaypee Brothes Medical Publishers, New Delhi, India (Chapter 31).

Rao, G.N., 2010. Textbook of Forensic Medicine & Toxicology. Jaypee Brothes Medical Publishers, New Delhi, India (Chapter 33).

CHAPTER 5

Eaton, D.L., Gilbert, S.G., 2013. Principles in toxicology. In: Klaassen, C.D. (Ed.), Casarett and Doull's Toxicology: The Basic Science of Poisons, eighth ed. McGraw-Hill, New York, pp. 11–45.

Gilbert, S.G., 2004. A Small Dose of Toxicology: The Health Effects of Common Chemicals. CRC Press, p. 266.

Gupta, P.K., 2010. Natural laws concerning toxicology. In: Gupta, P.K. (Ed.), Modern Toxicology: Basis of Organ and Reproduction Toxicity, vol. 1. second reprint, PharmaMed Press, Hyderabad, India, pp. 17–70.

LeBlanc, G.A., 2010. Acute toxicity. In: Hodgson, E.A. (Ed.), A Textbook of Modern Toxicology, fourth ed. John Wiley, New Jersey, pp. 213–224.

Semler, D.E., 1992. The rat toxicology. In: Gad, S.C., Chengelis, C.P. (Eds.), Animal Models in Toxicology. Marce Dekkar Inc., pp. 21–164.

CHAPTER 6

Baynes, R.E., 2010. Human health risk assessment. In: Hodgson, E.A. (Ed.), A Textbook of Modern Toxicology, fourth ed. John Wiley, New Jersey, pp. 423–437.

Faustman, E.M., Omenn, G.S., 2013. Risk assessment. In: Klaassen, C.D. (Ed.), Casarett and Doull's Toxicology: The Basic Science of Poisons, eighth ed. McGraw-Hill, New York, pp. 107–128.

Hodgson, E.A., 2010. Future considerations for environmental and human health. In: Hodgson, E.A. (Ed.), A Textbook of Modern Toxicology, fourth ed. John Wiley, New Jersey, pp. 521–524.

Shea, D., 2010. Environmental risk assessment. In: Hodgson, E.A. (Ed.), A Textbook of Modern Toxicology, fourth ed. John Wiley, New Jersey, pp. 501–517.

CHAPTER 7

Baynes, R.E., Hodgson, E., 2010. Absorption and distribution of toxicants. In: Hodgson, E.A. (Ed.), A Textbook of Modern Toxicology, fourth ed. John Wiley, New Jersey, pp. 77–109.

Gupta, P.K., 2010. Absorption, distribution, & excretion of xenobiotics. In: Gupta, P.K. (Ed.), Modern Toxicology: Basis of Organ and Reproduction Toxicity, vol. 1. second reprint, PharmaMed Press, Hyderabad, India, pp. 71–94.

LeBlanc, G.A., 2010. Elimination of toxicants. In: Hodgson, E.A. (Ed.), A Textbook of Modern Toxicology, fourth ed. John Wiley, New Jersey, pp. 203–211.

Lehman-McKeeman, L.D., 2013. Absorption, distribution, and excretion of toxicants. In: Klaassen, C.D. (Ed.), Casarett and Doull's Toxicology: The Basic Science of Poisons, eighth ed. McGraw-Hill, New York, pp. 131–160.

CHAPTER 8

Krishnamurti, C.R., 2010. Biotransformation of xenobiotics. In: Gupta, P.K. (Ed.), Modern Toxicology: Basis of Organ and Reproduction Toxicity, vol. 1. second reprint, PharmaMed Press, Hyderabad, India, pp. 95–129.

Patkinson, A., Ogilivie, B.W., 2013. Biotransformation of xenobiotics. In: Klaassen, C.D. (Ed.), Casarett and Doull's Toxicology: The Basic Science of Poisons, eighth ed. McGraw-Hill, New York, pp. 161–305.

Rose, R.L., Hodgson, E., 2010. Metabolism of toxicants. In: Hodgson, E.A. (Ed.), A Textbook of Modern Toxicology, fourth ed. John Wiley, New Jersey, pp. 111–148.

Rose, R.L., Hodgson, E., 2010. Chemical and physiological influences on xenobiotic metabolism. In: Hodgson, E.A. (Ed.), A Textbook of Modern Toxicology, fourth ed. John Wiley, New Jersey, pp. 163–201.

Rose, R.L., Levi, P.E., 2010. Reactive metabolites. In: Hodgson, E.A. (Ed.), A Textbook of Modern Toxicology, fourth ed. John Wiley, New Jersey, pp. 149–161.

CHAPTER 9

Ehrnebo, M., 2010. Kinetic analysis of xenobiotics. In: Gupta, P.K. (Ed.), Modern Toxicology: Basis of Organ and Reproduction Toxicity, vol. 1. second reprint, PharmaMed Press, Hyderabad, India, pp. 130–151.

Shen, D.D., 2013. Toxicokinetics. In: Klaassen, C.D. (Ed.), Casarett and Doull's Toxicology: The Basic Science of Poisons, eighth ed. McGraw-Hill, New York, pp. 305–326.

van der Merwe, D., Gehring, R., Buur, J.L., 2012. Toxicokinetics. In: Gupta, R.C. (Ed.), Veterinary Toxicology: Basic and Clinical Principles, second ed. Academic Press/ Elsevier, Amsterdam, pp. 37–47.

CHAPTER 10

Hodgson, E., 2010. Prevention of toxicity. In: Hodgson, E.A. (Ed.), A Textbook of Modern Toxicology, fourth ed. John Wiley, New Jersey, pp. 411–421.

Murphy, M.J., 2012. Toxicology and the law. In: Gupta, R.C. (Ed.), Veterinary Toxicology: Basic and Clinical Principles, second ed. Academic Press/Elsevier, Amsterdam, pp. 187–206.

Post, L.O., 2012. Regulatory considerations in veterinary toxicology. In: Gupta, R.C. (Ed.), Veterinary Toxicology: Basic and Clinical Principles, second ed. Academic Press/ Elsevier, Amsterdam, pp. 117–134.

Vettorazzi, G., 2010. Reproduction toxicity and teratogenicity. In: Gupta, P.K. (Ed.), Modern Toxicology: Basis of Organ and Reproduction Toxicity, vol. 1. second reprint, PharmaMed Press, Hyderabad, India, pp. 340–393.

CHAPTER 11

Choudhuri, S., Arvidson, K., Chanderbhan, R., 2012. Carcinogenesis: mechanisms and models. In: Gupta, R.C. (Ed.), Veterinary Toxicology: Basic and Clinical Principles, second ed. Academic Press/Elsevier, Amsterdam, pp. 406–425.

Cunny, H., Hodgson, E., 2010. Toxicity testing. In: Hodgson, E.A. (Ed.), A Textbook of Modern Toxicology, fourth ed. John Wiley, New Jersey, pp. 353–396.

Ernest, H., LeBlanc, G.A., Meyer, S.A., Smart, R.C., 2010. Introduction to biochemical and molecular methods in toxicology. In: Hodgson, E.A. (Ed.), A Textbook of Modern Toxicology, fourth ed. John Wiley, New Jersey, pp. 13–22.

CHAPTER 12

Branch, S., 2010. Teratogenesis. In: Hodgson, E.A. (Ed.), A Textbook of Modern Toxicology, fourth ed. John Wiley, New Jersey, pp. 251–259.

Cunny, H., Hodgson, E., 2010. Toxicity testing. In: Hodgson, E.A. (Ed.), A Textbook of Modern Toxicology, fourth ed. John Wiley, New Jersey, pp. 353–396.

Evans, T.J., 2012. Reproductive toxicity and endocrine disruption. In: Gupta, R.C. (Ed.), Veterinary Toxicology: Basic and Clinical Principles, second ed. Academic Press/ Elsevier, Amsterdam, pp. 288–318.

Gupta, R.C., 2012. Placental toxicity. In: Gupta, R.C. (Ed.), Veterinary Toxicology: Basic and Clinical Principles, second ed. Academic Press/Elsevier, Amsterdam, pp. 319–336.

Muhammad, F., Riviere, J.E., 2012. Dermal toxicity. In: Gupta, R.C. (Ed.), Veterinary Toxicology: Basic and Clinical Principles, second ed. Academic Press/Elsevier, Amsterdam, pp. 337–350.

Rogers, J.M., Jaclock, R.J., 2013. Developmental toxicology. In: Klaassen, C.D. (Ed.), Casarett and Doull's Toxicology: The Basic Science of Poisons, eighth ed. McGraw-Hill, New York, pp. 415–452.

Vettorazzi, G., 2010. Reproduction toxicity and teratogenicity. In: Gupta, P.K. (Ed.), Modern Toxicology: Basis of Organ and Reproduction Toxicity, vol. 1. second reprint, PharmaMed Press, Hyderabad, India, pp. 340–393.

CHAPTER 13

Oldham, J.W., 1997. Genetic toxicology. In: Sipes, G., McQueen, C.A., Gandolfi, A.J. (Eds.), Comprehensive Toxicology, vol. 2. Pergamon Press, pp. 133–144.

Preston, R.J., Hoffmann, G.R., 2013. Genetic toxicology. In: Klaassen, C.D. (Ed.), Casarett and Doull's Toxicology: The Basic Science of Poisons, eighth ed. McGraw-Hill, New York, pp. 381–413.

Smart, R.C., 2010. Chemical carcinogenesis. In: Hodgson, E.A. (Ed.), A Textbook of Modern Toxicology, fourth ed. John Wiley, New Jersey, pp. 225–250.

CHAPTER 14

Anadón, A., Martínez-Larrañaga, M.R., Castellano, V., 2012. Regulatory aspects for the drugs and chemicals used in food-producing animal in the European Union. In: Gupta, R.C. (Ed.), Veterinary Toxicology: Basic and Clinical Principles, second ed. Academic Press/Elsevier, Amsterdam, pp. 135–155.

Branch, S., 2010. Reproductive system. In: Hodgson, E.A. (Ed.), A Textbook of Modern Toxicology, fourth ed. John Wiley, New Jersey, pp. 343–349.

Sharma, R., 2012. Safety evaluation of new molecular entities for pharmaceutical development. In: Gupta, R.C. (Ed.), Veterinary Toxicology. Basic and Clinical Principles, second ed. Academic Press/Elsevier, Amsterdam, pp. 156–167.

CHAPTER 15

Anadón, A., Martínez-Larrañaga, M.R., Castellano, V., 2012. Regulatory aspects for the drugs and chemicals used in food-producing animal in the European Union. In: Gupta, R.C. (Ed.), Veterinary Toxicology: Basic and Clinical Principles, second ed. Academic Press/Elsevier, Amsterdam, pp. 135–155.

Gupta, P.K., Kannan, K., 2010. Immunosupression. In: Gupta, P.K. (Ed.), Modern Toxicology: The Adverse Effects of Xenobiotics, vol. 3. second reprint, PharmaMed Press, Hyderabad, India, pp. 135–200.

Mehrotra, N.K., 2010a. Immune system. In: Gupta, P.K. (Ed.), Modern Toxicology: The Adverse Effects of Xenobiotics, vol. 3. second reprint, PharmaMed Press, Hyderabad, India, pp. 1–59.

Mehrotra, N.K., 2010b. Hypersensitivity and occupational allergens. In: Gupta, P.K. (Ed.), Modern Toxicology: The Adverse Effects of Xenobiotics, vol. 3. second reprint, PharmaMed Press, Hyderabad, India, pp. 60–134.

Mishra, N.C., Sopori, M.L., 2012. Immunotoxicity. In: Gupta, R.C. (Ed.), Veterinary Toxicology: Basic and Clinical Principles, second ed. Academic Press/Elsevier, Amsterdam, pp. 364–382.

Selgrade, M.K., 2010. Immunotoxicity. In: Hodgson, E.A. (Ed.), A Textbook of Modern Toxicology, fourth ed. John Wiley, New Jersey, pp. 327–342.

Sharma, R., 2012. Safety evaluation of new molecular entities for pharmaceutical development. In: Gupta, R.C. (Ed.), Veterinary Toxicology: Basic and Clinical Principles, second ed. Academic Press/Elsevier, Amsterdam, pp. 156–167.

CHAPTER 16

Lawrence, W.H., 2010. Toxicology of synthetic biomaterials. In: Gupta, P.K. (Ed.), Modern Toxicology: The Adverse Effects of Xenobiotics, vol. 2. second reprint, PharmaMed Press, Hyderabad, India, pp. 362–397.

Mohannan, P.V., 2006. Regulatory aspects on biomaterials and medical devices safety testing. In: Mohannan, P.V. (Ed.), Good Laboratory Practice and Regulatory Issues. Education Book Centre, Mumbai, India, pp. 155–162.

CHAPTER 17

Gupta, P.K., 1986. Pesticides in the Indian Environment. Interprint, New Delhi.

Gupta, P.K., 1988a. Veterinary Toxicology. Cosmo Publications, New Delhi, India (Chapter 6).

Gupta, P.K., 1988b. Veterinary Toxicology. Cosmo Publications, New Delhi, India (Chapter 9).

Gupta, P.K., 2010a. Epidemiology of anticholinesterase pesticides: India. In: Satoh, T., Gupta, R.C. (Eds.), Anticholinesterase Pesticides: Metabolism, Neurotoxicity, and Epidemiology. John Wiley & Sons, USA, pp. 417–431.

Gupta, P.K., 2010b. Pesticides. In: Gupta, P.K. (Ed.), Modern Toxicology: The Adverse Effects of Xenobiotics, vol. 2. second reprint, PharmaMed Press, Hyderabad, India, pp. 1–60.

Gupta, P.K., 2012. Toxicity of herbicides. In: Gupta, R.C. (Ed.), Veterinary Toxicology: Basic and Clinical Principles, second ed. Academic Press/Elsevier, Amsterdam, pp. 631–652.

Gupta, P.K., Agarwal, M., 2012. Toxicity of fungicides. In: Gupta, R.C. (Ed.), Veterinary Toxicology: Basic and Clinical Principles, second ed. Academic Press/Elsevier, Amsterdam, pp. 653–670.

Gupta, P.K. Herbicides and fungicides. In: Gupta, R.C. (Ed.), Reproductive and Developmental Toxicology, second ed. Academic Press/Elsevier, Amsterdam, in press.

Lucio, G.C., 2013. Toxic effects of pesticides. In: Klaassen, C.D. (Ed.), Casarett and Doull's Toxicology: The Basic Science of Poisons, eighth ed. McGraw-Hill, New York, pp. 883–930.

CHAPTER 18

Garland, T., 2012. Arsenic. In: Gupta, R.C. (Ed.), Veterinary Toxicology: Basic and Clinical Principles, second ed. Academic Press/Elsevier, Amsterdam, pp. 499–502.

Gupta, P.K., 1988. Veterinary Toxicology. Cosmo Publications, New Delhi, India (Chapter 7).

Gupta, R.C., 2012. Mercury. In: Gupta, R.C. (Ed.), Veterinary Toxicology: Basic and Clinical Principles, second ed. Academic Press/Elsevier, Amsterdam, pp. 537–543.

Hooser, S.B., 2012. Cadmium. In: Gupta, R.C. (Ed.), Veterinary Toxicology: Basic and Clinical Principles, second ed. Academic Press/Elsevier, Amsterdam, pp. 503–507.

Liu, J., Goyer, R.A., Waalkes, M.P., 2013. Toxic effects of metals. In: Klaassen, C.D. (Ed.), Casarett and Doull's Toxicology: The Basic Science of Poisons, eighth ed. McGraw-Hill, New York, pp. 931–980.

Pillay, V.V., 2008. Comprehensive Medical Toxicology, second ed. Paras Medical Publisher, Hyderabad, India.

Squibb, K.S., Kardish, R.M., Carmichael, N.G., Fowler, B.A., 2010. Metal toxicity. In: Gupta, P.K. (Ed.), Modern Toxicology: The Adverse Effects of Xenobiotics, vol. 2. second reprint, PharmaMed Press, Hyderabad, India, pp. 61–130.

Thompson, L.J., 2012. Copper. In: Gupta, R.C. (Ed.), Veterinary Toxicology: Basic and Clinical Principles, second ed. Academic Press/Elsevier, Amsterdam, pp. 510–512.

CHAPTER 19

Barceloux, D.G., Bond, G.R., Krenzelok, E.P., et al., 2002. American Academy of Clinical Toxicology practice guidelines on the treatment of methanol poisoning. J. Toxicol. Clin. Toxicol. 40, 415–446.

Bird, M.G., Greim, H., Snyder, R., Rice, J.M., 2005. International symposium: recent advances in benzene toxicity. Chem-Biol. Interact 153–154, 1–5.

Bruckner, J.V., Anand, S.S., Warren, D.A., 2013. Toxic effects of solvents and vapors. In: Klaassen, C.D. (Ed.), Casarett and Doull's Toxicology: The Basic Science of Poisons, eighth ed. McGraw-Hill, New York, pp. 981–1050.

Sills, R.C., Morgan, D.L., Harry, G.J., 1998. Carbon disulfide neurotoxicity in rats: introduction and study design. Neurotoxicology 19, 83–88.

Sills, R.C., Harry, G.J., Valentine, W.M., Morgan, D.L., 2005. Interdisciplinary neurotoxicity inhalation studies: carbon disulfide and carbonyl sulfide research in F344 rats. Toxicol. Appl. Pharmacol. 207, S245–S250.

CHAPTER 20

Brenne, E.D., Stevenson, D.W., Twiggr, R.W., 2003. Cycads: evolutionary innovations and the role of plant-derived neurotoxins. Trends Plant Sci. 8 (9), 446–452, doi:10.1016/S1360-1385(03)00190-0.

Rao, G.N., 2010. Textbook of Forensic Medicine & Toxicology. Jaypee Brothes Medical Publishers, New Delhi, India (Chapter 34).

U.S. Congress, Office of Technology Assessment, Neurotoxicity, 1990. Identifying and Controlling Poisons of the Nervous System. OTA-BA-436 (U.S. Government Printing Office, April 1990, Washington, DC). OTA-BA-436 NTIS order #PB90-252511.

CHAPTER 21

Ansford, A.J., Morris, H., 1981. Fatal oleander poisoning. Med. J. Aust. 1, 360–361 [PubMed].

Frohne, D.P., Fander, H.J., 1984. A Colour Atlass of Poisonous Plants. Wolfe Publishing LTD, London, p. 190.

Khan, I., Kant, C., Sanwaria, A., Meen, L., 2010. Acute cardiac toxicity of *Nerium oleander/indicum* poisoning (kaner) poisoning. Heart Views 11 (3), 115–116. Available from: http://dx.doi.org/10.4103/1995-705X.76803.

Pillay, V.V., 2008. Comprehensive Medical Toxicology, second ed. Paras Medical Publisher, Hyderabad, India (Chapter 15).

Rao, G.N., 2010. Textbook of Forensic Medicine & Toxicology. Jaypee Brothes Medical Publishers, New Delhi, India (Chapter 35).

CHAPTER 22

Bruckner, V., Anand, S.S., Warren, D.A., 2013. Toxic effects of solvents and vapors. In: Klaassen, C.D. (Ed.), Casarett and Doull's Toxicology: The Basic Science of Poisons, eighth ed. McGraw-Hill, New York, pp. 981–1052.

Cope, R., 2012. Toxic gases. In: Gupta, R.C. (Ed.), Veterinary Toxicology: Basic and Clinical Principles, second ed. Academic Press/Elsevier, Amsterdam, pp. 719–734.

Dixon, R.L., 2010. Environmental toxicology. In: Gupta, P.K. (Ed.), Modern Toxicology: The Adverse Effects of Xenobiotics, vol. 2. second reprint, PharmaMed Press, Hyderabad, India, pp. 398–446.

Rao, G.N., 2010. Textbook of Forensic Medicine & Toxicology. Jaypee Brothes Medical Publishers, New Delhi, India (Chapter 36).

CHAPTER 23

Pillay, V.V., 2008. Comprehensive Medical Toxicology, second ed. Paras Medical Publisher, Hyderabad, India (Chapter 5).

Rao, G.N., 2010. Textbook of Forensic Medicine & Toxicology. Jaypee Brothes Medical Publishers, New Delhi, India (Chapter 32).

CHAPTER 24

Bischoff, K., 2012. Toxicity of drugs of abuse. In: Gupta, R.C. (Ed.), Veterinary Toxicology: Basic and Clinical Principles, second ed. Academic Press/Elsevier, Amsterdam, pp. 468–492.
Bischoff, K., Mukai, M., 2012. Toxicity of over-the-counter drugs. In: Gupta, R.C. (Ed.), Veterinary Toxicology: Basic and Clinical Principles, second ed. Academic Press/Elsevier, Amsterdam, pp. 443–468.
Gupta, P.K., 1988. Veterinary Toxicology. Cosmo Publications, New Delhi, India (Chapter 8).
Papich, M.G., 1990. Toxicosis from over-the-counter human drugs. Vet. Clin. North Am. Small Anim. Pract. 20, 431–451.
Pillay, V.V., 2008. Comprehensive Medical Toxicology, second ed. Paras Medical Publisher, Hyderabad, India (Chapter 21).
Rao, G.N., 2010. Textbook of Forensic Medicine & Toxicology. Jaypee Brothes Medical Publishers, New Delhi, India (Chapter 40).

CHAPTER 25

Gupta, P.K., 2010. Common poisons. In: Gupta, P.K. (Ed.), Modern Toxicology: The Adverse Effects of Xenobiotics, vol. 3. second reprint, PharmaMed Press, Hyderabad, India, pp. 265–328.
Pillay, V.V., 2008. Comprehensive Medical Toxicology, second edition Paras Medical Publisher, Hyderabad, India (Chapter 11).
Rao, G.N., 2010. Textbook of Forensic Medicine & Toxicology. Jaypee Brothes Medical Publishers, New Delhi, India (Chapter 37).

CHAPTER 26

Gupta, P.K., 1988. Veterinary Toxicology. Cosmo Publications, New Delhi, India (Chapter 5).
Norton, S., 2013. Toxic effects of plants. In: Klaassen, C.D. (Ed.), Casarett and Doull's Toxicology: The Basic Science of Poisons, eighth ed. McGraw-Hill, New York, pp. 1103–1116.
Pillay, V.V., 2008. Comprehensive Medical Toxicology, second ed. Paras Medical Publisher, Hyderabad, India (Chapter 18).
Rao, G.N., 2010. Textbook of Forensic Medicine & Toxicology. Jaypee Brothes Medical Publishers, New Delhi, India (Chapter 33).
Sharma, R.P., Salunkhe, D.K., 2010. Animal and plant toxins. In: Gupta, P.K. (Ed.), Modern Toxicology: The Adverse Effects of Xenobiotics, vol. 2. second reprint, PharmaMed Press, Hyderabad, India, pp. 252–316.

CHAPTER 27

Gupta, P.K., 1988. Veterinary Toxicology. Cosmo Publications, New Delhi, India (Chapter 4).

Gupta, P.K., Singh, Y.P., 2010. Mycotoxins. In: Gupta, P.K. (Ed.), Modern Toxicology: The Adverse Effects of Xenobiotics, vol. 2. second reprint, PharmaMed Press, Hyderabad, India, pp. 317–341.

Pillay, V.V., 2008. Comprehensive Medical Toxicology, second ed. Paras Medical Publisher, Hyderabad, India (Chapter 19).

Rao, G.N., 2010. Textbook of Forensic Medicine & Toxicology. Jaypee Brothes Medical Publishers, New Delhi, India (Chapter 39).

Sharma, R.P., Salunkhe, D.K., 2010. Animal and plant toxins. In: Gupta, P.K. (Ed.), Modern Toxicology: The Adverse Effects of Xenobiotics, vol. 2. second reprint, PharmaMed Press, Hyderabad, India, pp. 252–316.

Thompson, L.J., 2012. Enterotoxins. In: Gupta, R.C. (Ed.), Veterinary Toxicology: Basic and Clinical Principles, second ed. Academic Press/Elsevier, Amsterdam, pp. 950–952.

CHAPTER 28

Gupta, P.K., 1988. Veterinary Toxicology. Cosmo Publications, New Delhi, India (Chapter 5).

Gwaltney-Brant, S.M., Dunayer, E., Youssef, H., 2012. Terrestrial zootoxins. In: Gupta, R.C. (Ed.), Veterinary Toxicology: Basic and Clinical Principles, second ed. Academic Press/ Elsevier, Amsterdam, pp. 969–992.

Manual, M., 2006. Bites and Stings. Merck Research Laboratories, Merck & Co. Inc, pp. 2638–2651.

Pillay, V.V., 2008. Comprehensive Medical Toxicology, second ed. Paras Medical Publisher, Hyderabad, India (Chapter 20).

Rao, G.N., 2010. Textbook of Forensic Medicine & Toxicology. Jaypee Brothes Medical Publishers, New Delhi, India (Chapter 33).

Sharma, R.P., Salunkhe, D.K., 2010. Animal and plant toxins. In: Gupta, P.K. (Ed.), Modern Toxicology: The Adverse Effects of Xenobiotics, vol. 2. second reprint, PharmaMed Press, Hyderabad, India, pp. 252–316.

Watkins III, J.B., 2013. Properties and toxicities of animal venoms. In: Klaassen, C.D. (Ed.), Casarett and Doull's Toxicology: The Basic Science of Poisons, eighth ed. McGraw-Hill, New York, pp. 1083–1102.

CHAPTER 29

Kotsonis, F.N., Burdock, G.A., 2013. Food toxicology. In: Klaassen, C.D. (Ed.), Casarett and Doull's Toxicology: The Basic Science of Poisons, eighth ed. McGraw-Hill, New York, pp. 1191–1236.

Manual, M., 2006. Bites and Stings. Merck Research Laboratories, Merck & Co. Inc, pp. 2638–2651.

Pillay, V.V., 2008. Comprehensive Medical Toxicology, second ed. Paras Medical Publisher, Hyderabad, India (Chapter 19).

CHAPTER 30

Gupta, P.K., 1988. Veterinary Toxicology. Cosmo Publications, New Delhi, India (Chapter 10).

Harley, N.H., 2013. Health effects of radiation and radioactive materials. In: Klaassen, C.D. (Ed.), Casarett and Doull's Toxicology: The Basic Science of Poisons, eighth ed. McGraw-Hill, New York, pp. 1053–1083.

Rebois, R.V., Ray, K., 2012. Ionizing radiation and radioactive materials in health and disease. In: Gupta, R.C. (Ed.), Veterinary Toxicology: Basic and Clinical Principles, second ed. Academic Press/Elsevier, Amsterdam, pp. 1391–1405.

CHAPTER 31

Branch, S., 2010. Forensic and clinical toxicology. In: Hodgson, E.A. (Ed.), A Textbook of Modern Toxicology, fourth ed. John Wiley, New Jersey, pp. 399–409.

Pillay, V.V., 2008. Comprehensive Medical Toxicology, second ed. Paras Medical Publisher, Hyderabad, India (Chapter 3).

Poklis, A., 2013. Analytic/forensic toxicology. In: Klaassen, C.D. (Ed.), Casarett and Doull's Toxicology: The Basic Science of Poisons, eighth ed. McGraw-Hill, New York, pp. 1237–1255.

Rao, G.N., 2010. Textbook of Forensic Medicine & Toxicology. Jaypee Brothes Medical Publishers, New Delhi, India (Chapter 31).

CHAPTER 32

Branch, S., 2010. Forensic and clinical toxicology. In: Hodgson, E.A. (Ed.), A Textbook of Modern Toxicology, fourth ed. John Wiley, New Jersey, pp. 399–409.

Jain, A.V., Arnold, B.S., 2012. Basic concepts of analytical toxicology. In: Gupta, R.C. (Ed.), Veterinary Toxicology: Basic and Clinical Principles, second ed. Academic Press/Elsevier, Amsterdam, pp. 1321–1334.

Leidy, R.B., 2010a. Toxicant analysis and quality assurance principles. In: Hodgson, E.A. (Ed.), A Textbook of Modern Toxicology, fourth ed. John Wiley, New Jersey, pp. 23–28.

Leidy, R.B., 2010b. Analytical methods in toxicology. In: Hodgson, E.A. (Ed.), A Textbook of Modern Toxicology, fourth ed. John Wiley, New Jersey, pp. 441–461.

Pillay, V.V., 2008. Comprehensive Medical Toxicology, second ed. Paras Medical Publisher, Hyderabad, India (Chapter 4).

Poklis, A., 2013. Analytic/forensic toxicology. In: Klaassen, C.D. (Ed.), Casarett and Doull's Toxicology: The Basic Science of Poisons, eighth ed. McGraw-Hill, New York, pp. 1237–1255.

Rao, G.N., 2010. Textbook of Forensic Medicine & Toxicology. Jaypee Brothes Medical Publishers, New Delhi, India (Chapter 31).

CHAPTER 33

Branch, S., 2010. Forensic and clinical toxicology. In: Hodgson, E.A. (Ed.), A Textbook of Modern Toxicology, fourth ed. John Wiley, New Jersey, pp. 399–409.

Cantilena Jr., L.R., 2013. Clinical toxicology. In: Klaassen, C.D. (Ed.), Casarett and Doull's Toxicology: The Basic Science of Poisons, eighth ed. McGraw-Hill, New York, pp. 1257–1271.

Gupta, P.K., 1988. Veterinary Toxicology. Cosmo Publications, New Delhi, India (Chapter 11).

Pillay, V.V., 2008. Comprehensive Medical Toxicology, second ed. Paras Medical Publisher, Hyderabad, India (Chapter 2).

Rao, G.N., 2010. Textbook of Forensic Medicine & Toxicology. Jaypee Brothes Medical Publishers, New Delhi, India (Chapter 31).

CHAPTER 34

Gupta, P.K., 1988a. Veterinary Toxicology. Cosmo Publications, New Delhi, India (Chapter 14).

Gupta, P.K., 1988b. Veterinary Toxicology. Cosmo Publications, New Delhi, India (Chapter 15).

Gupta, P.K., 2010a. Principles of non-specific therapy. In: Gupta, P.K. (Ed.), Modern Toxicology: The Adverse Effects of Xenobiotics, vol. 3. second reprint, PharmaMed Press, Hyderabad, India, pp. 210–243.

Gupta, P.K., 2010b. Mechanism of antidotal therapy. In: Gupta, P.K. (Ed.), Modern Toxicology: The Adverse Effects of Xenobiotics, vol. 3. second reprint, PharmaMed Press, Hyderabad, India, pp. 244–264.

Manual, M., 2006. Poisoning. Merck Research Laboratories, Merck & Co. Inc., pp. 2651–2695.

Pillay, V.V., 2008. Comprehensive Medical Toxicology, second ed. Paras Medical Publisher, Hyderabad, India (Chapter 2).

Rao, G.N., 2010. Textbook of Forensic Medicine & Toxicology. Jaypee Brothes Medical Publishers, New Delhi, India (Chapter 31).

Index

Note: Page numbers followed by "*f*" and "*t*" refer to figures and tables, respectively.

B

C

D

E

N

T

Printed in the United States
By Bookmasters